Social Determinants
of Health in Surgery

Social Determinants of Health in Surgery

A Primer for the Practicing Surgeon

Edited by

SAMILIA OBENG-GYASI, MD, MPH
Division of Surgical Oncology, Department of Surgery,
The Ohio State University Wexner Medical Center,
James Cancer Hospital, Columbus, OH, United States

TIMOTHY M. PAWLIK, MD, PHD, MPH, MTS, MBA
Division of Surgical Oncology, Department of Surgery,
The Ohio State University Wexner Medical Center,
James Cancer Hospital, Columbus, OH, United States

ELSEVIER

Notices

Practitioners and researchers must always rely on their own experience and knowledge in evaluating and using any information, methods, compounds or experiments described herein. Because of rapid advances in the medical sciences, in particular, independent verification of diagnoses and drug dosages should be made. To the fullest extent of the law, no responsibility is assumed by Elsevier, authors, editors or contributors for any injury and/or damage to persons or property as a matter of products liability, negligence or otherwise, or from any use or operation of any methods, products, instructions, or ideas contained in the material herein.

Publisher: Sarah E. Barth
Acquisitions Editor: Jessica L.McCool
Editorial Project Manager: Kristi Anderson
Production Project Manager: Selvaraj Raviraj
Cover Designer: Matthew Limbert

3251 Riverport Lane
St. Louis, Missouri 63043

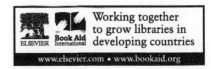

List of Contributors

Adeseye Adekeye, MD, PhD
Department of Surgery
Thomas Jefferson University
Philadelphia, PA, United States

Nicolás Ajkay, MD, MBA, FACS
Associate Professor of Surgery
Breast Surgical Oncology
University of Louisville
Louisville, KY, United States

Benjamin G. Allar, MD, MPH
Center for Surgery and Public Health
Department of Surgery
Brigham and Women's Hospital
Harvard Medical School
Boston, MA, United States

Barbara L. Andersen, PhD
Distinguished University Professor
Department of Psychology
The Ohio State University
Columbus, OH, United States

Elizabeth R. Berger, MD, MS
Department of Surgery
Yale School of Medicine
New Haven, CT, United States

Smilow Cancer Center
Yale New Haven Health System
New Haven, CT, United States

Cancer Outcomes, Public Policy
    and Effectiveness Research Center
Yale School of Medicine
New Haven, CT, United States

J.L. Campbell, MD
Louisiana State University- Louisiana Children's
    Medical Center Cancer Center
New Orleans, LA, United States

J.C. Chen, MD
Division of Surgical Oncology
Department of Surgery
The Ohio State University Wexner Medical Center
James Cancer Hospital
Columbus, OH, United States

Steven W. Cole, PhD
Professor of Psychiatry & Biobehavioral Sciences and
    Medicine,
UCLA School of Medicine
Los Angeles, CA, United States

Angelena Crown, MD
Deputy Director of Breast Surgery
True Family Women's Cancer Center
Swedish Cancer Institute
Seattle, WA, United States

Melissa B. Davis, PhD
Director, Institute of Translational Genomic Medicine
Georgia Research Alliance Distinguished Investigator
Associate Professor (interim) of Microbiology
    Biochemistry and Immunology
Morehouse School of Medicine
Atlanta, GA, United States

Scientific Director
International Center for the Study of Breast
    Cancer Subtypes

Pranam Dey, BS
Department of Surgery
Yale School of Medicine
New Haven, CT, United States

Hiba Dhanani, MD, ScM
Center for Surgery and Public Health
Department of Surgery
Brigham and Women's Hospital
Harvard Medical School, Boston, MA, United States

Adrian Diaz
Department of Surgery
The Ohio State University
Columbus, OH, United States

Center for Healthcare Outcomes and Policy
University of Michigan, Ann Arbor, MI, United States

Oluwadamilola M. Fayanju, MD, MA, MPHS
Division of Breast Surgery
Department of Surgery, Perelman School of Medicine
The University of Pennsylvania
Philadelphia, PA, United States

Rena Rowan Breast Center
Abramson Cancer Center
Penn Medicine
Philadelphia, PA, United States

Leonard Davis Institute of Health Economics (LDI)
The University of Pennsylvania
Philadelphia, PA, United States

Penn Center for Cancer Care Innovation
Abramson Cancer Center
Philadelphia, PA, United States

Rachel A. Greenup, MD, MPH
Department of Surgery
Yale School of Medicine
New Haven, CT, United States

Smilow Cancer Center
Yale New Haven Health System
New Haven, CT, United States

Cancer Outcomes, Public Policy, and Effectiveness
Research Center, Yale School of Medicine
New Haven, CT, United States

Adil H. Haider, MD, MPH, FACS
Center for Surgery and Public Health
Brigham and Women's Hospital
Harvard T.H. Chan School of Public Health
Boston, MA, United States

Aga Khan University
Karachi, Pakistan

Chanita Hughes Halbert, PhD
Department of Population and Public Health Sciences
University of Southern California
Los Angeles, CA, United States

Norris Comprehensive Cancer Center
University of Southern California
Los Angeles, CA, United States

Andrew M. Ibrahim
Center for Healthcare Outcomes and Policy
University of Michigan
Ann Arbor, MI, United States

Department of Surgery
University of Michigan, Ann Arbor, MI, United States

Taubman College of Architecture & Urban Planning
University of Michigan, Ann Arbor, MI, United States

Yoshiko Iwai, MS
University of North Carolina School of Medicine
Chapel Hill, NC, United States

Kathie Ann Joseph, MD, MPH
Professor of Surgery and Population Health
NYU Grossman School of Medicine
New York, NY, United States

NYU Langone Health Institute for Excellence in
    Health Equity, New York, NY, United States

Mira L. Katz, PhD, MPH
Professor Division of Health Behavior and Health
    Promotion, College of Public Health
The Ohio State University
Columbus, OH, United States

Kirsten C. Lung, MD
Department of Surgery
Thomas Jefferson University
Philadelphia, PA, United States

Lisa Ann Newman, MD, MPH, FACS, FASCO, FSSO
Professor of Surgery, Chief
Division of Breast Surgery Director
Interdisciplinary Breast Program
Executive Director and Founder
International Center for the Study of
    Breast Cancer Subtypes
Weill Cornell Medicine/New York Presbyterian
    Hospital Network, Weill Cornell Medicine
Department of Surgery New York, NY, United States

Samilia Obeng-Gyasi, MD, MPH
Division of Surgical Oncology
Department of Surgery
The Ohio State University Wexner Medical Center
James Cancer Hospital, Columbus, OH, United States

Gezzer Ortega, MD, MPH
Center for Surgery and Public Health
Department of Surgery
Brigham and Women's Hospital
Harvard Medical School, Boston, MA, United States

Kylie R. Park
Department of Psychology
The Ohio State University
Columbus, OH, United States

Timothy M. Pawlik, MD, PhD, MPH, MTS, MBA
Division of Surgical Oncology
Department of Surgery, The Ohio State University
Wexner Medical Center, James Cancer Hospital
Columbus, OH, United States

Hiram C. Polk, Jr., MD
Department of Surgery
Division of Surgical Oncology
University of Louisville School of Medicine
Louisville, KY, United States

Ellie M. Proussaloglou, MD
Department of Surgery
Yale School of Medicine
New Haven, CT, United States

Smilow Cancer Center
Yale New Haven Health System
New Haven, CT, United States

Cancer Outcomes, Public Policy
    and Effectiveness Research Center
Yale School of Medicine
New Haven, CT, United States

Namra Qadeer Shaikh, MBBS
Dean's Office
Aga Khan University
Karachi, Pakistan

Nicole L. Simone, MD
Department of Radiation Oncology
Thomas Jefferson University
Philadelphia, PA, United States

John H. Stewart, IV, MD, MBA
Louisiana State University- Louisiana Children's
    Medical Center Cancer Center
New Orleans, LA, United States

Foreword

At the core of the book *Social Determinants of Health* is the role of the physician best demonstrated by the quote of Sir William Osler, "the good physician treats the disease, the great physician treats the patient who happens to have that disease." This statement foreshadows the necessary and critical understanding of social determinants and the impact that they have on the patients' health disparities and the delivery of care they receive. Many of these patients live in impoverished settings, who often are underrepresented minorities in healthcare in America. One of the most significant challenges for American Healthcare is addressing health disparities. The problem we saw highlighted best during the COVID-19 pandemic with the differential suffering of those who lived with disparities and significant social determinants of health. These social determinants are the factors that affect healthcare outcomes that are driven by either racial or ethnic differences that do not relate to medical-related factors. These determinants are the circumstances in which people are born, grow up, live, and work and the health systems that are put in place to deal with their illnesses. Determinants of health also relate to clinical care, genes, and biology but are the minority factors that determine health outcomes. Behaviors are largely driven by the educational, social, and economic factors and physical environment that make up the vast majority of the outcomes of health. These factors bolster the understanding that one's zip code versus genetic code is still the greatest determinant of your health outcome. It is crucial for the "great" (competent) physician to understand these social determinants in the context of their impact on their patient who happens to have diseases that are often driven by them. The impact of social determinants and their cost to American Healthcare is framed by the economic instability, the limited physical environment for both exercise and safety, a lack of quality education, food insecurity, the lack of full integration within communities, persistent discrimination, as well as limited access to health systems. All of these factors are critical for surgeons and physicians alike, to understand their implications and the healthcare outcomes of the patients they serve. Unfortunately, this is a burden we have ignored too long. This book provides the opportunity to look at each of these significant determinants, provides a basis for understanding and their impact, as well as the research that has been accomplished around this, demonstrating in many ways how we may address these determinants and improve disparities. Finally, we must avoid the misconception of this being a zero-sum game. In fact, we will create better healthcare for all both by taking down barriers and by creating more effective, efficient, and cost-effective healthcare systems by addressing these social determinants.

Selwyn Vickers

Preface

The COVID-19 pandemic revealed the magnitude and breadth of long-simmering structural inequalities and systemic inequities in health and healthcare in the United States. Specifically, individuals from socially and economically marginalized groups (e.g., Black people and individuals with low socioeconomic status) had a higher incidence and worse mortality from the virus than their counterparts from privileged backgrounds. Further, the virus highlighted how differences in social determinants of health, social risks, and health-related social needs between socially and economically privileged populations and those experiencing marginalization and minoritization affected the diagnosis, treatment, and mortality from the virus. These Covid-related disparities, coupled with the civil unrest in 2020 due to the murders of unarmed Black men such as George Floyd, catapulted social determinants of health to the forefront of discourse within the medical community.

In the surgical field, the inequality and inequity highlighted by the virus increased interest in the relationships between social determinants of health and surgical care. Social determinants of health describe the intersection of governmental policy, sociocultural values, socioeconomic position, the healthcare system, biology, and psychosocial support within the context of everyday living and working conditions. Over the past 3 years, the surgical literature has seen a significant proliferation of studies examining structural (e.g., Medicaid expansion) and intermediary (e.g., neighborhood contextual factors) determinants of health and their implications for surgical management and outcomes. However, this burgeoning interest in social determinants of health within the field of surgery has revealed knowledge gaps in existing theoretical and conceptual frameworks that inform this type of research.

In this book, we leverage the expertise of renowned surgeon—scientist and academic scholars to provide surgeons and the medical community with a robust armamentarium of theories, conceptual frameworks, and a review of existing research on social determinants of health to inform future research in this area. Further, we were intentional in mainly including scholars from historically and intentionally excluded groups in surgery and academia who have built and are building legacies of robust and exceptional equity-focused scholarship and research.

As we recover from the COVID-19 pandemic, high-quality health equity research is needed to unpack the long-term implications of the pandemic on surgical care. We hope that the chapters in this book will serve as a roadmap to ask, interrogate, and solve research questions focused on social determinants of health with an eye toward health equity.

Samilia Obeng-Gyasi, MD, MPH

Timothy Pawlik, MD, PhD, MPH, MTS, MBA

Contents

CHAPTER 1

Social Determinants of Health in Surgery Overview

ANGELENA CROWN, MD • KATHIE-ANN JOSEPH, MD, MPH

INTRODUCTION

Health outcomes are mediated by the intersection of socioeconomic and environmental factors with healthcare.[1] Although life expectancy and disease outcomes have improved over time, it is important to note these improvements have not been equal across all populations, with significant disparities observed across race, ethnicity, and socioeconomic status.[2,3] The World Health Organization defines social determinants of health as the "conditions in which people are born, grow, work, live, and age, and the wider set of forces and systems shaping the conditions of daily life."[4]

Multiple factors drive disparities in health outcomes; variation in life expectancy has been thought to be modulated by the superimposition of socioeconomic and race/ethnicity with behavioral and metabolic risk factors as well as by differences in access to care.[3] Together, these forces insidiously erect barriers to preventative care and screening and compromise the quality of medical care and availability of treatment options. Additionally, social determinants of health have been implicated in surgical outcomes with lower socioeconomic status, underinsurance, race and ethnicity, education, and geography influencing outcomes.[5-7] This textbook will develop a framework for understanding social determinants of health and elucidate how they underpin disparities in surgical outcomes as well as describe interventions to improve outcomes and research strategies for measuring progress.

ACCESS TO CARE

Access to care has been implicated as a critical modulator of healthcare disparities. Preventative care and health screening are associated with a lower frequency of emergent diagnosis and surgery, which are, in turn, associated with reduced morbidity and mortality.[7,8] In a study of patients presenting for evaluation by the acute case surgery service at a level 1 trauma hospital, Hambright et al. found that adherence to preventative screenings and interventions, including mammography, colonoscopy, and pneumococcal vaccinations, was only 57%.[9] When patients had a primary care doctor, the adherence rate was 60% versus 27% when patients did not have a primary care doctor.[9] Education beyond high school has been associated with increased adherence to preventative screenings.[10] Multiple studies have demonstrated that access to preventative screening and adherence to preventative screening recommendations are also impacted by race and ethnicity, with rates of screening colonoscopy higher in non-Hispanic populations rather than Hispanic populations.[9-11] These data have inspired targeted interventions by primary care programs, with some programs reporting significant improvements.[12]

Reduced access to care results in barriers to screening, delays in diagnostic workup, and is associated with more advanced disease and worse oncologic outcomes.[13-15] Income and insurance status are linked to screening, with low-income and underinsured patients being less likely to receive screening and having a greater likelihood of late-stage diagnosis.[16,17] Quality of screening is also impacted by socioeconomic status, education, and race and ethnicity, with studies of breast cancer screening demonstrating that digital mammography and supplemental breast ultrasound use lower among disadvantaged groups.[18,19] Notably, when African American women undergo screening, they are more likely to be done at lower resourced and nonaccredited facilities and have longer intervals between mammograms and follow-up imaging.[20] These trends have been implicated in the findings that regional disease is present in approximately 33% of African American women compared with 25% of Caucasian American women.[21]

Lack of access to preventative care is implicated in the diagnosis and treatment of gallbladder disease.[7,8]

Treatment of cholecystitis in the emergency setting, rather than in the elective setting, is associated with increased morbidity and mortality.[7,8] Moreover, insurance status and race have also been implicated in access to cholecystectomy, with Medicaid insurance being associated with a lower rate of surgery being performed at the index hospitalization for acute cholecystitis as well as a reduced rate of laparoscopic surgery when surgery was performed.[22]

Safety net hospitals disproportionately care for patients from disadvantaged backgrounds who are most affected by the social risk factors of poverty, food insecurity, and unstable housing. As a result, these hospitals serve a significant number of uninsured patients and patients on Medicaid.[23] While studies evaluating surgical outcomes in safety net hospitals have demonstrated mixed results, with similar mortality rates in major vascular operations but increased morbidity and mortality following ventral hernia repairs, colectomies, and Whipple operations.[24,25] In a study of nonfederally funded California hospitals, hospitals with higher rates of Medicaid-insured and uninsured patients had a higher rate of patients with perforated appendicitis as well as a lower rate of laparoscopic surgery, again demonstrating the higher disease acuity associated with being underinsured and not being able to access care in a timely fashion.[26] What does appear to be clear is that access to care does not fully explain disparities in surgical outcomes. Factors including geographic location, physician communication, discrimination, and logistical challenges have also been implicated in these disparities.[27]

POVERTY AND INSURANCE

Studies have demonstrated that poverty may account for 6% of US mortality.[28] The difference in life expectancy between the most wealthy 1% and the poorest 1% is estimated at 14.6 years for men and 10.1 years for women, with a trend of increasing disparities over time.[29] Lower socioeconomic status is inextricably linked to a lack of adequate insurance coverage, significantly limiting access to care. US census data report higher rates of poverty among African Americans and Hispanics (19.5% and 17.0%, respectively) compared with non-Hispanic Whites and Asians (8.2% and 8.1%, respectively).[30] Paralleling these findings, African Americans and Hispanics have the highest uninsured rates (10.4% and 18.3%, respectively) compared with non-Hispanic Whites and Asians (5.4% and 5.9%, respectively).[31] In the United States, socioeconomic status strongly correlates with race and ethnicity, and both low socioeconomic status and minority race are independent predictors of surgical mortality.[15,32,33] Further, Diaz et al. found that Black patients from lower socioeconomic status have a 58%–60% increased odds of 30-day mortality as well as a markedly higher risk of 30-day mortality than White patients from any socioeconomic status.[5]

Medicaid expansion under the Affordable Care Act resulted in increased coverage for racial and ethnic minorities. National Cancer Database (NCDB) data demonstrated that this expansion resulted in improvements in time to definitive care for breast, colon, lung, and prostate cancers, but this did not translate into improved timeliness of care at minority servicing hospitals on a hospital level.[34] Medicaid expansion also failed to increase the receipt of definitive treatment for patients with these cancers, indicating that having insurance is not the only barrier to obtaining definitive cancer care.[34]

Lower socioeconomic status has been associated with increased surgical mortality.[15,32] Additionally, comorbidities, including diabetes and hypertension, are more prevalent among patients from lower socioeconomic status, increasing the risk of complications following elective surgery.[35] Factors including access barriers, care at lower-quality and underresourced hospitals, presence of comorbidities, socioeconomic factors, and disease severity have been proposed as potential drivers of these disparities.[32,33,36]

There has been increased interest in applying tools such as the Social Vulnerability Index (SVI) to surgical outcomes.[7] The SVI incorporates data relating to socioeconomic status, household composition and disability, minority status and language, as well as housing and transportation, into a composite measure.[37] Carmichael et al. found that the use of the SVI in a multivariable model, including age, sex, and chronicity of symptoms, resulted in a similar performance to a more complex model, including race, insurance status, access to primary care, and interpreter needs.[7]

Studies in colorectal surgery have demonstrated that both poverty and race are associated with increased rates of emergent colorectal cancer diagnosis and emergency colorectal surgery as well as reduced access to clinical trials.[27,38] One study using SEER data from 1992 to 2005 found that poverty was only associated with higher rates of emergent diagnosis and surgery among African Americans, suggesting that African Americans experiencing poverty face additional barriers to colorectal cancer screening and treatment.[27] In contrast, poverty was not associated with higher rates of emergent diagnosis and surgery among White patients.

What does appear to be clear is that access to care does not fully explain disparities in colorectal cancer outcomes. Factors including physician communication, discrimination, and logistical challenges have also been implicated in these disparities.[27]

In the breast cancer literature, multiple studies have shown that uninsured women and those with government insurance are at increased risk of advanced breast cancer, treatment delays, and risk of death from breast cancer compared with those with private insurance.[39–43] Lack of adequate insurance has been implicated in delays in diagnosis, need for more intensive treatment, including receipt of chemotherapy and need for mastectomy, and treatment-associated morbidity and poor quality of life.[44,45] These more intensive treatments are subsequently risk factors for future unemployment, which further erodes economic resources.[46,47] Underinsurance can also contribute to financial hardship due to high out-of-pocket costs for treatment.[48,49]

FOOD AND HOUSING INSECURITY

Lack of insurance and government insurance is also associated with higher rates of unmet social needs.[50] Relative to patients with private insurance, patients with Medicaid and no insurance reported higher rates of food insecurity (46% vs. 39% vs. 10%), housing instability (43% and 51% vs. 19%), and delayed care due to transportation concerns (11% and 5% vs. 1%).[50] Race and ethnicity were also associated with differences in rates of unmet social needs, with non-Hispanic Black and Hispanic patients reporting higher rates of unmet social needs compared with non-Hispanic White patients, including food insecurity (32% and 29% vs. 13%), housing instability (33% and 38% vs. 19%), and delayed care due to transportation concerns (6% and 5% vs. 3%).[50] Each unmet social need was an independent predictor of poor health among surgical patients, highlighting the importance of these factors in health disparities and identifying potential targets for intervention.

Housing instability has been associated with reduced access to screening and higher stages of presentation among women with breast cancer.[51] Indeed, homelessness has been associated with lower rates of breast cancer screening and more advanced stages at diagnosis.[51,52] Degree of housing instability appears to have correlated with screening rates with women who are temporarily residing with other people ("doubling up") and women in transitional housing having improved access to social support resources and higher rates of mammographic screening compared with those living in shelters or on the streets.[53]

SYSTEMIC RACISM AND ALLOSTATIC LOAD

The legacy of centuries of systemic racism and accompanying chronic activation of physiologic stress responses, termed allostatic load, has been implicated in poor health outcomes among African Americans.[54–56] While studies exploring racial disparities rarely mention the word "racism," the role of racism in driving disparities in health outcomes is being recognized and reported.[57] The effects of racism permeate all socioeconomic variables, not limited to wealth generation, transportation, access to medical care, education and employment opportunities, and housing. Allostatic load is defined as the heightened neural and neuroendocrine responses to chronic environmental stressors, which are, in turn, associated with poorer health outcomes.[58,59] Maladaptive changes in the cardiovascular, and gastrointestinal systems, as well as in metabolic rates and development of immunosuppression, may also occur.[59] These changes have been measured through stress hormone and glucose levels, blood pressure, body mass index, and waist–hip ratios.[60,61]

Allostatic load is inversely related to socioeconomic status, with increased allostatic load reported among people for disadvantaged socioeconomic backgrounds; higher allostatic load also varies with race and ethnicity, with African Americans carrying significantly higher allostatic loads relative to Caucasians.[26,27,62,63] Furthermore, racial discrimination and social inequalities have been associated with increased allostatic load.[63–65]

Increased allostatic load has been associated with chronic conditions and mortality.[61,66,67] Studies have shown that chronic stress is associated with reduced cancer immunosurveillance and increased inflammation, which promotes tumor invasion and angiogenesis; these factors, in turn, can have deleterious effects on tumor biology and oncologic outcomes.[54,68]

Higher levels of poor sleep, alcohol consumption, and smoking have been linked to higher allostatic load.[69–71] Additionally, comorbidities including cardiovascular disease, diabetes, depression, and anxiety can impact surgical outcomes.[72–76]

EDUCATION

The highest levels of education are associated with mortality rates 2.5 times lower relative to the lowest education levels.[77] According to the 2017 census bureau statistics, the majority of individuals in the US population without health insurance coverage had a high school education or less.[78] The poverty rates and proportions of the population that lack health insurance are two to three times higher among minority racial and ethnic groups such as African Americans and

Hispanic/Latino Americans.[79] Those who did not complete high school made up 27% of the uninsured population in the United States.[78] Education is inversely associated with cancer mortality.[80] Using data from the 2001 National Center for Health Statistics, Albano et al. found that the relative risks for all all-cancer mortality comparing the three lowest educational categories with the three highest education categories were 2.38 (95% CI = 2.33−2.43) for Black men, 2.24 (95% CI = 2.23−2.26) for White men, 1.43 (95% CI = 1.41−1.46) for Black women, and 1.76 (95% CI = 1.75−1.78) for White women.[80] Morality rates were higher among Black patients than among White patients at similar education levels, highlighting that education likely interacts with other variables including income, access to care, and spousal socioeconomic status.[80] Another alarming finding in this study was that a higher percentage of Black patients were in the three lowest educational categories (53% of Black patients vs. 40% of White patients); as a result, the interaction between of education and mortality has a disproportionate impact on Black patients.[80] While previous studies have demonstrated that level of education is frequently overestimated on death certificates compared with previous self-report, most commonly listing people as high-school graduates when they had less than a high school education.[81] This misclassification was more common in death certificates of Black patients (50%) than among White patients; while these discrepancies could underestimate impact of education on mortality among those who complete high school and those who do not, comparing compound outcomes of the lowest three education levels versus highest three education levels should be less sensitive to this limitation.[81]

REPRESENTATION IN MEDICINE

Disparities in surgical outcomes have multiple interrelated drivers, including socioeconomic factors and comorbidities compounded by barriers to care; a diverse workforce is necessary to critically evaluate these factors and meet the needs of an increasingly diverse US population. Medical school admission and graduation rates do not reflect the current population trends. Hispanics and Blacks comprise 18.7% and 12.1% of the US population, respectively, but only make up 6.8% and 8.1%, respectively, of medical students.[82,83] Despite investment in pipeline programs and national initiatives to increase diversity in medicine and the adoption of holistic admissions, rates of underrepresented minorities in medicine remain alarmingly low and fail to keep pace with the changing demographics of the US population.[83−87] Black men remain strikingly

underrepresented, making up only 2.9% of medical students in 2019.[88]

This underrepresentation has consequences for healthcare outcomes, as underrepresented minority physicians have repeatedly been shown to provide disproportionate care to vulnerable populations, including uninsured, non−English-speaking, and underrepresented minority patients.[89−91] Indeed, Marrast et al. found that underrepresented minority doctors provided care to 54% of underrepresented minority patients and for 70% of non−English-speaking patients.[89]

White medical students also benefit from racial and ethnic diversity in the medical student body, reporting increased preparedness to care for underrepresented minority populations and strong attitudes endorsing equitable healthcare access.[92] Despite these positive effects, this has not translated into increased rates of White medical students electing to serve underrepresented minority communities.[92] The finding that 49% of underrepresented minority students elect to practice in underserved communities compared with 19% of White students again highlights the disproportionate work that underrepresented minorities perform in these communities.

Racial concordance between underrepresented minority patients and physicians has repeatedly been associated with improved rates of accessing healthcare and adhering to medical recommendations.[91,93−95] Further, improvements in communication, a feeling of respect, and higher quality of care have been reported by underrepresented minority patients when they are treated by racially concordant physicians.[93,96,97] Lack of racial and ethnic diversity in medicine has significant repercussions and has been implicated in the propagation of healthcare disparities. Studies have demonstrated that racial discordance between physicians and patients is associated with patients perceiving lower quality of care and poorer communication.[93,96] Conversely, racial concordance predicts improved doctor−patient communication and higher rates of perceiving a physician as excellent and respectful.[93,96] It is also associated with higher rates of accessing preventative and necessary care.[93] As a result, recruitment and retention of physicians from underrepresented minority groups is pivotal to improving the patient experience and maximizing utilization of preventative and necessary care and could potentially help to improve rates of adherence to prescribed medical treatments, and avoid the need for emergency surgery.

Diversity is especially lacking in surgery, with a recent study evaluating trends in racial and ethnic diversity in general surgery residency, surgical oncology fellows, and surgical faculty in the United States from 2011/2012 to 2019/2020, demonstrating that underrepresented minority residents comprised only 5% of surgical residents.[98] Interestingly, this study demonstrated that having more women faculty was associated with an increase in underrepresented minority fellows (84% increase in underrepresented minority fellows for every 100% increase in women faculty), suggesting that the recruitment and retention of women surgeons may not only increase gender diversity in surgery but may indirectly improve racial and ethnic diversity as well.[98]

Black women surgical trainee applicants have increased from 2.2% to 3.5% ($P < .001$) between 2005 and 2018.[99] There was no statistical difference in Black men surgical trainee applicants (3.7% −4.6%). While surgery residency matriculation and the proportion of graduates remained similar among Black women (2.4% vs. 2.3% and 1.7 vs. 2.2%, respectively), it decreased significantly among Black men (3.0% vs. 2.4% $P = .04$) as did the proportion of surgery residency graduates (4.3% vs. 2.7%, $P = .03$). These trends highlight the significant underrepresentation of Black surgery trainees that will propagate as this cohort of surgical trainees becomes faculty.

Diversity among faculty and medical students is critically important to promoting an understanding of cultural and spiritual beliefs across different backgrounds.[100] Biases, both implicit and unconscious, compromise communication and clinical decision-making. In addition to improving the recruitment and retention of physicians from underrepresented minority groups, there is significant opportunity to improve cultural competence and communication efforts for physicians of all backgrounds to improve surgical outcomes.

REFERENCES

1. The case for more active policy attention to health promotion. *Health Aff*. 2002;21(2):78−93.
2. Harper S, Lynch J, Burris S, Davey Smith G. Trends in the black-white life expectancy gap in the United States, 1983-2003. *JAMA*. 2007;297(11):1224−1232.
3. Dwyer-Lindgren L, Bertozzi-Villa A, Stubbs RW, et al. Inequalities in life expectancy among US counties, 1980 to 2014: temporal trends and key drivers. *JAMA Intern Med*. 2017;177(7):1003−1011.
4. World Health Organization (WHO). Social Determinants of Health. https://www-who-int.offcampus.lib.washington.edu/health-topics/social-determinants-of-health#tab=tab_1. Accessed January 10, 2023.
5. Diaz A, Hyer JM, Barmash E, Azap R, Paredes AZ, Pawlik TM. County-level social vulnerability is associated with worse surgical outcomes especially among minority patients. *Ann Surg*. 2021;274(6):881−891.
6. Hyer JM, Tsilimigras DI, Diaz A, et al. High social vulnerability and "textbook outcomes" after cancer operation. *J Am Coll Surg*. 2021;232(4):351−359.
7. Carmichael H, Moore A, Steward L, Velopulos CG. Using the social vulnerability index to examine local disparities in emergent and elective cholecystectomy. *J Surg Res*. 2019;243:160−164.
8. Havens JM, Peetz AB, Do WS, et al. The excess morbidity and mortality of emergency general surgery. *J Trauma Acute Care Surg*. 2015;78(2):306−311.
9. Hambright G, Agrawal V, Sladek PL, Slonim SM, Truitt MS. Acute care surgery: trauma, critical care, emergency general surgery ... and preventative health? *Am J Surg*. 2016;212(5):803−806.
10. National Center for Health Statistics. *Health, United States, 2014: With Special Feature on Adults Aged 55-64*. Hyattsville, MD: U.S. Government Printing Office; 2015.
11. Miranda-Diaz C, Betancourt E, Ruiz-Candelaria Y, Hunter-Mellado RF. Barriers for compliance to breast, colorectal, and cervical screening cancer tests among hispanic patients. *Int J Environ Res Publ Health*. 2016;13(1). ijerph13010021-ijerph13010021.
12. Ruggeri CE, Reed RE, Coyle B, Stoltzfus J, Fioravanti G, Tehrani R. Closing the gap: a resident-led quality improvement project to improve colorectal cancer screening in primary care community clinics. *J Grad Med Educ*. 2020;12(1):104−108.
13. Lannin DR, Mathews HF, Mitchell J, Swanson MS, Swanson FH, Edwards MS. Influence of socioeconomic and cultural factors on racial differences in late-stage presentation of breast cancer. *JAMA*. 1998;279(22):1801−1807.
14. Miles RC, Onega T, Lee CI. Addressing potential health disparities in the adoption of advanced breast imaging technologies. *Acad Radiol*. 2018;25(5):547−551.
15. Patel AK. Disparities in access to screening for breast cancer: current state and potential solutions. *J Am Coll Radiol*. 2022;19(10):1119−1120.
16. O'Malley AS, Forrest CB, Mandelblatt J. Adherence of low-income women to cancer screening recommendations. *J Gen Intern Med*. 2002;17(2):144−154.
17. Yedjou CG, Sims JN, Miele L, et al. Health and racial disparity in breast cancer. *Adv Exp Med Biol*. 2019;1152:31−49.
18. Lee CI, Zhu W, Onega T, et al. Comparative access to and use of digital breast tomosynthesis screening by women's race/ethnicity and socioeconomic status. *JAMA Netw Open*. 2021;4(2):e2037546.
19. Ezratty C, Vang S, Brown J, Margolies LR, Jandorf L, Lin JJ. Racial/ethnic differences in supplemental imaging for breast cancer screening in women with dense breasts. *Breast Cancer Res Treat*. 2020;182(1):181−185.
20. Molina Y, Silva A, Rauscher GH. Racial/ethnic disparities in time to a breast cancer diagnosis: the mediating effects of healthcare facility factors. *Med Care*. 2015;53(10):872−878.

21. *United States Cancer Statistics: 1999-2013 Incidence and Mortality Web-Based Report*. Atlanta: U.S. Dept of Health and Human Services, Cernters for Disease Control and Prevention and National Cancer Institute; 2016.

22. Greenstein AJ, Moskowitz A, Gelijns AC, Egorova NN. Payer status and treatment paradigm for acute cholecystitis. *Arch Surg*. 2012;147(5):453–458.

23. Crown A, Ramiah K, Siegel B, Joseph K-A. The role of safety net hospitals in reducing disparities in breast cancer care. *Ann Surg Oncol*. 2022. https://doi.org/10.1245/s10434-022-11576-3. Epub ahead of print. PMID: 35357616.

24. Hoehn RS, Wima K, Vestal MA, et al. Effect of hospital safety-net burden on cost and outcomes after surgery. *JAMA Surgery*. 2016;151(2):120–128.

25. Eslami MH, Rybin D, Doros G, Farber A. Care of patients undergoing vascular surgery at safety net public hospitals is associated with higher cost but similar mortality to nonsafety net hospitals. *J Vasc Surg*. 2014;60(6):1627–1634.

26. Won RP, Friedlander S, Lee SL. Outcomes and costs of managing appendicitis at safety-net hospitals. *JAMA Surgery*. 2017;152(11):1001–1006.

27. Pruitt SL, Davidson NO, Gupta S, Yan Y, Schootman M. Missed opportunities: racial and neighborhood socioeconomic disparities in emergency colorectal cancer diagnosis and surgery. *BMC Cancer*. 2014;14(1):927.

28. Pappas G, Queen S, Hadden W, Fisher G. The increasing disparity in mortality between socioeconomic groups in the United States, 1960 and 1986. *N Engl J Med*. 1993;329(2):103–109.

29. Chetty R, Stepner M, Abraham S, et al. The association between income and life expectancy in the United States, 2001-2014. *JAMA*. 2016;315(16):1750–1766.

30. Shrider E, Kollar M, Chen F, Semega J. *Income and Poverty in the United States: 2020*. U.S. Census Bureau; 2021:60–273. Current Population Reports.

31. Keisler-Starkey K, Brunch LN. *Health Insurance Coverage in the United States: 2020*. U.S. Census Bureau; 2021:60–274. Current Population Reports.

32. Bennett KM, Scarborough JE, Pappas TN, Kepler TB. Patient socioeconomic status is an independent predictor of operative mortality. *Ann Surg*. 2010;252(3):552–557. discussion 557-558.

33. Osborne NH, Upchurch Jr GR, Mathur AK, Dimick JB. Explaining racial disparities in mortality after abdominal aortic aneurysm repair. *J Vasc Surg*. 2009;50(4):709–713.

34. Nguyen D-D, Paciotti M, Marchese M, et al. Effect of medicaid expansion on receipt of definitive treatment and time to treatment initiation by racial and ethnic minorities and at minority-serving hospitals: a patient-level and facility-level analysis of breast, colon, lung, and prostate cancer. *JCO Oncology Practice*. 2021;17(5):e654–e665.

35. Centers for Disease Control and Prevention. CDC health disparities and inequalities report—United States, 2013. *MMWR Morb Mortal Wkly Rep*. 2013;62(3):1–186.

36. Roetzheim RG, Pal N, Gonzalez EC, Ferrante JM, Van Durme DJ, Krischer JP. Effects of health insurance and race on colorectal cancer treatments and outcomes. *Am J Publ Health*. 2000;90(11):1746–1754.

37. Flanagan BE, Gregory EW, Hallisey EJ, Heitgerd JL, Lewis B. A social vulnerability index for disaster management. *J Homel Secur Emerg Manag*. 2011;8:1–22.

38. Duma N, Vera Aguilera J, Paludo J, et al. Representation of minorities and women in oncology clinical trials: review of the past 14 years. *J Oncol Pract*. 2018;14(1):e1–e10.

39. Berrian JL, Liu Y, Lian M, Schmaltz CL, Colditz GA. Relationship between insurance status and outcomes for patients with breast cancer in Missouri. *Cancer*. 2021;127(6):931–937.

40. Ayanian JZ, Kohler BA, Abe T, Epstein AM. The relation between health insurance coverage and clinical outcomes among women with breast cancer. *N Engl J Med*. 1993;329(5):326–331.

41. Pan HY, Walker GV, Grant SR, et al. Insurance status and racial disparities in cancer-specific mortality in the United States: a population-based analysis. *Cancer Epidemiol Biomark Prev*. 2017;26(6):869–875. A Publication of the American Association for Cancer Research, Cosponsored by the American Society of Preventive Oncology.

42. Samiian L, Sharma P, Van Den Bruele AB, Smotherman C, Vincent M, Crandall M. The effect of insurance and race on breast cancer tumor biology and short-term outcomes. *Am Surg*. 2018;84(7):1223–1228.

43. Kantor O, Wang ML, Bertrand K, et al. Racial and socioeconomic disparities in breast cancer outcomes within the AJCC pathologic prognostic staging system. *Ann Surg Oncol*. 2021;29(1):686–696. https://doi.org/10.1245/s10434-021-10527-8. PMID: 34331158.

44. Ko NY, Hong S, Winn RA, Calip GS. Association of insurance status and racial disparities with the detection of early-stage breast cancer. *JAMA Oncol*. 2020;6(3):385–392.

45. Ganz PA, Desmond KA, Leedham B, Rowland JH, Meyerowitz BE, Belin TR. Quality of life in long-term, disease-free survivors of breast cancer: a follow-up study. *J Natl Cancer Inst*. 2002;94(1):39–49.

46. Carlsen K, Ewertz M, Dalton SO, Badsberg JH, Osler M. Unemployment among breast cancer survivors. *Scand J Publ Health*. 2014;42(3):319–328.

47. Jagsi R, Hawley ST, Abrahamse P, et al. Impact of adjuvant chemotherapy on long-term employment of survivors of early-stage breast cancer. *Cancer*. 2014;120(12):1854–1862.

48. Liu C, Maggard-Gibbons M, Weiser TG, Morris AM, Tsugawa Y. Impact of the affordable care Act insurance marketplaces on out-of-pocket spending among surgical patients. *Ann Surg*. 2021;274(6):e1252–e1259.

49. Chhabra KR, Sheetz KH, Nuliyalu U, Dekhne MS, Ryan AM, Dimick JB. Out-of-Network bills for privately insured patients undergoing elective surgery with in-network primary surgeons and facilities. *JAMA*. 2020;323(6):538–547.

50. Taylor KK, Neiman PU, Bonner S, Ranganathan K, Tipirneni R, Scott JW. Unmet social health needs as a driver of inequitable outcomes after surgery: a cross-

sectional analysis of the national health interview survey. *Ann Surg.* 2022. https://doi.org/10.1097/SLA.0000000000005689. PMID: 36017938; PMCID: PMC10122453.

51. Baggett TP, Chang Y, Porneala BC, Bharel M, Singer DE, Rigotti NA. Disparities in cancer incidence, stage, and mortality at boston health care for the homeless program. *Am J Prev Med.* 2015;49(5):694–702.

52. Asgary R, Garland V, Sckell B. Breast cancer screening among homeless women of New York city shelter-based clinics. *Wom Health Issues.* 2014;24(5):529–534.

53. Kosog K, Earle M, Stellon E, et al. Identifying an association between socio-demographic factors and breast cancer screening adherence in a federally qualified health centre sample in the United States. A retrospective, cross sectional study. *Health Soc Care Community.* 2020; 28(5):1772–1779.

54. Obeng-Gyasi S, Tarver W, Carlos RC, Andersen BL. Allostatic load: a framework to understand breast cancer outcomes in Black women. *NPJ Breast Cancer.* 2021;7(1): 100.

55. Beckie TM. A systematic review of allostatic load, health, and health disparities. *Biol Res Nurs.* 2012;14(4): 311–346.

56. Mathew A, Doorenbos AZ, Li H, Jang MK, Park CG, Bronas UG. Allostatic load in cancer: a systematic review and mini meta-analysis. *Biol Res Nurs.* 2021;23(3): 341–361.

57. Loehrer AP, Cevallos PC, Jiménez RT, Wong SL. Reporting on race and racial disparities in breast cancer: the neglect of racism as a driver of inequitable care. *Ann Surg.* 2023;277(2):329–334.

58. McEwen BS, Stellar E. Stress and the individual. Mechanisms leading to disease. *Arch Intern Med.* 1993; 153(18):2093–2101.

59. Guidi J, Lucente M, Sonino N, Fava GA. Allostatic load and its impact on health: a systematic review. *Psychother Psychosom.* 2020;90:11.

60. Seeman TE, Singer BH, Rowe JW, Horwitz RI, McEwen BS. Price of adaptation–allostatic load and its health consequences. MacArthur studies of successful aging. *Arch Intern Med.* 1997;157(19):2259–2268.

61. Seeman TE, McEwen BS, Rowe JW, Singer BH. Allostatic load as a marker of cumulative biological risk: MacArthur studies of successful aging. *Proc Natl Acad Sci U S A.* 2001; 98(8):4770–4775.

62. Cobb RJ, Thomas CS, Laster Pirtle WN, Darity Jr WA. Self-identified race, socially assigned skin tone, and adult physiological dysregulation: assessing multiple dimensions of "race" in health disparities research. *SSM Popul Health.* 2016;2:595–602.

63. Geronimus AT, Hicken M, Keene D, Bound J. "Weathering" and age patterns of allostatic load scores among blacks and whites in the United States. *Am J Publ Health.* 2006;96(5):826–833.

64. Schwartz JA. Long-term physical health consequences of perceived inequality: results from a twin comparison design. *Soc Sci Med.* 2017;187:184–192.

65. O'Campo P, Schetter CD, Guardino CM, et al. Explaining racial and ethnic inequalities in postpartum allostatic load: results from a multisite study of low to middle income woment. *SSM Popul Health.* 2016;2:850–858.

66. Mattei J, Demissie S, Falcon LM, Ordovas JM, Tucker K. Allostatic load is associated with chronic conditions in the Boston Puerto Rican Health Study. *Soc Sci Med.* 2010;70(12):1988–1996.

67. Robertson T, Beveridge G, Bromley C. Allostatic load as a predictor of all-cause and cause-specific mortality in the general population: evidence from the Scottish Health Survey. *PLoS One.* 2017;12(8):e0183297.

68. Antoni MH, Dhabhar FS. The impact of psychosocial stress and stress management on immune responses in patients with cancer. *Cancer.* 2019;125(9):1417–1431.

69. Sotos-Prieto M, Bhupathiraju SN, Falcón LM, Gao X, Tucker KL, Mattei J. A healthy lifestyle score is associated with cardiometabolic and neuroendocrine risk factors among Puerto Rican adults. *J Nutr.* 2015;145(7): 1531–1540.

70. Clark AJ, Dich N, Lange T, et al. Impaired sleep and allostatic load: cross-sectional results from the Danish Copenhagen Aging and Midlife Biobank. *Sleep Med.* 2014;15(12):1571–1578.

71. Forrester SN, Leoutsakos JM, Gallo JJ, Thorpe Jr RJ, Seeman TE. Association between allostatic load and health behaviours: a latent class approach. *J Epidemiol Community Health.* 2019;73(4):340–345.

72. Gillespie SL, Anderson CM, Zhao S, et al. Allostatic load in the association of depressive symptoms with incident coronary heart disease: the Jackson Heart Study. *Psychoneuroendocrinology.* 2019;109:104369.

73. Steptoe A, Hackett RA, Lazzarino AI, et al. Disruption of multisystem responses to stress in type 2 diabetes: investigating the dynamics of allostatic load. *Proc Natl Acad Sci U S A.* 2014;111(44):15693–15698.

74. Juster RP, Marin MF, Sindi S, et al. Allostatic load associations to acute, 3-year and 6-year prospective depressive symptoms in healthy older adults. *Physiol Behav.* 2011; 104(2):360–364.

75. Kobrosly RW, van Wijngaarden E, Seplaki CL, Cory-Slechta DA, Moynihan J. Depressive symptoms are associated with allostatic load among community-dwelling older adults. *Physiol Behav.* 2014;123:223–230.

76. Sabbah W, Watt RG, Sheiham A, Tsakos G. Effects of allostatic load on the social gradient in ischaemic heart disease and periodontal disease: evidence from the Third National Health and Nutrition Examination Survey. *J Epidemiol Community Health.* 2008;62(5):415–420.

77. National Center for Health Statistics. *Health, United States, 1998, with Socioeconomic Status and Health Chartbook.* Hyattsville, Md: NCHS; 1998. Pub. no. (PHS)98-1232.

78. Bureau USC. 2013-2017 American Community Survey 5-Year Estimates.

79. U.S. National Institutes of Health NCI. SEER Training Modules, Breast.

80. Albano JD, Ward E, Jemal A, et al. Cancer mortality in the United States by education level and race. *J Natl Cancer Inst.* 2007;99(18):1384−1394.

81. Sorlie PD, Johnson NJ. Validity of education information on the death certificate. *Epidemiology.* 1996;7(4): 437−439.

82. Bureau UC. *2020 Census Redistricting Data (Public Law 94-171) Summary File.* 2020.

83. Association of American Medical Colleges. In: *2021 FACTS: Enrollment, Graduates, and MD-PhD Data.* 2021.

84. Liaison Committee on Medical Education (LCME) Standards on Diversity.

85. Glazer GDJ, Michaels J, et al. *Holistic Admissions in the Health Professions: Findings from a National Survey.* Urban Universities for HEALTH; 2014.

86. Lett E, Murdock HM, Orji WU, Aysola J, Sebro R. Trends in racial/ethnic representation among U.S. Medical students. *JAMA Netw Open.* 2019;2(9). e1910490-e1910490.

87. Boatright DH, Samuels EA, Cramer L, et al. Association between the liaison committee on medical education's diversity standards and changes in percentage of medical student sex, race, and ethnicity. *JAMA.* 2018;320(21): 2267−2269.

88. Morris DB, Gruppuso PA, McGee HA, Murillo AL, Grover A, Adashi EY. Diversity of the national medical student body — four decades of inequities. *N Engl J Med.* 2021;384(17):1661−1668.

89. Marrast LM, Zallman L, Woolhandler S, Bor DH, McCormick D. Minority physicians' role in the care of underserved patients: diversifying the physician workforce may Be key in addressing health disparities. *JAMA Intern Med.* 2014;174(2):289−291.

90. Komaromy M, Grumbach K, Drake M, et al. The role of black and Hispanic physicians in providing health care for underserved populations. *N Engl J Med.* 1996; 334(20):1305−1310.

91. Moy E, Bartman BA. Physician race and care of minority and medically indigent patients. *JAMA.* 1995;273(19): 1515−1520.

92. Saha S, Guiton G, Wimmers PF, Wilkerson L. Student body racial and ethnic composition and diversity-related outcomes in US medical schools. *JAMA.* 2008; 300(10):1135−1145.

93. Saha S, Komaromy M, Koepsell TD, Bindman AB. Patient-physician racial concordance and the perceived quality and use of health care. *Arch Intern Med.* 1999; 159(9):997−1004.

94. Saha S, Taggart SH, Komaromy M, Bindman AB. Do patients choose physicians of their own race? *Health Aff.* 2000;19(4):76−83.

95. Schoenthaler A, Montague E, Baier Manwell L, Brown R, Schwartz MD, Linzer M. Patient-physician racial/ethnic concordance and blood pressure control: the role of trust and medication adherence. *Ethn Health.* 2014;19(5): 565−578.

96. Shen MJ, Peterson EB, Costas-Muniz R, et al. The effects of race and racial concordance on patient-physician communication: a systematic review of the literature. *J Racial Ethn Health Disparities.* 2018;5(1):117−140.

97. Laveist TA, Nuru-Jeter A. Is doctor-patient race concordance associated with greater satisfaction with care? *J Health Soc Behav.* 2002;43(3):296−306.

98. Yu AYL, Iwai Y, Thomas SM, Beasley GM, Sudan R, Fayanju OM. Diversity among surgical faculty, residents, and oncology fellows from 2011/2012 to 2019/2020. *Ann Surg Oncol.* 2022;29(5):2763−2765. https://doi.org/10.1245/s10434-021-11170-z. PMID: 35119546; PMCID: PMC9092460.

99. Keshinro A, Butler P, Fayanju O, et al. Examination of intersectionality and the pipeline for black academic surgeons. *JAMA Surgery.* 2022;157(4):327−334. https://doi.org/10.1001/jamasurg.2021.7430. PMID: 35138327; PMCID: PMC8829744.

100. Daley S, Wingard DL, Reznik V. Improving the retention of underrepresented minority faculty in academic medicine. *J Natl Med Assoc.* 2006;98(9):1435−1440.

CHAPTER 2

Internalizing Social Determinants of Health: The Ecosocial and Weathering Theories

J.C. CHEN, MD • TIMOTHY M. PAWLIK, MD, PHD, MPH, MTS, MBA • SAMILIA OBENG-GYASI, MD, MPH

AN INTRODUCTION TO SOCIAL EPIDEMIOLOGY

Healthy People 2030 emphasizes the need to focus on the social determinants of health (SDH), specifically with the goal to "create social, physical, and economic environments that promote attaining the full potential for health and well-being for all."[1] Social determinants of health refer to the nonmedical conditions and environments where people live, work, and play that ultimately impacts their health outcomes.[2] The study of sociostructural factors on the distribution of health and disease is called social epidemiology.[2] Although research evaluating the impact of SDH on health outcomes has only recently expanded, the notion that social conditions influence health originated at the beginning of the 19th century.[2] Villerme, Virchow, and Chadwick all examined the relationship between poor socioenvironmental conditions and disease.[2] However, the advent of the germ theory, in which germs were considered the major cause of disease, overshadowed the impact of social conditions until social epidemiology resurfaced in the 1980s.[2]

Since then, several models and theories have emerged to help explain the pathophysiology behind different population health distributions and health inequities. The germ theory introduced the dominant theory behind disease development—biomedical individualism, whereby (1) disease is fully attributable to individual-level biology, exposures, behaviors and, as such, is amenable to interventions through the healthcare system, (2) sociodemographic and contextual variables are considered secondary to biological causes of disease, and (3)

populations and their diseases reflect the sum of individual-level phenomena.[2,3] Differences in disease distribution by race, ethnicity, and gender are attributed to innate genetics, biology, and cultural preferences. The "web of causation" was then introduced to challenge the concept of single "agents" causing disease and, instead, emphasize the complexity and intersections of risk factors that ultimately lead to disease.[3] Additionally, the host–agent–environment epidemiological model became commonplace, describing the necessity for an external agent (e.g., infectious pathogen), susceptible host (e.g., human), and environment (e.g., extrinsic factors providing the opportunity for exposure) to produce disease.[4]

Alternative theories, such as the psychosocial theory, propose that disease occurs due to mutual stressful interactions between social, individual, and biological factors in multilevel, interactive environments.[2] The stress induced from these factors is then suggested to alter neuroendocrine function, leaving certain populations more susceptible to both physical and psychiatric diseases.[2] More modern concepts, such as allostatic load (AL), stem from the psychosocial theory.[5] Allostatic load relies on the fundamental concept of allostasis, where body systems achieve homeostasis after exposure to stressors.[6] Allostatic load, on the other hand, refers to the physiologic "wear and tear" induced from chronic overstimulation of the hypothalamic–pituitary–adrenal (HPA) axis and sympathetic–adrenal–medullary (SAM) pathway, leading to dysfunctional cardiovascular, metabolic, and immune

Social Determinants of Health in Surgery. https://doi.org/10.1016/B978-0-443-12366-5.00007-3

systems.[6] Social capital and cohesion are proposed as the most promising interventions for decreasing risk of disease according to the psychosocial theory.[2]

Another theoretical framework focuses on upstream–downstream effects, also known as "the political economy of health" or the "social production of disease," where economic and political determinants serve as structural barriers to people living healthy lives.[5] Specifically, society's priorities of capital accumulation lead to economic and political decisions that create, enforce, and perpetuate economic and social privilege and inequity, which is considered the fundamental cause of health inequities.[5] Recognizing nonbehavioral causes of health issues arose in response to criticisms of the dominant "blame-the-victim" "lifestyle" theories that persistently emphasized individuals' responsibilities in "choosing healthy lifestyles" without considering alternative factors contributing to health outcomes.[5,7] Interventions call for redistributive policies that reduce poverty and income inequality, termed "healthy public policies," as well as community empowerment for social change.[5] However, this upstream framework primarily describes how social factors either accelerate or hinder "normal" biological processes, only superficially discussing the interaction between social and biological factors.[3]

ECOSOCIAL THEORY

As such, Nancy Krieger developed the ecosocial theory in 1994 to incorporate multiple existing theories. Specifically, the ecosocial theory is composed of four key elements: embodiment, pathways of embodiment, the cumulative interplay of exposure, susceptibility, resistance, and agency and accountability, which are further described in Table 2.1.[3,8] The ecosocial theory considers biology and society as an "intertwining ensemble" in which individuals are situated within social groups whose everyday lives are shaped by the dominant society's economic and political priorities, which aim to benefit those individuals claiming superiority, ultimately leading to oppression and discrimination.[3,8] These discriminatory effects impact individuals' physical and social environments (i.e., pathways of embodiment), which are ultimately internalized (i.e., embodiment) from the cellular level throughout the individual and household within their lifetime.[3,8] Krieger, however, also emphasizes the need to consider the historical context of all levels (i.e., individual, intergenerational, societal, ecological), which will influence individuals' initial susceptibility and subsequent response to the oppression (i.e., cumulative interplay of exposure, susceptibility, resistance) (Fig. 2.1).[3,8]

TABLE 2.1
The Four Key Constructs of the Ecosocial Theory (Embodiment, Pathways of Embodiment, the Cumulative Interplay Among Exposure, Susceptibility, and Resistance, and Accountability and Agency) are Further Described in This Table.

KEY ELEMENTS OF THE ECOSOCIAL THEORY	
Elements	**Definition**
Embodiment	The biological incorporation of the physical and social environment through biologic mechanisms within our life span
Pathways of embodiment	Various ways that economic and political priorities impact social, biological, environmental conditions and interact with the body: - Economic and social deprivation - Exogenous hazards (toxic substances, pathogens, hazardous conditions) - Social trauma (discrimination and mental/physical/sexual trauma) - Targeted marketing of harmful commodities (tobacco, illicit drugs) - Inadequate/degrading healthcare - Ecosystem degradation (e.g., forcing indigenous populations from native land)
Cumulative interplay among exposure, susceptibility, and resistance	History, lifetime experiences, spatiotemporal factors, interactions that lead to different exposures, susceptibilities, and resistances for different social groups
Accountability and agency	State and social systems are responsible for disease distribution given their power to enforce, enable, or condone discrimination and redress the effects

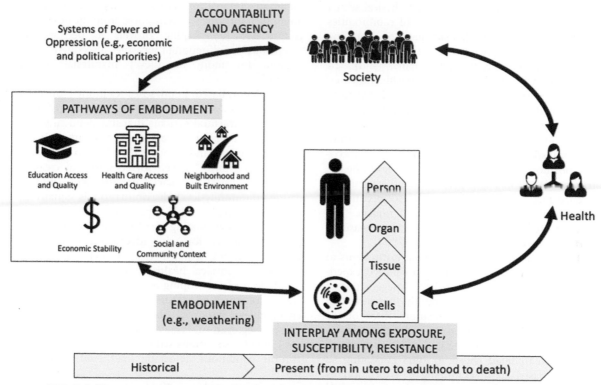

FIG. 2.1 The ecosocial theory posits that the dominant society's systems of power and oppression lead to discrimination impacting people's physical and social environments. This discrimination is internalized, which, in conjunction with historical context, leads to the current distribution of health inequities.

Nevertheless, the ecosocial theory posits that society's social system and the states that employ these priorities are responsible (i.e., agency and accountability) for generating the inequitable living and working conditions that have led to the current distribution of disease.[3,8]

Krieger's ecosocial theory challenges biomedical individualism and the construct that health outcomes are simply "natural" or "individually innate."[3] Rather, concepts such as race are social constructs created to racialize biology, demarcate groups, and generate inequities that are a consequence or expression of racism.[9] Inequitable social conditions are not "natural" but constructed from people who had a purpose (and are thereby accountable) in mind.[3] Krieger situates health behaviors in their social context, arguing that the health effects pathologically induced from the collective phenomena of discrimination and oppression cannot be reduced to individual attributes.[3] Patterns of disease represent the biological

consequences (from gene expression to physiological changes to behavioral development) of living and working conditions that are assigned from society's economic and political priorities.[8] The ecosocial theory therefore not only addresses *what* drives social inequities in health but also *who* creates these injustices.[9] As such, Krieger emphasizes that research on interventions should focus not just on the healthcare system, public health departments, and individuals, but also the broader determinants of health through widespread social action.[3]

DISCRIMINATION: AN EMBODIMENT PATHWAY

Krieger proposes that oppression is expressed through multiple "pathways of embodiment."[9] Namely, discrimination leads to economic and social deprivation, the creation of exogenous hazards (e.g., toxic substances, pathogens, hazardous conditions), social trauma (discrimination, mental/physical/sexual trauma), targeted marketing of harmful commodities (e.g., tobacco, illicit drugs), inadequate or degrading healthcare, and ecosystem degradation (e.g., exiling indigenous populations from their native land).[9] To study the impact of oppression on health, however, three approaches have been recommended: (1) indirectly through inference, (2) directly through self-reported measures, and (3) through institutional/population-based measures.[10] Indirect approaches involve adjusting studies for confounders and socioeconomic position, yet still seeing discrepancies in health outcomes among social groups.[10] While this persistent difference may be due to inadequate socioeconomic measurements or unmeasured confounders, the remaining difference may also reflect unmeasured noneconomic aspects of discrimination.[10]

Direct approaches use measurement instruments to inquire explicitly about patients' self-reported experiences with discrimination.[9,10] In 1999, Krieger reported on 20 studies in the public health literature that measured self-reported discrimination, three-fourths of which focused on race, three on gender, three on sexual orientation, and one on disability.[10] Williams et al. published an updated review in 2003 evaluating 53 population-based studies examining the association between racial discrimination and health indicators.[11] Multiple studies have noted positive associations between racial discrimination and psychological distress, major depression, anxiety, early substance use, psychosis, and anger.[11] Similarly, studies demonstrated positive associations with poorer self-perceived health status, blood pressure, cardiovascular outcomes, cigarette smoking, and alcohol use.[11] Since then, multiple reviews and metaanalyses have reported consistent associations between self-reported racial discrimination and poorer mental health with weaker relationships to poorer physical health.[12]

A variety of instruments have been developed to assess exposure to self-perceived racism, such as the Schedule of Racist Events, Racism and Life Experience Scales, Experiences of Discrimination, Perceived Racism Scale, Everyday Discrimination Scale, Perceived Ethnic Discrimination Questionnaire, Multidimensional Inventory of Black Identity, and the Nadanolitization scale.[12] However, these individual-level measures are limited by survey design and participant recall bias, which may underestimate the effects of racial discrimination on health and ultimately lead to mixed results.[13] Krieger cautions that differing self-reports of discrimination may be due to (1) internalized oppression, where

members internalize negative views and messages about their intrinsic worth imposed from the dominant culture and (2) shaping answers to be "socially acceptable."[10] Self-reported measures also often fail to account for more macrolevel manifestations of racism.[13]

Population-based approaches examine structural discrimination, which refers to the interaction of multiple macrostructural systems that independently and jointly assert bias to create discriminatory policies, practices, beliefs, and resource distribution to people in a social group.[14] Given society's role in creating disparate physical and social environments, investigating community-level discrimination is equally as crucial as individual-level experiences.[15] A recent systematic review evaluating area-level racial prejudice reported an association with adverse birth outcomes, increased cardiovascular disease, poorer self-reported mental and physical health, and higher mortality.[13] Similarly, a recent scoping review evaluating exposure clusters of structural racism (e.g., access to healthcare, civil and legal system discrimination, housing and residential segregation, incarceration, structural violence, etc.) noted associations with infant health outcomes, chronic conditions, allostatic load, and quality of life.[14]

Area-level racial prejudice has been examined using the General Social Survey, Project Implicit, Google Trends, and Twitter.[13] Additionally, at least 73 measurement scales or indices of structural racism have been created with the Index of Concentration of Extremes, Dissimilarity Index, Everyday Discrimination Scale, Experience of Discrimination Scale, Five Segregation Scale, Index of Race Related Stress, Isolation Index, and Perceived Racism Scale considered the most commonly used.[14] Residential housing patterns as an expression of structural racism are the most commonly evaluated, specifically through measurements of racial residential segregation and redlining.[16] However, methodological challenges are still reported. The majority of studies investigating structural racism are cross-sectional, leading to limitations in temporality and inferences for causality.[14] Existing measures of structural racism also primarily examine single dimensions of structural racism (i.e., housing, education, employment, incarceration).[17] However, this approach fails to capture the multidimensional nature of structural racism wherein mutually reinforcing systems drive health inequities.[17] Additionally, the extent of reinforcement among forms of structural racism is not examined.[18]

INCORPORATING THE ECOSOCIAL THEORY INTO SURGICAL RESEARCH

There is a paucity of research on the impact of discrimination, whether individual or structural, on surgical conditions and outcomes. However, several factors merit consideration for anyone planning to pursue future research incorporating the impact of discrimination (Box 2.1). Specifically, the majority of research uses race as a proxy for structural racism without properly discussing that the differences seen in racialized groups are a result of social exclusion rather than biological or cultural differences.[17] Variables evaluating structural racism are thereby preferred; otherwise, a clear distinction of the use of race as a reflection of structural racism is needed.[17] Additionally, individuals' lives are rarely shaped by a single system of oppression, rather by multiple overlapping systems warranting the need to apply an intersectional lens to future studies.[17,18] Incorporating mixed methods approaches will also provide opportunities to incorporate community voices and provide richer information about lived experiences of

structural racism, enabling connections between structural factors and individual outcomes.[17,18] As reinforced within the ecosocial theory, there is also a necessity to inquire about experiences in different situations, among close friends and family; delineate the duration, intensity, and frequency of exposures; and incorporate time-dependent exposure across the life course.[9,10,17] Additionally, Krieger advocates for the inclusion of nativity, as people born and raised outside of the United States may not be impacted until they learn how race is leveraged to discriminate against individuals in the United States (US).[9]

WEATHERING HYPOTHESIS

The weathering hypothesis provides an example of embodiment. In 1992, Arline Geronimus noticed different neonatality mortality rates among White, Black, and Puerto Rican individuals as they aged.[19] Specifically, White mothers were noted to have higher neonatal mortality rates during their teen years that decreased with increasing age.[19] Contrastingly, Black and Puerto Rican teenagers had low neonatal mortality rates that increased with maternal age (Fig. 2.2).[19] These data contradicted the dominant developmental paradigm, which suggested that neonatal mortality risks during teenage childbearing years would be outgrown if childbearing was delayed.[19] Instead, Geronimus noticed similar patterns (i.e., low Black–White disparities during teenage years that increased throughout childbearing ages) across biomedical, biobehavioral, and external causes that were linked to social class and racialized groups, suggesting a social commonality.[19] This finding led to the creation of the weathering theory, which hypothesizes that cumulative experiences of social, economic, and political exclusion (i.e., discrimination) lead to more rapid health deterioration.[19] Black women are then forced to cope with social injustice in a prolonged and effortful manner and remediate their poorer health, ultimately leading to an even greater physical toll.[19] Taken altogether, Black women's biological age quickly exceeds their chronological age compared with White women, leading to earlier onset of chronic diseases, disability, and death (Fig. 2.3).[19,20]

Geronimus posits that the effects of weathering start in infancy, whereby unequal infant health outcomes are compounded by the impedance of healthy childhood development and the cumulation of health insults throughout young and middle adulthood (e.g., persistent psychosocial stress from repeated social and economic adversity, high efforts necessary to cope with stress, exposure to environmental hazards, neighborhood deprivation, medical underservice, family

---

BOX 2.1
Factors to Consider When Incorporating the Ecosocial Theory and/or Weathering Hypothesis into Surgical Research

ECOSOCIAL THEORY
1. Refrain from using race as a proxy for structural racism—delineate that differences in racialized groups do not reflect biological or cultural differences.
2. Consider evaluating multiple systems of oppression with an intersectional lens.
3. Consider a mixed methods approach with both quantitative and qualitative data.
4. Inquire about experiences in different situations, among close friends and family, duration/intensity/ frequency of exposures, time-dependent exposure across the life course.
5. Consider including nativity.

WEATHERING HYPOTHESIS
1. Evaluate associations of the weathering hypothesis with surgical disease.
2. Investigate the applicability of the weathering hypothesis to other marginalized communities.
3. Shift from individual risk factors to structurally rooted biopsychosocial stressors.
4. Address underling social inequalities producing health inequities.
5. Eliminate current messages and practices stigmatizing marginalized communities.

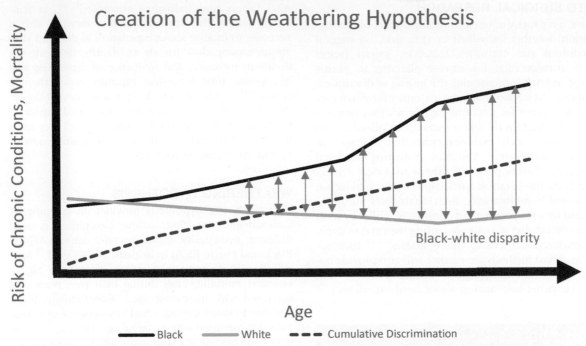

FIG. 2.2 Multiple biomedical, biobehavioral, and external causes were noted to have low black–White disparities (depicted in *blue*) during teenage years that rapidly increased with age, corresponding to the cumulative experiences of discrimination (dashed *red* line). This led to the creation of the weathering hypothesis.

disruption from early death, disability, incarceration, homelessness, and internal frustration and rage at racial injustice affecting sense of belonging), ultimately translating to earlier onset of chronic conditions and extremely shortened life expectancies.[19–23] In fact, early adversity in juvenile years has been suggested to prime individuals to perceive events as threatening, heighten sensitivity, and enhance the effect of discrimination in adulthood.[24] As such, even if individuals are able to escape marginalization in later stages, they are already left at a disadvantage compared with their White counterparts.[19,20,24]

MECHANISMS BEHIND THE WEATHERING HYPOTHESIS

Studies suggest weathering may be induced through multiple pathways. Social adversity (i.e., loneliness, bereavement, economic hardship, low social rank, repeat social defeat) has more recently been established as a predictor of inflammation.[25] The sympathetic nervous system normally activates the inflammatory system to address threatening conditions.[25] However,

persistent exposure to discrimination creates a social environment with a constant threat of hostility and disrespect, leading to chronic activation of β-adrenergic responsive transcription factors and gene transcription of proinflammatory cytokines.[25] Chronic inflammation has been directly implicated in the pathophysiology of chronic diseases.[25]

Allostatic load (AL) expands on the inflammatory pathway, suggesting that stress similarly chronically activates both the HPA axis and the SAM pathway.[26] Consequently, responding chemical messengers lead to physiologic dysregulation in the cardiovascular, metabolic, inflammatory, and neuroendocrine systems, which ultimately manifests as chronic diseases.[26] Geronimus reported that Black individuals have higher AL at all ages compared with White people.[27] Differences were small during teenage years but quickly increased with age (largest gap between ages 35–64) and were higher among women compared with men.[27] Additionally, 50% of Black women had high AL by age 45, whereas White women reached similar levels as they approached 60 years of age.[27] Lower socioeconomic status (SES) was also associated with higher AL, but White

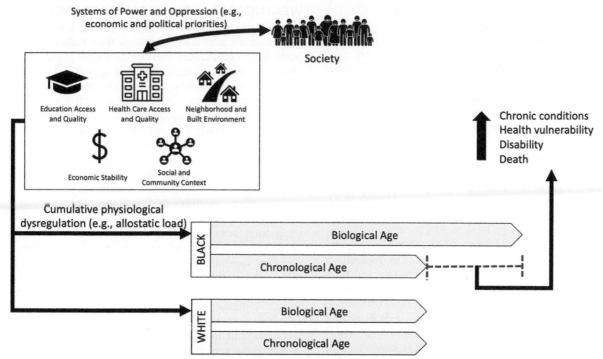

FIG. 2.3 The weathering hypothesis suggests that cumulative experiences of discrimination lead to accelerated biological aging relative to chronological age, ultimately causing earlier onset of chronic conditions, greater health vulnerability, disability, and mortality.

people with low SES were still less likely to have high AL compared with Black people with higher SES, suggesting that SES only serves as a "porous shield" from lived experiences of structural racism within the Black community.[21,27]

Activation of the HPA axis and the sympathetic nervous system have also been linked to peripheral blood leukocyte telomere length, a marker of cellular aging.[28] Telomeres are repeated DNA sequences that cap the ends of chromosomes to support chromosomal stability.[29] Psychosocial and physiologic stressors have been associated with oxidative stress and consequential telomere shortening.[29,30] Specifically, racial discrimination is associated with accelerated telomere shortening, leading to an estimated biological age 7.5 years older than chronological age.[29] Peripheral blood leukocytes have also been used to measure DNA methylation of CpG sites associated with aging.[31] Most of these sites are associated with oxidative stress, DNA damage, tissue degradation, and age-related conditions (e.g., cognitive decline, all-cause mortality).[31,32] Psychosocial stress similarly impacts epigenetic changes as one-third of the CpG sites are located in glucocorticoid response elements, leading to transcription of stress-response

genes.[32] Black individuals are noted to have 10 times as many methylated CpG sites associated with aging relative to their White counterparts.[32] Further, racial discrimination, low education, limited income, and neighborhood disadvantage have been correlated with greater methylation.[31,32]

APPLICATION OF THE WEATHERING HYPOTHESIS

Most studies evaluating the weathering hypothesis have noted associations with birth outcomes, such as neonatal and infant mortality, preterm birth, birth weight, size for gestational age, intrauterine growth retardation, and rates of spontaneous abortion.[33,34] However, data also support an association between the weathering hypothesis and body mass index, rates of hypertension, stroke, cardiovascular disease, diabetes, functional limitations, longevity, self-reported health, and cognition (e.g., episodic memory, working memory capacity, executive function).[33,35] Some studies have also noted that financial pressure and depressive symptoms moderate the rate of biological aging, rather than standard risk factors such as education and health-related behaviors.[36,37] For example, chronic conditions have been seen in Black women in their 20–30s with health-induced functional limitations by 35 years of age and disability rates comparable with White women at 55 years of age.[20] Black women with per capita incomes less than $3900 exhibit accelerated aging, specifically through financial hardship and pressures, whereas those with incomes above $15,000 experience decelerated aging.[37] In turn, Black women have an over 50% increased odds of mortality between 15 and 29 years of age compared with White women when death at this age is otherwise seen as unlikely.[19] Studies have also evaluated the applicability of the weathering hypothesis to Mexican and Latinx populations.[21] However, nativity frequently moderates this relationship as foreign-born and recently arrived immigrants tend to have better health than US-born populations.[21] Conversely, Mexican and Latinx individuals who have lived in the United States longer and have had to engage with social institutions controlled by the dominant White population are more attuned to the dehumanizing ideologies, negative prejudices, and stereotypes associated with US racial hierarchies.[21] While most research has historically focused on income and education levels, the aforementioned studies suggest that addressing the larger structural relationships between racial discrimination and inequitable health outcomes is necessary.[19]

The role of psychosocial stress in the weathering hypothesis has led to studies evaluating the impact of social factors on slowing biological age acceleration. Black individuals with greater social strain have faster rates of accelerated aging.[36] In contrast, individuals with greater social support, social participation, and social ties have slower rates of accelerated aging.[36] Supportive relationships, particularly positive romantic relationships with couple functioning (defined by effective communication, relationship confidence, relationship satisfaction, and perceived partner support), can buffer epigenetic aging.[38] Supportive family environments (assessed through perceived parental emotional support, parent–child conflict, and home organization) similarly buffer the impact of racial discrimination on epigenetic aging in adolescents.[39] Additionally, living in neighborhoods with greater cohesion or racial/ethnic densities leads to decreased "othering" encounters, enhanced identity safety, risk-pooling protections, and deeply rooted coethnic social ties that allow for sharing of counternarratives, all of which slow biological age acceleration.[21,36]

WEATHERING IN SURGICAL RESEARCH

To the best of our knowledge, no studies specifically evaluating the relationship between the weathering hypothesis and surgical diseases currently exist in the literature. However, in triple negative (ER-/PR-/HER2-) breast cancer, a subtype twice as prevalent in Black versus White women, Geronimus advocates to shift the focus from identifying genetic risk factors associated with African ancestry (i.e., individual risk factors) to social and behavior factors related to structurally rooted biopsychosocial stressors (Box 2.1).[40] Otherwise, strategies intended to alleviate disparities are likely to be rendered insufficient.[20] Further work is also needed to evaluate the applicability of the weathering hypothesis to other marginalized communities. Although identifying local stressors and providing stress-abatement techniques may help *ameliorate* accelerated health deterioration, Geronimus suggests that the only way to *eliminate* racial health inequities is to "get political" and address the underlying social inequalities producing them.[20] Specifically, social policies are necessary to eliminate current cultural messages and practices that stigmatize and discredit the Black community.[25] Understanding the factors that currently shape the public sentiment on race (i.e., structural racism) is needed, as current ideologies affect clinical judgment, fuel distrust within the healthcare system, and weaken support for initiatives meant to help improve the health of marginalized communities.[20]

Highlights

- Social epidemiology examines the impact of sociostructural factors on population health and disease.
- Several models and theories have emerged to help explain the pathophysiology behind different population health distributions and health inequities.
- The ecosocial theory considers biology and society as an "intertwining ensemble" in which individuals are situated within social groups whose everyday lives are shaped by the dominant society's economic and political priorities.
- The weathering theory hypothesizes that cumulative experiences of social, economic, and political exclusion (i.e., discrimination) lead to more rapid health deterioration.
- Individuals' lives are rarely shaped by a single system of oppression, rather by multiple overlapping systems warranting the need to apply an intersectional lens to future studies.

REFERENCES

1. 2030 HP. Social Determinants of Health. US Department of Health and Human Services, Office of Disease Prevention and Health Promotion. https://health.gov/healthypeople/priority-areas/social-determinants-health. Accessed January 20, 2023.

2. Honjo K. Social epidemiology: definition, history, and research examples. *Environ Health Prev Med.* September 2004;9(5):193–199. https://doi.org/10.1007/BF02898100.

3. Krieger N. Epidemiology and the web of causation: has anyone seen the spider? *Soc Sci Med.* 1994;39(7):887–903. https://doi.org/10.1016/0277-9536(94)90202-X.

4. Smith MN. The best possible condition for nature to act upon host-agent environment relationships. *Am Assoc Occup Health Nurs.* 1986;34(3):120–121.

5. Krieger N. Theories for social epidemiology in the 21st century: an ecosocial perspective. *Int J Epidemiol.* 2001;30(4):668–677. https://doi.org/10.1093/ije/30.4.668.

6. McEwen BS. Stress, adaptation, and disease. Allostasis and allostatic load. *Ann N Y Acad Sci.* May 01, 1998;840:33–44. https://doi.org/10.1111/j.1749-6632.1998.tb09546.x.

7. Green LW, Kreuter MW, Deeds SG, Partridge KB, Bartlett E. *Health Education Planning : A Diagnostic Approach.* 1980.

8. Krieger N. Proximal, distal, and the politics of causation: what's level got to do with it? *Am J Publ Health.* February 2008;98(2):221–230. https://doi.org/10.2105/AJPH.2007.111278.

9. Krieger N. Methods for the scientific study of discrimination and health: an ecosocial approach. *Am J Publ Health.* May 2012;102(5):936–944. https://doi.org/10.2105/AJPH.2011.300544.

10. Krieger N. Embodying inequality: a review of concepts, measures, and methods for studying health consequences of discrimination. *Int J Health Serv.* 1999;29(2):295–352. https://doi.org/10.2190/M11W-VWXE-KQM9-G97Q.

11. Williams DR, Neighbors HW, Jackson JS. Racial/ethnic discrimination and health: findings from community studies. *Am J Publ Health.* February 2003;93(2):200–208. https://doi.org/10.2105/ajph.93.2.200.

12. Paradies Y, Ben J, Denson N, et al. Racism as a determinant of health: a systematic review and meta-analysis. *PLoS One.* 2015;10(9):e0138511. https://doi.org/10.1371/journal.pone.0138511.

13. Michaels EK, Board C, Mujahid MS, et al. Area-level racial prejudice and health: a systematic review. *Health Psychol.* March 2022;41(3):211–224. https://doi.org/10.1037/hea0001141.

14. Ahmed K, Scretching D, Lane SD. Study designs, measures and indexes used in studying the structural racism as a social determinant of health in high income countries from 2000–2022: evidence from a scoping review. *Int J Equity Health.* 2023;22(1):4. https://doi.org/10.1186/s12939-022-01796-0.

15. Castle B, Wendel M, Kerr J, Brooms D, Rollins A. Public health's approach to systemic racism: a systematic literature review. *J Racial Ethn Health Disparities.* February 2019;6(1):27–36. https://doi.org/10.1007/s40615-018-0494-x.

16. Groos M, Wallace M, Hardeman R, Theall KP. Measuring inequity: a systematic review of methods used to quantify structural racism. *J Health Disparities Res Pract.* 2018;11(2):190–205.

17. Adkins-Jackson PB, Chantarat T, Bailey ZD, Ponce NA. Measuring structural racism: a guide for epidemiologists and other health researchers. *Am J Epidemiol.* March 24, 2022;191(4):539–547. https://doi.org/10.1093/aje/kwab239.

18. Hardeman RR, Homan PA, Chantarat T, Davis BA, Brown TH. Improving the measurement of structural racism to achieve antiracist health policy. *Health Aff.* February 2022;41(2):179–186. https://doi.org/10.1377/hlthaff.2021.01489.

19. Geronimus AT. The weathering hypothesis and the health of African-American women and infants: evidence and speculations. *Ethn Dis.* 1992;2(3):207–221.

20. Geronimus AT. Understanding and eliminating racial inequalities in women's health in the United States: the role of the weathering conceptual framework. *J Am Med Women's Assoc.* 2001;56(4):133–136.

21. Geronimus AT, Pearson JA, Linnenbringer E, et al. Weathering in detroit: place, race, ethnicity, and poverty as conceptually fluctuating social constructs shaping variation in allostatic load. *Milbank Q.* December 2020;98(4):1171–1218. https://doi.org/10.1111/1468-0009.12484.

22. Schmeer KK, Tarrence J. Racial-ethnic disparities in inflammation: evidence of weathering in childhood? *J Health Soc Behav.* September 2018;59(3):411–428. https://doi.org/10.1177/0022146518784592.

23. Lei MK, Beach SRH, Simons RL. Biological embedding of neighborhood disadvantage and collective efficacy: influences on chronic illness via accelerated cardiometabolic age. *Dev Psychopathol.* December 2018;30(5):1797–1815. https://doi.org/10.1017/S0954579418000937.

24. Simons RL, Lei MK, Beach SRH, et al. Discrimination, segregation, and chronic inflammation: testing the weathering explanation for the poor health of Black Americans. *Dev Psychol.* October 2018;54(10):1993–2006. https://doi.org/10.1037/dev0000511.

25. Simons RL, Lei MK, Klopack E, Zhang Y, Gibbons FX, Beach SRH. Racial discrimination, inflammation, and chronic illness among african American women at midlife: support for the weathering perspective. *J Racial Ethn Health Disparities.* April 2021;8(2):339–349. https://doi.org/10.1007/s40615-020-00786-8.

26. Seeman TE, Singer BH, Rowe JW, Horwitz RI, McEwen BS. Price of adaptation–allostatic load and its health consequences. MacArthur studies of successful aging. *Arch Intern Med.* October 27, 1997;157(19):2259–2268.

27. Geronimus AT, Hicken M, Keene D, Bound J. "Weathering" and age patterns of allostatic load scores among blacks and whites in the United States. *Am J Publ Health.* May 2006;96(5):826–833. https://doi.org/10.2105/AJPH.2004.060749.

28. Geronimus AT, Pearson JA, Linnenbringer E, et al. Race-ethnicity, poverty, urban stressors, and telomere length in a detroit community-based sample. *J Health Soc Behav.* June 2015;56(2):199–224. https://doi.org/10.1177/0022146515582100.

29. Chae DH, Wang Y, Martz CD, et al. Racial discrimination and telomere shortening among african Americans: the coronary artery risk development in young adults (CARDIA) study. *Health Psychol.* March 2020;39(3):209–219. https://doi.org/10.1037/hea0000832.

30. Geronimus AT, Hicken MT, Pearson JA, Seashols SJ, Brown KL, Cruz TD. Do US black women experience stress-related accelerated biological aging?: a novel theory and first population-based test of black-white differences in telomere length. *Hum Nat.* March 10, 2010;21(1): 19–38. https://doi.org/10.1007/s12110-010-9078-0.

31. Simons RL, Lei MK, Klopack E, Beach SRH, Gibbons FX, Philibert RA. The effects of social adversity, discrimination, and health risk behaviors on the accelerated aging of African Americans: further support for the weathering hypothesis. *Soc Sci Med.* August 2021;282:113169. https://doi.org/10.1016/j.socscimed.2020.113169.

32. Noren Hooten N, Pacheco NL, Smith JT, Evans MK. The accelerated aging phenotype: the role of race and social determinants of health on aging. *Ageing Res Rev.* January 2022; 73:101536. https://doi.org/10.1016/j.arr.2021.101536.

33. Forde AT, Crookes DM, Suglia SF, Demmer RT. The weathering hypothesis as an explanation for racial disparities in health: a systematic review. *Ann Epidemiol.* May 2019;33: 1–18.e3. https://doi.org/10.1016/j.annepidem.2019.02.011.

34. Frazier T, Hogue CJR, Bonney EA, Yount KM, Pearce BD. Weathering the storm; a review of pre-pregnancy stress and risk of spontaneous abortion. *Psychoneuroendocrinology.* June 2018;92:142–154. https://doi.org/10.1016/j.psyneuen.2018.03.001.

35. Letang SK, Lin SS, Parmelee PA, McDonough IM. Ethnoracial disparities in cognition are associated with multiple socioeconomic status-stress pathways. *Cogn Res Princ Implic.* October 09, 2021;6(1):64. https://doi.org/10.1186/s41235-021-00329-7.

36. Forrester SN, Whitfield KE, Kiefe CI, Thorpe RJ. Navigating black aging: the biological consequences of stress and depression. *J Gerontol B Psychol Sci Soc Sci.* November 23, 2022;77(11):2101–2112. https://doi.org/10.1093/geronb/gbab224.

37. Simons RL, Lei MK, Beach SR, et al. Economic hardship and biological weathering: the epigenetics of aging in a U.S. sample of black women. *Soc Sci Med.* February 2016;150:192–200. https://doi.org/10.1016/j.socscimed.2015.12.001.

38. Lei MK, Lavner JA, Carter SE, Adesogan O, Beach SRH. Relationship intervention indirectly buffers financial strain's effect on biological aging among Black adults. *J Fam Psychol.* June 2022;36(4):502–512. https://doi.org/10.1037/fam0000926.

39. Brody GH, Miller GE, Yu T, Beach SR, Chen E. Supportive family environments ameliorate the link between racial discrimination and epigenetic aging: a replication across two longitudinal cohorts. *Psychol Sci.* April 2016;27(4): 530–541. https://doi.org/10.1177/0956797615626703.

40. Linnenbringer E, Gehlert S, Geronimus AT. Black-white disparities in breast cancer subtype: the intersection of socially patterned stress and genetic expression. *AIMS Public Health.* 2017;4(5):526–556. https://doi.org/10.3934/publichealth.2017.5.526.

CHAPTER 3

Allostatic Load—Measurement Issues in Cancer Patients and Other Populations

CHANITA HUGHES HALBERT, PHD

INTRODUCTION

An emerging hypothesis about disparities in cancer risk and outcomes among disparity populations is that psychological and social stressors impact biological processes that play a role in the initiation and progression of disease.[1] Allostatic load is an indicator of biological dysregulation in response to psychological and social stress that is used to measure the impact of these stressors on biological functioning.[2−4] AL is an index that is determined based on physiological biomarkers such as immune (C-Reactive protein), neuroendocrine (cortisol), metabolic (HbAIc), and autonomic (systolic and diastolic blood pressure) functioning[4] also implicated in chronic diseases that are leading causes of morbidity and mortality among minority men. Several studies have examined racial differences in allostatic load, and this work has shown that individuals from disparity populations have greater allostatic load compared with those from other groups.[5−7] For this reason, allostatic load has been examined as a mechanism of cancer health disparities[3,8,9] and is now being included as one of the pathways through which the social environment contributes to racial disparities in cancer risk and outcomes in emerging conceptual models of minority health and cancer health disparities.[10] Nevertheless, important empirical questions remain about allostatic load because of inconsistencies in how this biomarker has been measured across studies and disease types and limited data about the longitudinal effects of allostatic load on disease risk and outcomes.[11] Moreover, few efforts have been made to integrate calculation of allostatic load into clinical or public health practice; therefore, the utility of using allostatic load as a framework to improve cancer health disparities and other domains in minority health is unknown. The purpose of this chapter is to review allostatic load theory and describe key issues in measuring allostatic load in community and clinical samples. This chapter also presents findings from studies on allostatic load in cancer populations and includes a case example of how allostatic load was used as the framework to guide transdisciplinary translational research on precision medicine research within the context of cancer health disparities along with a discussion of priorities for future research on allostatic load.

ALLOSTATIC LOAD THEORY AND CONCEPTUAL DEVELOPMENT

Allostatic load was first described by McEwen and Stellar as part of their work to describe the relationship between stress and disease risk.[12] This work was foundational because it identified physiological systems that are activated as part of the stress response and made important distinctions between homeostasis and allostasis within the context of risk of developing chronic and acute diseases. McEwen and Stellar also introduced the concept of allostatic load as the cumulative result of physiological wear and tear across multiple systems, organs, and tissues and set the stage for future research that described the conceptual basis of this construct and investigations on the nature and distribution of allostatic load across diverse populations.[12] According to these conceptual models, for instance, allostatic load can result when (1) there is repeated exposure to stressors, (2) adaptation to chronic stressors is reduced; (3) stress responses continue after the stressor has been alleviated; or (4) allostatic responses are not able to manage the stressor.[12,13]

Several aspects of allostatic load theory are relevant to minority health and cancer health disparities. First, this construct is based on the premise of physiological efforts to maintain stability when faced with challenges or stressors. The economic, social, and psychological challenges experienced by African Americans as a result of racism and discrimination are well documented,[14] and these stressors, and the challenges that result from these sociopolitical factors, are included as precursors to physical and mental health outcomes in early conceptual models of health disparities.[15] Further, stress exposure has been proposed as a central factor in health disparities, and allostatic load is one physical outcome included in conceptual models that are based on the stress process.[15] In addition, many of the diseases for which there are racial disparities in risk and outcomes have been linked with stress responses (e.g., hypertension, cardiovascular disease) and are hormone dependent (e.g., breast cancer, prostate cancer). Data from animal studies have shown that exposure to social stressors (e.g., isolation) is associated with an increased likelihood of developing mammary tumors that are histologically similar to those that develop among African American women.[16] This research has also shown that animals who had a dysregulated cortisol response in which hormonal levels do not decrease, or return to normal levels following stress exposure, are most likely to develop disease.[16] Cortisol is the primary hormone that is responsible for the stress response; previous research has shown that African Americans have a dysregulated cortisol response because of exposure to chronic social and psychological stressors (e.g., low limited financial resources, racial discrimination). Using data from the Midlife in the US Study (MIDUS), Cohen et al. found that the typical diurnal rhythm of cortisol differs between African Americans and whites.[17] Compared with whites, African Americans had lower cortisol levels in the morning and higher hormonal levels at the end of the day. Racial differences in cortisol were independent of SES factors, but low SES (e.g., education and income) was associated with a dysregulated cortisol response that was characterized by higher levels of cortisol during the evening among African Americans.[17] Similar findings were reported in a recent analysis that compared diurnal cortisol slopes between African American and White men in the MIDUS II study; African American men were more likely than White men to exhibit blunted cortisol responses.[18] In other work, Webb Hooper demonstrated that cortisol levels are lower at critical timepoints in the trajectory of a smoking cessation intervention (e.g., at baseline, end of treatment) among African Americans (vs. white).[19] Cortisol slopes (from baseline, end of treatment, and 1-month follow-up) were also flattered among African American smokers compared with White smokers in this study.[19] Lastly, allostatic load was

higher among participants in the MIDUS II study who reported pervasive discrimination, but the association between allostatic load and discrimination was stronger among African American relative to whites.[20]

ALLOSTATIC LOAD IN CANCER POPULATIONS

Cancer is an important clinical context to advance scientific knowledge about allostatic load and guide the development of strategies to enhance minority health and reduce cancer health disparities through cancer care delivery and community and population health approaches. This is because the drivers of minority health and cancer health disparities (e.g., biological factors, social and behavioral variables, psychological characteristics) contribute to allostatic load and allostatic load biomarkers are indicators of the chronic conditions for which there are racial disparities among diverse populations. For instance, physiological responses to social, psychological, and clinical stressors that are reflected in allostatic load scores are manifested and measured in clinical healthcare systems in which decisions about early detection, treatment, and management are influenced by the clinician's interpretation of biomarkers and indicators of risk and disease progression.

Empirical data about the nature and distribution of allostatic load among cancer patients have been generated through the inclusion and analysis of biomarker data in several large-scale studies that include the MacArthur Foundation Study on Successful Aging, the National Health and Nutrition Examination Study (NHANES), and MIDUS.[21] Allostatic load biomarkers have also been collected as part of institutional cohort studies.[22] For instance, Parente and colleagues used NHANES data to examine racial disparities in allostatic load and found that African American women with breast cancer in NHANES had higher allostatic load compared with those who did not have a personal history of disease. There were no differences in allostatic load among White women who had breast cancer and those who did not a personal history of disease.[23] Using data from the cohort in the Women's Circle of Health Follow-Up Study, Xing and colleagues found that prediagnostic levels of allostatic load were associated with larger tumors that were poorly differentiated among African American women.[24] This team also determined allostatic load profiles that were based on inflammatory biomarkers or lipid/metabolic biomarkers using medical records and found that patients who had higher inflammatory-based allostatic load before their diagnosis reported poorer functional well-being and overall quality of life.[24] Similar findings were reported by Shen et al. who used data from an institutional cohort of breast cancer patients to examine the association between allostatic load and neighborhood deprivation.[22] This group found that African American breast cancer patients were likely to reside in areas with high levels of area deprivation and had higher-grade breast cancer and tumors that were poorly differentiated. Patients who lived in areas with high levels of area deprivation also had higher allostatic load and lower global levels of DNA methylation. African American prostate cancer patients were also more likely than White prostate cancer patients to live in areas with high levels of social deprivation[25]; however, racial differences in allostatic load have not yet been examined extensively among prostate cancer patients even though there are several examples of the toxic social stressors that African American men face. Stabellini et al.[26] examined the association between allostatic load and cardiovascular outcomes among prostate cancer patients who were identified from an institutional repository and found that 6.6% of patients (n = 5261) had a major cardiac event following their diagnosis and with each 1-point increase in allostatic load; there was a 27% increased risk of having a major cardiac event within 60 days of being diagnosed. When measured as a time-varying exposure, the risk of having a major cardiac event increased 31% within 1 year of being diagnosed with this disease.[26] In work that examined the association between allostatic load and resilience among African American and White men at increased risk for adverse prostate cancer outcomes, Halbert et al. found that allostatic load was higher among men who reported they were able to bounce back following challenges or stressors (e.g., were more resilient) compared with those who reported less resilience.[27] Lastly, in a recent metaanalysis that included 30,769 subjects from studies (n = 4) that were included in a systematic review of allostatic load and cancer, there was a 9% increased risk of mortality from cancer with a 1-unit increase in allostatic load.[28]

As empirical data are being generated about the association between allostatic load and cancer risk and outcomes, an important next step is to translate these finding into evidence-based interventions. Rosemberg et al. conducted a scoping review of interventions that targeted allostatic load by improving stress responses and decreasing exposure to stressors through approaches that included cognitive behavioral therapy, mind–body approaches (e.g., tai chi), and health behavior interventions.[29] There were improvements in allostatic load in four of the six studies that were included in the review; however, it is important to note that only six studies met the inclusion for the scoping review. Nevertheless, demonstrating that allostatic load, as a cumulative index of physiological

wear and tear, is amenable to change, and these changes can be measured as part of diverse types of interventions has clinical and public health significance.

MEASUREMENT ISSUES IN ALLOSTATIC LOAD

The utility of using allostatic load as a predictor of cancer risk in prospective studies or as an outcome of cancer care services, psychosocial programs, and other types of interventions will depend on the ability to measure allostatic load consistently and with validity across studies.[30,31] Consistent with allostatic load theory, the measurement of this variable is based on the physiological systems that are activated and impacted in the stress response system. McEwen and Seeman[32] first established methods and principles for measuring allostatic load as part of the MacArthur Foundation Study on Aging, and several subsequent studies used these methods to obtain data on allostatic load biomarkers as part of population-based cohorts (e.g., NHANES).[21,32] Nevertheless, several concerns have been raised about the variability in the algorithms that are used to calculate allostatic load and differences in the biomarkers that are included in these formulations across studies. For instance, Carbone and colleagues found that heart rate, blood pressure (diastolic and systolic), HDL cholesterol, and C-reactive protein are measured most often in studies (n = 395) that were included in a scoping review of measurement issues in allostatic load.[21] Cortisol, body mass index, total cholesterol, and waist-to-hip ration were measured in about two-thirds of studies. With respect to the methods for calculating allostatic load, 52.5% of studies used a sample distribution strategy in which participants in the highest risk quartile are coded as having a dysregulated value for each individual biomarker. These values are then summed to generate a single score for allostatic load. One reason for using the sum of high-risk quartiles method is because some of the allostatic load biomarkers (e.g., cortisol) do not have established clinical cutoffs that can be used to establish dysregulation. Further, biomarkers such as cortisol and DHEAS may also not be routinely measured as part of healthcare delivery, and the resources that are needed to collect and process biospecimens and the costs associated with analyzing samples to determine allostatic load biomarkers may be prohibitive in clinic-, community-, and population-based studies on cancer health disparities. As a result, there is considerable variability in the allostatic load biomarkers that are assessed as part of studies, and consensus has not been reached about the minimal set of biomarkers that should be included in algorithms that are used to calculate this variable.[21]

CASE EXAMPLE: TRANSDISCIPLINARY COLLABORATIVE CENTER IN PRECISION MEDICINE AND MINORITY MEN'S HEALTH

The operationalization and measurement of allostatic load are critical areas that need to be addressed to realize the promise of using this variable to predict and impact disease risk and outcomes, especially among diverse populations.[30] These issues were considered as part of a Transdisciplinary Collaborative Center in Precision Medicine and Minority Men's Health that was established with funding from the National Institute on Minority Health and Health Disparities and the National Cancer Institute.[33] A specific goal for this center is to determine the utility of using allostatic load as a framework for integrating diverse types of data to increase the precision of approaches for addressing racial disparities in health outcomes among minority men. To do this, three translational studies related to prostate cancer risk and outcomes were developed to examine the effects of allostatic load within the context of a disease that has a significant clinical and public health impact among men from diverse racial groups, is a priority condition for intervention among stakeholders (e.g., patients, community residents, and representatives from public health organizations), and is also relevant to other chronic conditions that disproportionately affect minority men in terms of morbidity and mortality.

Prostate cancer continues to be one of the leading causes of morbidity and mortality among men,[34] and previous studies have shown that the social environment is important to consider along with biological variables in prostate cancer risk and outcomes, especially among African American men.[35,36] While racial disparities in life expectancy continue to be examined as part of population-based surveillance efforts[37] and targeted interventions are being developed to improve healthcare and outcomes specifically among African American men,[38–40] the overall social context has not yet been integrated into surveillance efforts or interventions strategies. Thus, while there has been significant national coverage of the acute and chronic stressors that African American experience men experience since the police killing of George Floyd in 2020; the physiological impact of being exposed to these toxic social stressors has not yet been examined widely as part of cancer health disparities research, but the evidence base about stress, stress responses, and cancer-related outcomes among African American men in clinic and community-based samples is growing. Previous research has shown that greater neighborhood deprivation is associated with higher allostatic load; the positive association between allostatic load and neighborhood deprivation is most pronounced among men, African Americans, and those who did not have high levels of emotional support.[41] Further, the association between neighborhood deprivation and allostatic load was linked with risk exposure behaviors, poor social and physical environments, and stress associated with living in an underserved neighborhood.[41] Other work has shown that perceived stress is associated significantly with emotional and physical well-being and cancer-related psychological distress among African American and White men who were newly diagnosed with prostate cancer.[42,43] Hoyt et al. also showed that prostate cancer patients who used avoidant coping strategies had a greater dysregulated cortisol response.[44] However, there is a paucity of empirical data on the complex ways in which biological, social, psychological, and clinical factors interact together and contribute to poor outcomes among racially diverse men with specific disease risks and disparities in clinical outcomes.

Accordingly, this precision medicine center in minority men's health uses allostatic load as the framework for conducting transdisciplinary translational research to examine the synergistic effects between biological, social, psychological, and clinical determinants of prostate cancer risk and outcomes among African American and White men. Allostatic load was selected as the overarching framework for this center because it reflects the cumulative effects of stress exposure across multiple physiological systems and could be expanded to address other chronic diseases that disproportionately affect African American men in terms of morbidity and mortality (e.g., diabetes, hypertension) along with the primary research focus on prostate cancer. An additional reason for using allostatic load as the overarching framework for this precision medicine center is that the biomarkers for this variable are likely to be collected as part of oncology care and recorded in the electronic health record in diverse clinical settings (e.g., academic medical centers, federally qualified health centers) that provide healthcare to disparity populations. This was an important consideration because one of the overall goals of this center is to develop precision medicine approaches that can be implemented into diverse clinical and public health settings and programs. Center projects are addressing critical empirical questions to (1) characterize stress reactivity among prostate cancer survivors at high risk for recurrence based on individual variation in allostatic load, social factors, chronic socioeconomic stressors as part of a prostate cancer vaccine clinical trial (Project 1); (2) develop novel biomarkers for prostate cancer and identify immune modulators of disease and determine the relationship between prostate cancer biomarkers and allostatic load in a retrospective cohort of patients who were treated with radical prostatectomy (Project 2); and (3) examine the effects of vitamin D_3 supplementation on changes in gene expression in prostate tissue samples among African American and White men undergoing biopsy within the context of HPA axis functioning and allostatic load biomarkers (Project 3).

Information about the organizational structure of this center has been published previously[33]; the shared resources for administrative support, data integration, and dissemination and implementation strategies provided oversight of the collection and measurement of allostatic load biomarkers. Under the leaderships of investigators from academic medical centers and representatives from public health agencies and community-based organizations, a standardized social determinants survey was developed and implemented across center projects,[45] and procedures were implemented to abstract data on allostatic load biomarkers at timepoints that were relevant to the clinical focus of the research. For instance, Project 1 is examining racial differences in stress reactivity, and responses to a prostate cancer vaccine and allostatic load biomarkers were measured using samples that were collected at the baseline clinic visit for a clinical trial that was examining the effects of a poxvirus vaccine (PROSTVAC) on the cancer growth and immune responses among patients who were at increased risk for recurrence. In contrast, Project 2 included patients who were treated with radical prostatectomy and donated a prostate tissue sample to an institutional biorepository. Data on allostatic load biomarkers were abstracted from electronic health records for these patients using vital statistics that were obtained during the presurgical visit. Finally, Project 3 included men who were undergoing prostate biopsy at the Urology Clinic in Veteran's Affairs Health System, and samples were obtained at the baseline biopsy visit to measure allostatic load biomarkers. Because prospective samples were not available to measure allostatic load biomarkers in Project 2, we developed an allostatic load score that was based on the biomarkers available in the electronic health record (EHR). This EHR-derived allostatic load includes body mass index, systolic blood pressure, diastolic blood pressure, total cholesterol, serum glucose, and heart rate and was calculated to allow allostatic load to be compared across projects using a variable that calculated using the same biomarkers. As in previous reports,[21] our EHR-derived allostatic load variable was calculated

using a sample distribution approach and was informed by our previous research, which demonstrated that African American and White prostate cancer patients in our retrospective cohort had nonsignificant differences in comorbidity status for the conditions that are the basis for allostatic load biomarkers.[46] We used a sample distribution method to calculate allostatic load because participants in center projects resided in a geographic area that has high rates of chronic conditions and established clinical cutoffs for allostatic biomarkers related to these conditions may not be able to identify individuals who have levels of physiological dysregulation that place them at high risk for disease and poor outcomes. For instance, Babatunde et al. found that African American prostate cancer patients were about three times more likely than White prostate cancer patients to live in neighborhoods with high levels of deprivation.[25] While there were no differences in biochemical recurrence based on social deprivation levels, African American prostate cancer patients had a higher risk of biochemical recurrence compared with White prostate cancer patients.[25] Further, there were no differences in comorbidity status between African American and White prostate cancer patients included in our retrospective cohort study.[46] An important next step for our precision medicine center is to characterize the nature and distribution of allostatic load using geospatial methods that allow this variable to be visualized spatially along with analyses to build upon prior studies that measure neighborhood deprivation as a stress exposure variable along with other social determinants of health.

CONCLUSIONS AND FUTURE DIRECTIONS

Since allostatic load was first introduced into the literature by McEwen and others,[12,32,47] allostatic load has emerged as a framework for examining cancer risk and racial disparities in outcomes for breast, prostate, and other types of cancer.[33,48,49] The ability to use allostatic load as a reliable predictor of disease risk and to measure outcomes of cancer care and cancer-related interventions will depend on reaching consensus about the minimal number and type of biomarkers that should be included in calculating allostatic load.[21,30,50] Since allostatic load scores can be generated using structured and unstructured data that are available in the electronic health record, it will also be important to integrate automatic methods for integrating scoring algorithms into cancer care delivery. Methods from machine learning and artificial intelligence (e.g., natural language processing) are now being used to identify patients who have social determinants of health documented in their electronic health record[51]; future efforts are needed to automate the scoring of allostatic load biomarkers and to integrate scoring algorithms into practice while considering the advantages and disadvantages of alternative scoring methods (e.g., using established clinical cutoff, sample distribution methods).[21] Research teams are addressing these issues by using standard methods to measure allostatic load studies that have different specific aims, research designs, and study populations.[33,48] Halbert and colleagues have developed an EHR-derived measure of allostatic load as part of a precision medicine center in minority men's health,[33] and future studies will compare this variable across the trajectory of prostate cancer diagnosis, treatment, and recovery. New research is being funded by the American Cancer Society and the National Institutes of Health to increase the evidence base about the association between cancer risk and outcomes; it will be important for these studies to describe their allostatic load biomarkers and characterize when and how they were measured and scored to generate scores for this variable. Lastly, as efforts are made to increase the precision of allostatic load measurement in clinical, community, and population-based samples, it will also be important to examine longitudinal changes in allostatic load along with generating empirical data about the impact of clinical, psychosocial, and behavioral interventions on differences in allostatic load.

Highlights

- Psychological and social stressors impact biological processes that play a role in the initiation and progression of disease.
- Allostatic load is an indicator of biological dysregulation in response to psychological and social stress that is used to measure the impact of these stressors on biological functioning.
- Stress exposure has been proposed as a central factor in health disparities, and allostatic load is one physical outcome included in conceptual models that are based on the stress process.
- The measurement of allostatic load is based on the physiological systems that are activated and impacted in the stress response system.
- In the future, hopefully, there will be an increased ability to use allostatic load as a reliable predictor of disease risk and to measure outcomes of cancer care and cancer-related interventions.

REFERENCES

1. Gehlert S, Sohmer D, Sacks T, Mininger C, McClintock M, Olopade O. Targeting health disparities: a model linking upstream determinants to downstream interventions. *Health Aff*. 2008;27(2):339–349.
2. Seeman T, Epel E, Gruenewald T, Karlamangla A, McEwen BS. Socio-economic differentials in peripheral biology: cumulative allostatic load. *Ann N Y Acad Sci*. 2010;1186(1):223–239.
3. Szanton SL, Gill JM, Allen JK. Allostatic load: a mechanism of socioeconomic health disparities? *Biol Res Nurs*. 2005; 7(1):7–15.
4. Karlamangla A, Gruenewald T, Seeman T. Promise of biomarkers in assessing and predicting health. In: Wolfe B, Evans W, Seeman T, eds. *The Biological Consequences of Socioeconomic Inequalities*. Russell Sage Foundation; 2012: 38–62.
5. Murkey JA, Watkins BX, Vieira D, Boden-Albala B. Disparities in allostatic load, telomere length and chronic stress burden among African American adults: a systematic review. *Psychoneuroendocrinology*. June 2022;140:105730. https://doi.org/10.1016/j.psyneuen.2022.105730.
6. Kezios KL, Suglia SF, Doyle DM, et al. Comparing different operationalizations of allostatic load measured in mid-life and their patterning by race and cumulative life course socioeconomic status. *Psychoneuroendocrinology*. May 2022; 139:105689. https://doi.org/10.1016/j.psyneuen.2022.105689.
7. Akinyemiju T, Wilson LE, Deveaux A, et al. Association of allostatic load with all-cause and Cancer mortality by race and body mass index in the REGARDS cohort. *Cancers*. June 26, 2020;12(6). https://doi.org/10.3390/cancers12061695.
8. Duru OK, Harawa NT, Kermah D, Norris KC. Allostatic load burden and racial disparities in mortality. *J Natl Med Assoc*. 2012;104(1–2):89.
9. Hickson DA, Diez Roux AV, Gebreab SY, et al. Social patterning of cumulative biological risk by education and income among African Americans. *Am J Publ Health*. 2012;102(7):1362–1369.
10. Linnenbringer E, Gehlert S, Geronimus AT. Black-white disparities in breast cancer subtype: the intersection of socially patterned stress and genetic expression. *AIMS Public Health*. 2017;4(5):526–556. https://doi.org/10.3934/publichealth.2017.5.526.
11. Gallo LC, Fortmann AL, Mattei J. Allostatic load and the assessment of cumulative biological risk in biobehavioral medicine: challenges and opportunities. *Psychosom Med*. September 2014;76(7):478–480. https://doi.org/10.1097/psy.0000000000000095.
12. McEwen BS, Stellar E. Stress and the individual. Mechanisms leading to disease. *Arch Intern Med*. September 27, 1993;153(18):2093–2101.
13. Guidi J, Lucente M, Sonino N, Fava GA. Allostatic load and its impact on health: a systematic review. *Psychother Psychosom*. 2021;90(1):11–27. https://doi.org/10.1159/000510696.

14. Williams DR, Lawrence JA, Davis BA. Racism and health: evidence and needed research. *Annu Rev Publ Health*. April 1, 2019;40:105−125. https://doi.org/10.1146/annurev-publhealth-040218-043750.

15. Turner RJ. Understanding health disparities: the relevance of the stress process model. *Soc Ment Health*. 2013;3(3):170−186. https://doi.org/10.1177/2156869313488121.

16. Hermes GL, Delgado B, Tretiakova M, et al. Social isolation dysregulates endocrine and behavioral stress while increasing malignant burden of spontaneous mammary tumors. *Proc Natl Acad Sci U S A*. December 29, 2009;106(52):22393−22398. https://doi.org/10.1073/pnas.0910753106.

17. Cohen S, Schwartz JE, Epel E, Kirschbaum C, Sidney S, Seeman T. Socioeconomic status, race, and diurnal cortisol decline in the coronary artery risk development in young adults (CARDIA) study. *Psychosom Med*. Jan-Feb 2006;68(1):41−50. https://doi.org/10.1097/01.psy.0000195967.51768.ea.

18. Allen JO, Watkins DC, Chatters L, Geronimus AT, Johnson-Lawrence V. Cortisol and racial health disparities affecting black men in later life: evidence from MIDUS II. *Am J Men's Health*. Jul-Aug 2019;13(4):1557988319870969. https://doi.org/10.1177/1557988319870969.

19. Webb Hooper M. Racial/ethnic differences in physiological stress and relapse among treatment seeking tobacco smokers. *Int J Environ Res Publ Health*. August 25, 2019;16(17). https://doi.org/10.3390/ijerph16173090.

20. Van Dyke ME, Baumhofer NK, Slopen N, et al. Pervasive discrimination and allostatic load in African American and white adults. *Psychosom Med*. April 2020;82(3):316−323. https://doi.org/10.1097/psy.0000000000000788.

21. Carbone JT, Clift J, Alexander N. Measuring allostatic load: approaches and limitations to algorithm creation. *J Psychosom Res*. December 2022;163:111050. https://doi.org/10.1016/j.jpsychores.2022.111050.

22. Shen J, Fuemmeler BF, Guan Y, Zhao H. Association of allostatic load and All cancer risk in the SWAN cohort. *Cancers*. June 21, 2022;14(13). https://doi.org/10.3390/cancers14133044.

23. Parente V, Hale L, Palermo T. Association between breast cancer and allostatic load by race: national health and nutrition examination survey 1999-2008. *Psycho Oncol*. March 2013;22(3):621−628. https://doi.org/10.1002/pon.3044.

24. Xing CY, Doose M, Qin B, et al. Prediagnostic allostatic load as a predictor of poorly differentiated and larger sized breast cancers among black women in the Women's Circle of health follow-up study. *Cancer Epidemiol Biomarkers Prev*. January 2020;29(1):216−224. https://doi.org/10.1158/1055-9965.Epi-19-0712.

25. Babatunde OA, Pearce JL, Jefferson MS, et al. Racial distribution of neighborhood-level social deprivation in a retrospective cohort of prostate cancer survivors. *Diseases*. October 3, 2022;10(4). https://doi.org/10.3390/diseases10040075.

26. Stabellini N, Cullen J, Bittencourt MS, et al. Allostatic load and cardiovascular outcomes in males with prostate cancer. *JNCI Cancer Spectr*. March 1, 2023;7(2). https://doi.org/10.1093/jncics/pkad005.

27. Hughes Halbert C, Jefferson M, Ambrose L, Caulder S, Savage SJ. Resiliency and allostatic load among veterans at risk for adverse prostate cancer outcomes. *Ethn Dis*. 2020;30(Suppl 1):177−184. https://doi.org/10.18865/ed.30.S1.177.

28. Mathew A, Doorenbos AZ, Li H, Jang MK, Park CG, Bronas UG. Allostatic load in cancer: a systematic review and mini meta-analysis. *Biol Res Nurs*. July 2021;23(3):341−361. https://doi.org/10.1177/1099800420969898.

29. Rosemberg MS, Granner J, Li Y, Seng JS. A scoping review of interventions targeting allostatic load. *Stress*. September 2020;23(5):519−528. https://doi.org/10.1080/10253890.2020.1784136.

30. Li Y, Rosemberg MS. The promise of allostatic load rests upon strategic operationalization, scoring, and targeted interventions. *Psychoneuroendocrinology*. January 2021;123:104877. https://doi.org/10.1016/j.psyneuen.2020.104877.

31. Rodriquez EJ, Kim EN, Sumner AE, Nápoles AM, Pérez-Stable EJ. Allostatic load: importance, markers, and score determination in minority and disparity populations. *J Urban Health*. March 2019;96(Suppl 1):3−11. https://doi.org/10.1007/s11524-019-00345-5.

32. McEwen BS, Seeman T. Protective and damaging effects of mediators of stress. Elaborating and testing the concepts of allostasis and allostatic load. *Ann N Y Acad Sci*. 1999;896:30−47. https://doi.org/10.1111/j.1749-6632.1999.tb08103.x.

33. Halbert CH, Allen CG, Jefferson M, et al. Lessons learned from the medical university of South Carolina transdisciplinary collaborative center (TCC) in precision medicine and minority men's health. *Am J Men's Health*. Nov-Dec 2020;14(6):1557988320979236. https://doi.org/10.1177/1557988320979236.

34. Siegel RL, Miller KD, Wagle NS, Jemal A. Cancer statistics, 2023. *Ca - Cancer J Clin*. January 2023;73(1):17−48. https://doi.org/10.3322/caac.21763.

35. Zeigler-Johnson C, Morales KH, Glanz K, Spangler E, Mitchell J, Rebbeck TR. Individual- and neighborhood-level education influences the effect of obesity on prostate cancer treatment failure after prostatectomy. *Cancer Causes Control*. September 2015;26(9):1329−1337. https://doi.org/10.1007/s10552-015-0628-y.

36. Zeigler-Johnson CM, Tierney A, Rebbeck TR, Rundle A. Prostate cancer severity associations with neighborhood deprivation. *Prostate Cancer*. 2011;2011:846263. https://doi.org/10.1155/2011/846263.

37. De Ramos IP, Auchincloss AH, Bilal U. Exploring inequalities in life expectancy and lifespan variation by race/ethnicity and urbanicity in the United States: 1990 to 2019. *SSM Popul Health*. September 2022;19:101230. https://doi.org/10.1016/j.ssmph.2022.101230.

38. Dean DAL, Griffith DM, McKissic SA, Cornish EK, Johnson-Lawrence V. Men on the move-nashville:

feasibility and acceptability of a technology-enhanced physical activity pilot intervention for overweight and obese middle and older age African American men. *Am J Men's Health*. July 2018;12(4):798–811. https://doi.org/10.1177/1557988316644174.

39. Griffith DM, Jaeger EC. Mighty men: a faith-based weight loss intervention to reduce cancer risk in African American men. *Adv Cancer Res*. 2020;146:189–217. https://doi.org/10.1016/bs.acr.2020.01.010.

40. Rogers CR, Rogers TN, Matthews P, et al. Psychosocial determinants of colorectal Cancer screening uptake among African-American men: understanding the role of masculine role norms, medical mistrust, and normative support. *Ethn Health*. July 2022;27(5):1103–1122. https://doi.org/10.1080/13557858.2020.1849569.

41. Ribeiro AI, Amaro J, Lisi C, Fraga S. Neighborhood socioeconomic deprivation and allostatic load: a scoping review. *Int J Environ Res Publ Health*. May 28, 2018;15(6). https://doi.org/10.3390/ijerph15061092.

42. Halbert CH, Coyne J, Weathers B, et al. Racial differences in quality of life following prostate cancer diagnosis. *Urology*. September 2010;76(3):559–564. https://doi.org/10.1016/j.urology.2009.09.090.

43. Halbert CH, Wrenn G, Weathers B, Delmoor E, Ten Have T, Coyne JC. Sociocultural determinants of men's reactions to prostate cancer diagnosis. *Psycho Oncol*. May 2010;19(5):553–560. https://doi.org/10.1002/pon.1574.

44. Hoyt MA, Marin-Chollom AM, Bower JE, Thomas KS, Irwin MR, Stanton AL. Approach and avoidance coping: diurnal cortisol rhythm in prostate cancer survivors. *Psychoneuroendocrinology*. 2014;49:182–186.

45. Halbert CH, Jefferson M, Allen CG, et al. Racial differences in patient portal activation and research enrollment among patients with prostate cancer. *JCO Clin Cancer Inform*. June 2021;5:768–774. https://doi.org/10.1200/cci.20.00131.

46. Jefferson M, Drake RR, Lilly M, Savage SJ, Tucker Price S, Hughes Halbert C. Co-Morbidities in a retrospective cohort of prostate cancer patients. *Ethn Dis*. 2020;30(Suppl 1):185–192. https://doi.org/10.18865/ed.30.S1.185.

47. McEwen BS. Stress, adaptation, and disease. Allostasis and allostatic load. *Ann N Y Acad Sci*. May 1, 1998;840:33–44. https://doi.org/10.1111/j.1749-6632.1998.tb09546.x.

48. Halbert CH, Jefferson MS, Danielson C, Froeliger B, Giordano A, Thaxton JE. An observational study and randomized trial of stress reactivity in cancer disparities. *Health Psychol*. September 2020;39(9):745–757. https://doi.org/10.1037/hea0000882.

49. Obeng-Gyasi S, Tarver W, Carlos RC, Andersen BL. Allostatic load: a framework to understand breast cancer outcomes in Black women. *NPJ Breast Cancer*. July 30, 2021;7(1):100. https://doi.org/10.1038/s41523-021-00309-6.

50. Rodriguez JM, Karlamangla AS, Gruenewald TL, Miller-Martinez D, Merkin SS, Seeman TE. Social stratification and allostatic load: shapes of health differences in the MIDUS study in the United States. *J Biosoc Sci*. September 2019;51(5):627–644. https://doi.org/10.1017/s0021932018000378.

51. Zhu VJ, Lenert LA, Bunnell BE, Obeid JS, Jefferson M, Halbert CH. Automatically identifying social isolation from clinical narratives for patients with prostate Cancer. *BMC Med Inf Decis Making*. March 14, 2019;19(1):43. https://doi.org/10.1186/s12911-019-0795-y.

CHAPTER 4

The Conserved Transcriptional Response to Adversity

Prepared for Social Determinants of Health in Surgery

STEVEN W. COLE, PHD

INTRODUCTION

Beginning in 2007,[1] a series of RNA profiling studies found that human beings who were exposed to adverse social conditions for extended periods of time showed a recurrent pattern of alterations in immune cell gene expression.[2,3] This pattern was characterized by increased expression of genes involved in inflammation (e.g., *IL1B*, *IL6*, IL8/*CXCL8*, COX2/*PTGS2*, and *TNF*) and decreased expression of genes involved in type I interferon—mediated innate antiviral responses (e.g., *IFI-*, *MX-*, and *OAS*-family genes). This same general pattern was observed across a variety of adverse social conditions such as loneliness, poverty, bereavement, and chronic stress, as well as in subsequent animal models that experimentally manipulated social adversity.[4–12] The consistency of these gene regulatory alterations across species and across different forms of adversity led to its characterization as a Conserved Transcriptional Response to Adversity (CTRA). Subsequent research has linked the CTRA to an array of chronic disease processes and health outcomes as well differential responses to medical and surgical therapies. This chapter reviews the CTRA's discovery and theoretical conceptualization, early laboratory analyses mapping its biological mechanisms, and more recent studies assessing its role in mediating social disparities in disease risk and treatment responses (including surgical and transplant outcomes). This chapter also highlights emerging behavioral and pharmacological interventions to block CTRA-mediated health risks, surveys some key issues in CTRA measurement, and summarizes several areas of ongoing CTRA research.

DISCOVERY OF THE CONSERVED TRANSCRIPTIONAL RESPONSE TO ADVERSITY

Epidemiologic studies have long documented social disparities in disease risk, stretching back at least to Virchow's 1848 analysis of poverty's effect on Typhus, and arguably a millennium earlier to Galen of Pergamon's observations linking patient social conditions to breast cancer in second-century Greece. However, the biological processes through which social factors influence disease development have only recently become a topic of significant scientific attention. In the late 1990s and early 2000s, the MacArthur Foundation convened a network of behavioral and biological scientists to analyze the pathways by which social factors such as poverty and social isolation influenced biological vulnerability to disease. Research on human genome function was surging in parallel with the completion of the human genome sequence and the development of massively parallel microarray assays that could quantify variations in the activity of all ~20,000 human genes simultaneously. Previous research in simple genomic systems such as viruses and experimental animal models had established that social conditions could causally affect RNA transcription and the expression of selected genes. These two strands of research intersected in the MacArthur network meetings, with behavioral scientists reasoning that there must be some molecular manifestation of the social gradients in disease they had observed, and biological scientists recognizing that recent advances in genomics had greatly enhanced the feasibility of

Social Determinants of Health in Surgery. https://doi.org/10.1016/B978-0-443-12366-5.00008-5

identifying such mechanisms. These considerations motivated a small pilot study examining the genome-wide RNA correlates of one of the best established psychosocial risk factors for disease—perceived social isolation, or loneliness.[1] Despite the limited statistical power available in this small proof-of-concept study, a clear pattern of biological differences emerged: immune cells from chronically lonely people showed relative upregulation of multiple genes involved in inflammation, and relative downregulation of multiple genes involved in type I interferon innate antiviral responses. These results paralleled earlier observations in mouse models of repeated social defeat, which found a similar proinflammatory bias,[6] and in monkey models of social stress, which found similar decrements in type I interferon activity.[13] These molecular differences also provided a clear explanation for the profile of disease risks associated with loneliness in epidemiological studies, with increased inflammation plausibly contributing to the elevated risk observed for cardiovascular and neoplastic diseases, and decreased antiviral response contributing to the elevated risk observed for viral infections and cellular immune responses. Bioinformatic analyses of these gene expression differences identified specific transcription control pathways that could potentially account for those molecular patterns through increased signaling from the sympathetic nervous system (SNS) and reduced signaling from glucocorticoid hormones that would normally inhibit inflammatory gene expression (paralleling observations of acquired glucocorticoid insensitivity in mouse models of repeated social defeat).

Biobehavioral health researchers quickly applied the analytic framework of the "lonely genes" study to other social—environmental risk factors ranging from chronic stress[14,15] and poverty[16,17] to bereavement[18] and post-traumatic stress disorder.[19,20] As is typical in genomics studies, only a small fraction of the specific individual genes that were differentially expressed in the loneliness study showed similar differential expression in analyses of other types of adversity. However, higher-order bioinformatics analyses identified two recurrent functional themes across the multiple studies: genes that were empirically upregulated in the context of adversity tended to include transcripts involved in inflammation, and genes that were empirically downregulated tended to include transcripts involved in type I interferon activity. Bioinformatic analyses of transcription factor activity also repeatedly indicated upregulated activity of SNS-responsive signaling pathways (e.g., the CREB family of transcription factors) and proinflammatory factors (e.g., NF-κB and AP-1), and downregulated

activity of interferon response factors (IRFs) and, more variably, the glucocorticoid receptor (GR). In light of these common functional characteristics of gene expression differences observed across distinct types of adversity and across species ranging from fish to primates, this pattern was characterized as a CTRA. Individual studies also identified varying patterns of unique transcriptomic effects specific to each type of social adversity. However, uniqueness is the norm in genomics findings, and so it was remarkable to observe the recurrence of a few consistent biological themes regarding gene function and upstream transcriptional control pathways across different species and different risk factors.

The conservation of the CTRA molecular profile across organisms and risk factors motivated a series of follow-up studies to identify the biological mechanisms involved and define their evolutionary adaptive value. Biochemical studies in cellular and animal models confirmed bioinformatic indications that β-adrenergic signaling played a key role in mediating the CTRA, both by altering gene transcription in existing immune cells and by altering bone marrow production of monocytes, granulocytes, and dendritic cells.[6,7,12] Transient changes in the prevalence of these short-lived "myeloid lineage" immune cells resulted in a proinflammatory/antiinterferon bias in the population structure of the circulating white blood cell pool (Fig. 4.1).

Teleologic analyses suggested that the CTRA's adaptive significance lay in its ability to pivot the basal antimicrobial stance of the innate immune system away from its default antiviral bias (mediated by type I interferons and cellular immune responses) and toward a more proinflammatory stance that would optimally defend against bacterial infections and wounding injury.[2,3] Under ancestral conditions, when threat experiences were often acute but transient, SNS activation of the CTRA molecular program allowed the immune system to anticipate changing microbial exposures and preempt bacterial infections while accelerating wound repair. Under contemporary conditions of more chronic low-grade threat or anxiety, however, the CTRA instead promotes chronic low-grade inflammation and thereby contributes to the development of cardiovascular, neurodegenerative, and neoplastic diseases, while chronically undermining cellular immune responses and antiviral defenses.[2,3]

HEALTH IMPLICATIONS

The CTRA transcriptome pattern was initially recognized due to the well-established role of inflammation

CTRA signal transduction

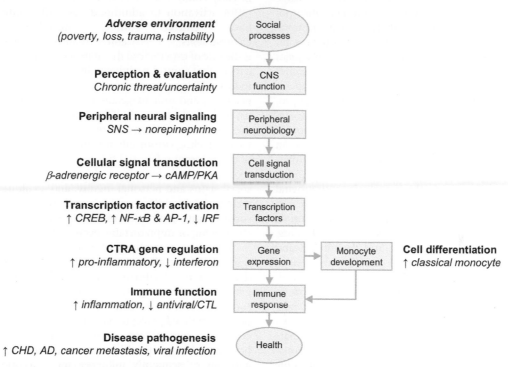

FIG. 4.1 CTRA Signal Transduction.   The "social signal transduction" pathway that drives CTRA gene expression involves extended exposure to adverse environmental conditions, which results in activation of evolutionarily conserved threat-response systems in the central nervous system (CNS), resulting in activation of fight-or-flight stress responses from the sympathetic nervous system (SNS) and release of the neurotransmitter, norepinephrine, from sympathetic nerve terminals. These signals are transduced by leukocyte beta-adrenergic receptors into activation of intracellular second messenger systems such as the cyclic-3′-5′-adenosine monophosphate/protein kinase A (cAMP/PKA) pathway, which exerts diverse effects on multiple transcription control pathways such as increased activity of the cAMP response element—binding factor (CREB) family, increased activity of the proinflammatory NF-κB/Rel and activator protein 1 (AP-1) transcription factor families, and decreased activity of interferon response factors (IRFs). Differential activation of these transcription factor families results in upregulated transcription of proinflammatory genes and downregulated transcription of type I interferon antiviral genes, resulting in downstream alterations in inflammatory and antiviral immune responses (including cytotoxic T lymphocytes; CTL) and consequent alterations in the risk of inflammation-related diseases such as coronary heart disease (CHD), Alzheimer's disease (AD), tumor development and metastasis, and viral infection. In addition to direct regulation of gene transcription in existing cells, SNS nerve fiber activation in the bone marrow also results in increased production of myeloid lineage immune cells (particularly classical monocytes), resulting in a proinflammatory bias in the circulating leukocyte pool.

in the pathogenesis of multiple chronic diseases and the key role of interferon responses in viral infections. During the basic definition of CTRA mechanisms, experimental animal models confirmed the relevance of the proinflammatory/antiinterferon transcriptome shift for disease pathogenesis in the context of cancer,[21] cardiovascular disease,[7] and viral infections.[9] More recent epidemiologic studies have confirmed that the CTRA is associated with increased risk or severity of multiple cardiovascular, metabolic, and neoplastic diseases,[17] and clinical studies have linked the CTRA to increased cancer progression[22,23] and poorer response to hematopoietic cell transplant in the context of cancer.[23–25] Several studies have also linked symptoms of chronic fatigue and depression to the proinflammatory and/or antiinterferon components of the CTRA.[26–29] Large population health cohort studies have recently incorporated prospective and longitudinal transcriptome assessments,[30,31] which will provide additional insight into the CTRA's predictive relationship to subsequent disease incidence and mortality, as those outcomes accumulate over decades of longitudinal follow-up.

Beyond its impact on disease development and progression, the CTRA can also affect the efficacy of therapeutic interventions for disease, including responses to medical, surgical, and transplantation therapies. An early example involved SNS inhibition of type I interferon activity in HIV-infected individuals, which undermined the efficacy of pharmacologic antiretroviral medications.[32] In the context of surgery, stress is well established to affect treatment outcomes via multiple pathways that include impaired wound healing, increased postsurgical infection, and the survival and progression of minimal residual disease in the context of tumor resection.[33,34] In the context of wound healing, for example, SNS-induced CTRA activation in wound-infiltrating monocytes/macrophages and neutrophils can prolong and amplify the initial inflammatory phase of wound response[35,36] and also dysregulate the subsequent epithelial–mesenchymal differentiation processes needed to successfully reconstitute healthy tissue.[37,38] In the context of cancer resection, SNS-induced CTRA activation within the local surgical milieu and systemic circulating immune cells both tend to promote the survival and growth of minimal residual disease and impair antitumor cellular immune responses, each of which increases the risk of disease recurrence and mortality.[21,34,39–42] Finally, in the context of tissue transplant therapies, CTRA activation can undermine tissue engraftment and increase the risk of posttransplant infections, thereby significantly reducing the therapeutic efficacy of the transplant and increasing the risk of disease relapse and mortality.[23–25]

SOCIAL DETERMINANTS OF HEALTH

In light of relationships between social processes, CTRA gene regulation, and disease risk, social epidemiologists have examined the CTRA as one mechanistic pathway that may contribute to the long-observed social disparities in disease risk. Several studies have documented variations in CTRA gene expression as a function of age, sex, race/ethnicity, socioeconomic status, and regional sociocultural contexts,[30,31] as well as neighborhood exposures to violence and social instability,[43,44] and experiences of discrimination on the basis of race

or sexual orientation.[45–48] Adverse social environments in early childhood are also associated with persisting CTRA activation in adulthood even after individuals have entered more favorable social environments.[14,49–51] Central to all of these pathways is the role of experienced threat in activating CNS neural circuits that control peripheral SNS activity and thereby induce CTRA gene expression. Subjective experiences of persistent and unmanageable threat constitute the key psychological trigger of CTRA gene regulation,[3,52] and the adverse social determinants of health all leave individuals feeling chronically threatened and/or uncertain of their present safety and future prospects. By contrast, secure social relationships, stable economic well-being, social status and personal dignity, and a culture of social trust and stability provide a sense of safety and personal security that buffers individual stress responses to challenging or unpredictable events.[3,52]

Individual perceptions of security, autonomy, and opportunity are all undermined by the adverse social determinants of health, including disadvantaged demographic identities (e.g., racial/ethnic, gender/sexuality), socioeconomic status, and cultural and political identities. Generalized perceptions of the social, cultural, and economic environment as safe and generative versus hostile and unpredictable typically form early in life and can subsequently influence the perception and interpretation of experiences over the remainder of the life span. Early life influences on "world view" and "social perception" allow childhood social conditions to influence CTRA biology and health years later in middle and older adulthood (i.e., above and beyond the contemporaneous social and environmental conditions that prevail later in life).[14,49–51] A central contribution of the CTRA paradigm to social epidemiology lies in its integrative synthesis of the connections between social environments, individual psychological experiences, neurobiological control of gene expression, and molecular mechanisms of health and disease.

INTERVENTIONS

The strong public policy interest in reducing social disparities in disease has motivated the search for effective interventions to block CTRA biology and its associated health risks. A root cause analysis suggests that large-scale changes to social, political, and economic conditions should provide the most comprehensive impact in reducing CTRA biology by increasing individual experiences of social security and reducing experiences of social threat across the population as a whole. However, no empirical data have yet shown that any large-scale policy change can significantly impact CTRA gene expression or associated health outcomes (because no large-scale policy studies have yet incorporated CTRA measures into their analyses). There is a great need for future policy research to incorporate molecular markers of multidisease vulnerability such as the CTRA because it is far from certain that intuitively appealing social interventions will actually have favorable health impacts, and there is clear potential for unintended harm to the health of disadvantaged populations. Previous research provides several examples in which intuitively appealing policy interventions (e.g., eliminating stable social hierarchies) can paradoxically increase individual stress and CTRA biology as individuals negotiate a more complex and unpredictable social environment that results.[9,13] As such, there is a great need for empirical assessment of the CTRA and other stress-related biomarkers and clinical outcomes in future social policy research.

Within the narrower domain of healthcare, several different intervention approaches have been examined as potential strategies for reducing CTRA biology and its attending health risks. One approach involves deploying pharmacologic β-adrenergic antagonists to block SNS induction of the CTRA in immune cells[40] and diseased tissues.[39,41,42] In the context of cancer surgery, for example, several "window of opportunity" trials have demonstrated that brief perisurgical β-blockade can reduce CTRA biology in both circulating immune cells (e.g., reduced inflammation and enhanced cellular immune parameters)[40] and diseased tissues (e.g., reductions in prometastatic, mesenchymal, and macrophage-related molecular profiles within primary tumor tissues).[39,41,42] Brief β-blockade protocols show similarly promising biological impacts in the context of hematopoietic cell transplantation for hematologic malignancy.[24] CTRA transcriptional alterations are mediated primarily by β_2-adrenergic receptors, so it is critical to select intervention agents in light of the distinction between selective β-antagonists (which predominately target β_1 receptors and may therefore not impact the CTRA) and nonselective β-antagonists (which are more likely to impact the CTRA due to their coverage of β_2-adrenergic receptors).

There is also great interest in blocking CTRA effects upstream of the SNS at the level of CNS processes involved in driving experienced threat, autonomic activity, and their downstream impact on gene regulation. One randomized controlled trial documented significant CTRA reductions in response to an atypical serotonin-boosting medication,[53] and several other trials have shown that wellness practices such as meditation,[54,55] yoga,[56] tai chi,[57] and cognitive

behavioral stress management[22,58] can downregulate CTRA gene expression under basal conditions and in highly threatening contexts such as exposure to warfare or diagnosis with cancer. Recent results also suggest that lifestyle modifications that extend beyond stress reduction to promote positive psychological processes such as value engagement and prosocial behavior (eudaimonic well-being) may also favorably impact CTRA profiles.[59–61]

A wide range of lifestyle, behavioral, and public policy modifications could potentially inhibit the CTRA, and which specific interventions are the most impactful may vary across individuals and population subgroups depending on their specific genetic background, life history, psychological makeup, cultural context, and socio-environmental conditions. It is difficult to accurately forecast which interventions will work best for any specific individual or subgroup, but it may be more feasible to empirically optimize CTRA reductions through "molecular biofeedback"—using machine learning analyses of intraindividual variations in gene expression assessed repeatedly over time. Development of highly automated RNA sequencing and analysis platforms that can provide near-real-time assessment of targeted gene sets raises the potential for a kind of "molecular biofeedback" in which an array of measured lifestyle or social contextual parameters can be empirically recorded during an observational "training period" and then sifted by machine learning to identify those parameters that show the strongest inverse relationship to CTRA biology, after which those candidate factors can be intentionally varied to verify causal influence and drive further feedback optimization.[2] This type of molecular biofeedback has the potential help motivate changes in lifestyle, behavior, and social conditions (including occupational, recreational, and residential "niches") decades before their effects manifest in the form of overt (and often irreversible) disease. Providing individuals and socially disadvantaged subgroups with timely insight into their own molecular well-being represents one of the most striking implications of our growing ability to map the molecular pathways by which psychological and social processes impact human physiology and health.

MEASUREMENT

Given the scientific, health, and policy relevance of the CTRA, there is growing interest in measuring this pattern in RNA transcriptome profiles collected in research and clinical settings. As shown in Fig. 4.2, the CTRA can be quantified at multiple levels of analysis

Multi-level assessment of the CTRA

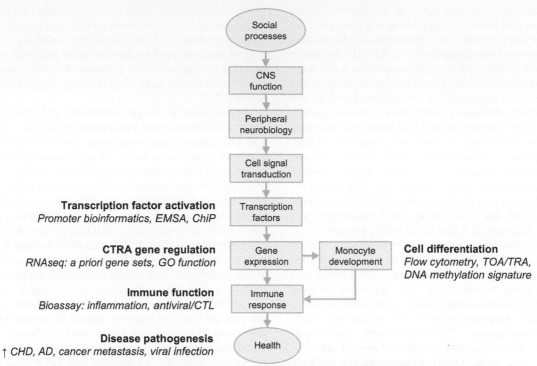

FIG. 4.2 Multilevel Assessment of the CTRA. The CTRA immunoregulatory pattern can be assessed at multiple levels of the "social signal transduction" cascade outlined in Fig. one, including upregulated activity of proinflammatory transcription factors and downregulated activity of antiviral transcription factors (e.g., through bioinformatic analyses of gene regulation, electrophoretic mobility-shift assays/EMSA, or chromatin immunoprecipitation/ChIP assays); upregulated expression of proinflammatory effector genes (e.g., *IL1B*, *IL6*, *IL8*, *TNF*) and downregulated expression of interferon response genes (e.g., *IFI-*, *MX-*, and *OAS*-family genes) as assessed by RNA sequencing (RNAseq) and Gene Ontology (GO) analyses; upregulated production of classical monocytes and downregulated prevalence of nonclassical monocytes (e.g., as assessed by flow cytometry, bioinformatic analysis of leukocyte transcriptome profiles by transcript origin analysis/TOA or transcriptome representation analysis/TRA, or cell type–specific DNA methylation signatures); upregulated functional bioassays of inflammation and/or downregulated antiviral or cytotoxic T lymphocyte (CTL) responses; or epidemiologic increases in CTRA-related diseases such as coronary heart disease (CHD), Alzheimer's disease (AD), metastatic cancer, and viral infections.

including "Gene Ontology" functional tagging of empirical differences in gene expression (i.e., testing for upregulation of inflammation-related gene annotations and downregulation of interferon-related gene annotations)[1,3]; assessment of transcription factors driving empirical differences in gene expression (i.e., testing for upregulation of proinflammatory mediators such as NF-κB and AP-1 and down-regulation of interferon-responsive IRFs)[1,3]; quantifying myeloid cell population dynamics (i.e., testing for upregulation of classical monocyte-related gene transcripts and downregulation of nonclassical monocyte-related

transcripts,[3,6,62] or DNA methylation profiles characteristic of myeloid cell upregulation[17]); and assessing a priori-defined sets of canonical inflammatory and interferon-related genes (e.g., the 53-gene CTRA "contrast score" used in several high-profile biobehavioral studies).[3,59,63–67] The CTRA could also be assessed at the level of its downstream impact on immune function (e.g., antimicrobial responses to a controlled bacterial or viral challenge, or a relevant molecular mimetic)[3,7,9,10] or protein-based assessments of cell prevalence (e.g., flow cytometric enumeration of classical and nonclassical monocytes).[3,6,7,9]

None of these approaches is perfect, and each comes with advantages and disadvantages in terms of cost, sensitivity, measurement reliability, and interpretive relevance for health. Most approaches tap only some aspects of the CTRA. For example, analyses of myeloid cell prevalence miss the impact of β-adrenergic signaling on existing cells; analyses of a priori-defined gene sets miss effects on genes outside the prespecified set; analyses of RNA or methylation profiles do not guarantee an impact on protein profiles or cellular function; functional assays do not capture the transcriptomic phenomenon originally identified as the CTRA and are often noisy and insensitive relative to molecular assays; functional bioassays and protein biomarkers do not enjoy the statistical advantages of RNA and methylation profiling that can efficiently assess 100s or 1000s of parameters and thus benefit from "law of large numbers" statistical smoothing; etc. The optimal approach for any given study depends on research objectives and technical feasibility, and each of the approaches listed before could be considered a valid indicator of the CTRA concept. The strongest approach is to assess the CTRA at multiple levels of analysis and integrate results across molecular, cellular, and functional measures.[11,30,64]

It is important to note that the CTRA is a physiological pattern and is not equivalent to any specific method of measuring that pattern. Just as there are multiple ways to measure other physiological patterns such as "depression," each of the approaches mentioned above represents one way of measuring the CTRA, but the CTRA is not equivalent to (or defined by) any one of those metrics. It has sometimes been assumed that the CTRA is defined by the 53-gene contrast used in several high-visibility studies.[63,64] However, that contrast score represents only one way of measuring the CTRA, and analytic and empirical analyses suggest that it may not be the most sensitive or reliable one. (Bioinformatic inferences of transcription factor activity derived from genome-wide transcriptome differences often prove most sensitive.) The 53-gene contrast score does have a major advantage in being easy to specify and compute, and so is often used due to its simplicity.

Pragmatic constraints on tissue sampling also influence CTRA measurement. Laboratory studies have verified that CTRA gene expression dynamics are mediated predominately in myeloid lineage immune cells (i.e., blood monocytes, tissue macrophages, and dendritic cells in both compartments),[6,9,12,14,15,62] which comprise ∼2%−10% of circulating leukocytes. CTRA-diagnostic genes are only weakly expressed in nonmyeloid blood cells, which makes it feasible to assess the CTRA in samples of whole blood (e.g., as captured by PAXgene or Tempus tubes, or in dried blood spots) and peripheral blood mononuclear cells (e.g., derived from Ficoll density gradient centrifugation) despite the presence of numerous other "contaminating" cell types (which simply lack any appreciable expression of the target mRNAs). It is also important to note that the CTRA is fundamentally a property of circulating myeloid lineage leukocytes, and would not be expected to appear in its canonical form in other types of tissue. However, myeloid cells regulate a wide variety of immunologic and inflammatory processes in other tissues, and so it is not uncommon to find distinct molecular profiles in other tissues that reflect the downstream impact of CTRA activation in circulating myeloid cells.[7,11,13,21,68,69]

PROSPECTS

The CTRA has emerged as one of the most theoretically comprehensive and empirically validated frameworks for understanding the social determinants of human health. However, it is important to note that the CTRA represents only one of many pathways through which social factors can affect human health, and multiple pathways likely operate in parallel to structure the overall social determinants on human health. Other pathways include differential exposure to physiological insults (e.g., violent injury; microbes; physicochemical toxins; etc.), differential access to physiological resources (e.g., nutrition; effective medical treatment; etc.), and differential activity of other stress-related physiological pathways (e.g., the hypothalamus−pituitary−adrenal axis). As such, the CTRA is best construed as one strand in a complex network of pathways through which social factors impact human biology to generate disparate health outcomes and longevity. Moreover, these multiple pathways undoubtedly interact with one another to produce synergistic effects that remain largely unexplored and constitute important topics for future research in social epidemiology.

Despite these limitations, the CTRA represents an important advance in our understanding of the social determinants of health by integrating traditionally distinct domains of research on individual stress biology, human functional genomics, molecular pathogenesis of disease, and social epidemiology. The first decade of research on the CTRA yielded rapid progress in characterizing its scope and nature, the cellular and molecular mechanisms involved, its evolutionary adaptive value, and its implications for health and disease. Translational studies are now identifying behavioral and pharmacologic strategies for mitigating the CTRA and reducing its adverse health impacts. Major areas of ongoing CTRA research involve defining the role of positive psychological processes and socioenvironmental resources in conferring resistance to CTRA development[11,20,59,61,63,64,66]; neuroimaging analyses of the CNS pathways involved in CTRA production (particularly the interplay between threat-response circuits involving the amygdala and reward circuits involving the ventral striatum and ventral tegmental area)[70,71]; behavioral metrics to help monitor the neural threat-response systems that drive the CTRA[67]; and the CTRA's potential use as a prospective biomarker of risk for a broad range of diseases involving inflammation, interferon, and cellular immune responses, which opens up new opportunities for personalized "molecular biofeedback" to optimize individual health trajectories, as well as new leading indicators of disease risk[17,30] that can help assess the impact of pharmacologic, behavioral, and policy interventions to advance health equity. As researchers seek to understand and ultimately mitigate social disparities in disease, the CTRA paradigm provides a useful genomic framework for understanding how macrolevel social and structural processes can impact the microlevel biology of health and disease, and thereby suggests new strategies to prevent disease and promote health equity for all members of society.

Highlights

- Social factors can influence human gene expression via neural regulation of gene transcription.
- The CTRA is one common transcriptional response to adverse social conditions.
- The CTRA involves increased expression of proinflammatory genes and decreased expression of type I interferon antiviral genes by circulating myeloid immune cells.
- CTRA gene regulation is mediated by β-adrenergic signaling from the sympathetic nervous system.
- The CTRA enhances development of cardiovascular, neoplastic, and neurodegenerative diseases, while undermining cellular immune responses and antiviral defenses.
- In the context of surgery, the CTRA undermines wound healing, impairs transplant engraftment, and promotes infection and cancer minimal residual disease and recurrence.
- The CTRA represents one major pathway through which social factors can influence the molecular mechanisms of disease and thereby structure health disparities.

ACKNOWLEDGEMENTS

Preparation of this chapter was supported by NIH grants R01-AG073053, R01-CA261752, UG3-CA260317, U19-AG051426, and P30-AG017265, and the Breast Cancer Research Foundation.

REFERENCES

1. Cole SW, Hawkley LC, Arevalo JM, Sung CY, Rose RM, Cacioppo JT. Social regulation of gene expression in human leukocytes. *Genome Biol.* 2007;8(R189):1−13.
2. Cole SW. Human social genomics. *PLoS Genet.* 2014; 10(8):e1004601.
3. Cole SW. The conserved transcriptional response to adversity. *Curr Opin Behav Sci.* 2019;28:31−37.
4. Cole SW, Arevalo JM, Ruggerio AM, Heckman JJ, Suomi S. Transcriptional modulation of the developing immune system by early life social adversity. *Proc Natl Acad Sci U S A.* 2012;109:20578−20583.
5. Tung J, Barreiro LB, Johnson ZP, et al. Social environment is associated with gene regulatory variation in the rhesus macaque immune system. *Proc Natl Acad Sci U S A.* 2012;109(17):6490−6495.
6. Powell ND, Sloan EK, Bailey MT, et al. Social stress up-regulates inflammatory gene expression in the leukocyte transcriptome via beta-adrenergic induction of myelopoiesis. *Proc Natl Acad Sci U S A.* 2013;110(41): 16574−16579.
7. Heidt T, Sager HB, Courties G, et al. Chronic variable stress activates hematopoietic stem cells. *Nat Med.* 2014;20(7): 754−758.
8. Korytar T, Nipkow M, Altmann S, Goldammer T, Kollner B, Rebl A. Adverse husbandry of maraena whitefish directs the immune system to increase mobilization of myeloid cells and proinflammatory responses. *Front Immunol.* 2016;7:631.
9. Cole SW, Capitanio JP, Chun K, Arevalo JM, Ma J, Cacioppo JT. Myeloid differentiation architecture of leukocyte transcriptome dynamics in perceived social isolation. *Proc Natl Acad Sci U S A.* 2015;112(49):15142−15147.
10. Snyder-Mackler N, Sanz J, Kohn JN, et al. Social status alters immune regulation and response to infection in macaques. *Science.* 2016;354(6315):1041−1045.
11. Cole SW, Cacioppo JT, Cacioppo S, et al. The Type I interferon antiviral gene program is impaired by lockdown and preserved by caregiving. *Proc Natl Acad Sci U S A.* 2021; 118(29).
12. McKim DB, Yin W, Wang Y, Cole SW, Godbout JP, Sheridan JF. Social stress mobilizes hematopoietic stem cells to establish persistent splenic myelopoiesis. *Cell Rep.* 2018;25(9):2552−2562.
13. Sloan EK, Capitanio JP, Tarara RP, Mendoza SP, Mason WA, Cole SW. Social stress enhances sympathetic innervation of primate lymph nodes: mechanisms and implications for viral pathogenesis. *J Neurosci.* 2007;27(33):8857−8865.

14. Miller GE, Chen E, Sze J, et al. A functional genomic finger-print of chronic stress in humans: blunted glucocorticoid and increased NF-kappaB signaling. *Biol Psychiatr.* 2008; 64(4):266—272. Epub 2008 Apr 2028.

15. Miller GE, Murphy MLM, Cashman R, et al. Greater in-flammatory activity and blunted glucocorticoid signaling in monocytes of chronically stressed caregivers. *Brain Behav Immun.* 2014;41:191—199.

16. Miller GE, Chen E, Fok AK, et al. Low early-life social class leaves a biological residue manifested by decreased gluco-corticoid and increased proinflammatory signaling. *Proc Natl Acad Sci U S A.* 2009;106(34):14716—14721.

17. Simons RL, Lei MK, Beach SRH, et al. An index of the ratio of inflammatory to antiviral cell types mediates the effects of social adversity and age on chronic illness. *Soc Sci Med.* 2017;185:158—165.

10. O'Connor MF, Schultze-Florey CR, Irwin MR, Arevalo JM, Cole SW. Divergent gene expression responses to compli-cated grief and non-complicated grief. *Brain Behav Immun.* 2014;37:78—83.

19. O'Donovan A, Sun B, Cole S, et al. Transcriptional control of monocyte gene expression in post-traumatic stress disorder. *Dis Markers.* 2011;30(2—3):123—132.

20. Kohrt BA, Worthman CM, Adhikari RP, et al. Psychological resilience and the gene regulatory impact of posttraumatic stress in Nepali child soldiers. *Proc Natl Acad Sci U S A.* 2016;113(29):8156—8161.

21. Sloan EK, Priceman SJ, Cox BF, et al. The sympathetic ner-vous system induces a metastatic switch in primary breast cancer. *Cancer Res.* 2010;70(18):7042—7052.

22. Antoni MH, Bouchard LC, Jacobs JM, et al. Stress manage-ment, leukocyte transcriptional changes and breast cancer recurrence in a randomized trial: an exploratory analysis. *Psychoneuroendocrinology.* 2016;74:269—277.

23. Knight JM, Rizzo JD, Logan BR, et al. Low socioeconomic status, adverse gene expression profiles, and clinical out-comes in hematopoietic stem cell transplant recipients. *Clin Cancer Res: An Off J Am Assoc Cancer Res.* 2016; 22(1):69—78.

24. Knight JM, Rizzo JD, Hari P, et al. Propranolol inhibits molecular risk markers in HCT recipients: a phase 2 ran-domized controlled biomarker trial. *Blood advances.* 2020;4(3):467—476.

25. Knight JM, Rizzo JD, Wang T, et al. Molecular correlates of socioeconomic status and clinical outcomes following he-matopoietic cell transplantation for leukemia. *JNCI Cancer Spectr.* 2019;3(4):pkz073.

26. Bower JE, Ganz PA, Irwin MR, Arevalo JM, Cole SW. Fa-tigue and gene expression in human leukocytes: increased NF-kappaB and decreased glucocorticoid signaling in breast cancer survivors with persistent fatigue. *Brain Behav Immun.* 2011;25(1):147—150.

27. Black DS, Cole SW, Christodoulou G, Figueiredo JC. Genomic mechanisms of fatigue in survivors of colorectal cancer. *Cancer.* 2018;124(12):2637—2644.

28. Xiao C, Beitler JJ, Higgins KA, et al. Differential regulation of NF-kB and IRF target genes as they relate to fatigue in

29. Mellon SH, Wolkowitz OM, Schonemann MD, et al. Alter-ations in leukocyte transcriptional control pathway activity associated with major depressive disorder and antidepres-sant treatment. *Transl Psychiatry.* 2016;6:e821.

30. Cole SW, Shanahan MJ, Gaydosh L, Harris KM. Population-based RNA profiling in Add Health finds social disparities in inflammatory and antiviral gene regulation to emerge by young adulthood. *Proc Natl Acad Sci U S A.* 2020;117(9):4601—4608.

31. Mann FD, Krueger RF, Clouston S, Cole S. Demographic correlates of inflammatory and antiviral gene expression in the study of Midlife in the United States (MIDUS). *Bio-demogr Soc Biol.* 2020;66(3—4):236—249.

32. Cole SW, Naliboff BD, Kemeny ME, Griswold MP, Fahey JL, Zack JA. Impaired response to HAART in HIV infected individuals with high autonomic nervous system activity. *Proceedings of the National Academy of Sciences of the USA.* 2001;98:12695—12700.

33. Gouin JP, Kiecolt-Glaser JK. The impact of psychological stress on wound healing: methods and mechanisms. *Immunol Allergy Clin.* 2011;31(1):81—93.

34. Horowitz M, Neeman E, Sharon E, Ben-Eliyahu S. Exploit-ing the critical perioperative period to improve long-term cancer outcomes. *Nat Rev Clin Oncol.* 2015;12(4): 213—226.

35. Cole S, Arevalo J, Takahashi R, et al. Computational iden-tification of gene-social environment interaction at the hu-man IL6 locus. *Proc Natl Acad Sci U S A.* 2010;107(12): 5681—5686.

36. Roy S, Khanna S, Yeh PE, et al. Wound site neutrophil tran-scriptome in response to psychological stress in young men. *Gene Expr.* 2005;12(4—6):273—287.

37. Liu H, Wang C, Xie N, et al. Activation of adrenergic recep-tor β2 promotes tumor progression and epithelial mesen-chymal transition in tongue squamous cell carcinoma. *Int J Mol Med.* 2018;41(1):147—154.

38. Shan T, Cui X, Li W, et al. Novel regulatory program for norepinephrine-induced epithelial-mesenchymal transi-tion in gastric adenocarcinoma cell lines. *Cancer Sci.* 2014;105(7):847—856.

39. Haldar R, Ricon-Becker I, Radin A, et al. Perioperative COX2 and β-adrenergic blockade improves biomarkers of tumor metastasis, immunity, and inflammation in colo-rectal cancer: a randomized controlled trial. *Cancer.* 2020; 126(17):3991—4001.

40. Haldar R, Shaashua L, Lavon H, et al. Perioperative inhibi-tion of beta-adrenergic and COX2 signaling in a clinical trial in breast cancer patients improves tumor Ki-67 expres-sion, serum cytokine levels, and PBMCs transcriptome. *Brain Behav Immun.* 2018;73:294—309.

41. Shaashua L, Shabat-Simon M, Haldar R, et al. Periopera-tive COX-2 and beta-adrenergic blockade improves meta-static biomarkers in breast cancer patients in a phase-II randomized trial. *Clin Cancer Res: Off J Am Assoc Cancer Res.* 2017;23(16):4651—4661.

patients with head and neck cancer. *Brain Behav Immun.* 2018;74:291—295.

42. Hiller JG, Cole SW, Crone EM, et al. Preoperative β-blockade with propranolol reduces biomarkers of metastasis in breast cancer: a phase II randomized trial. *Clin Cancer Res: Off J Am Assoc Cancer Res.* 2020;26(8):1803−1811.

43. Miller GE, Chen E, Finegood E, Shimbo D, Cole SW. Prospective associations between neighborhood violence and monocyte pro-inflammatory transcriptional activity in children. *Brain Behav Immun.* 2022;100:1−7.

44. Lee MJ, Rittschof CC, Greenlee AJ, et al. Transcriptomic analyses of black women in neighborhoods with high levels of violence. *Psychoneuroendocrinology.* 2021;127:105174.

45. Brown KM, Diez-Roux AV, Smith JA, et al. Social regulation of inflammation related gene expression in the multi-ethnic study of atherosclerosis. *Psychoneuroendocrinology.* 2020;117:104654.

46. Brown KM, Diez-Roux AV, Smith JA, et al. Expression of socially sensitive genes: the multi-ethnic study of atherosclerosis. *PLoS One.* 2019;14(4):e0214061.

47. Li MJ, Takada S, Okafor CN, Gorbach PM, Shoptaw SJ, Cole SW. Experienced homophobia and gene expression alterations in Black and Latino men who have sex with men in Los Angeles County. *Brain Behav Immun.* 2020; 83:120−125.

48. Thames AD, Irwin MR, Breen EC, Cole SW. Experienced discrimination and racial differences in leukocyte gene expression. *Psychoneuroendocrinology.* 2019;106:277−283.

49. Schwaiger M, Grinberg M, Moser D, et al. Altered stress-induced regulation of genes in monocytes in adults with a history of childhood adversity. *Neuropsychopharmacology: Off Pub Am College Neuropsychopharmacol.* 2016;41(10): 2530−2540.

50. Marie-Mitchell A, Cole SW. Adverse childhood experiences and transcriptional response in school-age children. *Dev Psychopathol.* 2022;34(3):875−881.

51. Bower JE, Kuhlman KR, Ganz PA, Irwin MR, Crespi CM, Cole SW. Childhood maltreatment and monocyte gene expression among women with breast cancer. *Brain Behav Immun.* 2020;88:396−402.

52. Slavich GM, Cole SW. The emerging field of human social genomics. *Clin Psychol Sci.* 2013;1(3):331−348.

53. Eyre H, Siddarth P, Cyr N, et al. Comparing the immune-genomic effects of vilazodone and paroxetine in late-life depression: a pilot study. *Pharmacopsychiatry.* 2017;50(6): 256−263.

54. Black DS, Cole SW, Irwin MR, et al. Yogic meditation reverses NF-kappaB and IRF-related transcriptome dynamics in leukocytes of family dementia caregivers in a randomized controlled trial. *Psychoneuroendocrinology.* 2012;38: 348−355.

55. Creswell JD, Irwin MR, Burklund LJ, et al. Mindfulness-Based Stress Reduction training reduces loneliness and pro-inflammatory gene expression in older adults: a small randomized controlled trial. *Brain Behav Immun.* 2012; 26(7):1095−1101.

56. Bower JE, Greendale G, Crosswell AD, et al. Yoga reduces inflammatory signaling in fatigued breast cancer survivors: a randomized controlled trial. *Psychoneuroendocrinology.* 2014;43:20−29.

57. Irwin M, Olmstead R, Breen E, et al. Tai Chi Chih reduces cellular and genomic markers of inflammation in breast cancer survivors with insomnia. *J Natl Cancer Inst.* 2014 (in press).

58. Antoni MH, Lutgendorf SK, Blomberg B, et al. Transcriptional modulation of human leukocytes by cognitive-behavioral stress management in women undergoing treatment for breast cancer. *Biol Psychiatr.* 2012;71(4): 366−372.

59. Nelson-Coffey SK, Fritz MM, Lyubomirsky S, Cole SW. Kindness in the blood: a randomized controlled trial of the gene regulatory impact of prosocial behavior. *Psychoneuroendocrinology.* 2017;81:8−13.

60. Seeman T, Merkin SS, Goldwater D, Cole SW. Intergenerational mentoring, eudaimonic well-being and gene regulation in older adults: a pilot study. *Psychoneuroendocrinology.* 2020;111:104468.

61. Regan A, Fritz MM, Walsh LC, Lyubomirsky S, Cole SW. The genomic impact of kindness to self vs. others: a randomized controlled trial. *Brain Behav Immun.* 2022;106: 40−48.

62. Cole SW, Hawkley LC, Arevalo JM, Cacioppo JT. Transcript origin analysis identifies antigen-presenting cells as primary targets of socially regulated gene expression in leukocytes. *Proc Natl Acad Sci U S A.* 2011;108(7): 3080−3085.

63. Fredrickson BL, Grewen KM, Algoe SB, et al. Psychological well-being and the human conserved transcriptional response to adversity. *PLoS One.* 2015;10(3):e0121839.

64. Fredrickson BL, Grewen KM, Coffey KA, et al. A functional genomic perspective on human well-being. *Proc Natl Acad Sci U S A.* 2013;110(33):13684−13689.

65. Cole SW, Levine ME, Arevalo JM, Ma J, Weir DR, Crimmins EM. Loneliness, eudaimonia, and the human conserved transcriptional response to adversity. *Psychoneuroendocrinology.* 2015;62:11−17.

66. Kitayama S, Akutsu S, Uchida Y, Cole SW. Work, meaning, and gene regulation: findings from a Japanese information technology firm. *Psychoneuroendocrinology.* 2016;72: 175−181.

67. Mehl MR, Raison CL, Pace TWW, Arevalo JMG, Cole SW. Natural language indicators of differential gene regulation in the human immune system. *Proc Natl Acad Sci U S A.* 2017;114(47):12554−12559.

68. Chun K, Capitanio JP, Lamkin DM, Sloan EK, Arevalo JM, Cole SW. Social regulation of the lymph node transcriptome in rhesus macaques (*Macaca mulatta*). *Psychoneuroendocrinology.* 2017;76:107−113.

69. Lutgendorf SK, Degeest K, Sung CY, et al. Depression, social support, and beta-adrenergic transcription control in human ovarian cancer. *Brain Behav Immun.* 2009;23(2): 176−183.

70. Ben-Shaanan TL, Schiller M, Azulay-Debby H, et al. Modulation of anti-tumor immunity by the brain's reward system. *Nat Commun.* 2018;9(1):2723.

71. Eisenberger NI, Cole SW. Social neuroscience and health: neurophysiological mechanisms linking social ties with physical health. *Nat Neurosci.* 2012;15(5):669−674.

CHAPTER 5

Finances as a Social Determinant of Health in Surgery

ELLIE M. PROUSSALOGLOU, MD • PRANAM DEY, BS •
RACHEL A. GREENUP, MD, MPH • ELIZABETH R. BERGER, MD, MS

INTRODUCTION

Cost in healthcare is a complex, multifaceted topic that affects every stakeholder differently. Understanding the financial implications of surgical care as a social determinant of health (SDH) has become an increasingly crucial aspect of this field of study. Patients undergoing surgery and perioperative care face rising costs of healthcare that impact their lives well beyond the acute recovery phase. The World Health Organization's (WHO) Commission on the Social Determinants of Health has defined SDH as "the conditions in which people are born, grow, live, work and age and the fundamental drivers of these conditions."[1] During the past two decades, a compelling body of evidence has demonstrated that socioeconomic factors such as income, wealth, and education are fundamental drivers of health outcomes. As the US healthcare system moves toward value-based care models incentivizing "well care" over "sick care," SDH are crucial components of efforts to enhance health outcomes and improve value-based care delivery. Characterizing the impact of finances as an SDH in the surgical patient will promote the provision of equitable, high-quality care to all, from initial diagnosis to post-op follow-up visit.

In this chapter, we will begin by exploring the key principles of health economics and how they impact national spending on healthcare in the United States. This will lead to a discussion of patient out-of-pocket (OOP) spending on both surgery and associated perioperative care and the resulting potential impact of the cost-related burden on patients, also known as the *financial toxicity* of surgical care.[2] We will then explore the indirect financial consequences of surgical care including bankruptcy and employment disruption.

Finally, we will define high-value surgical care and highlight the initiatives of the American College of Surgeons and other groups to recenter surgical care on high-value, low-cost, effective treatments. This summary of the complex topic of healthcare costs as related to surgical care will allow for a better understanding of how finances are an independent and vital SDH that requires additional research and attention in a coordinated attempt to minimize healthcare disparities.

A BRIEF OVERVIEW OF HEALTH ECONOMICS AND THE COMPLEXITY OF COST

Economics is the study of how societies choose to allocate scarce resources, given the combination of near unlimited demand for, and constrained supply of, valuable goods and services. Health economics, a field of study pioneered by Kenneth Arrow in the 1970s, aims to understand efficiency, trade-offs, value, and behavior in the production and consumption of healthcare.[3] Arrow's analysis highlights characteristics that differentiate the healthcare market from other markets, including (1) irregular and unpredictable demand as patients cannot predict when and how much medical care they will need; (2) an expectation that physicians act in their patients' best interests, with diagnosis and treatment based on science instead of personal interest; (3) uncertainty of treatment outcomes, even with modern medical advances; and (4) strict regulatory frameworks controlling supply and raising costs of hospital construction and expansion, drug and device development, and training of physician and allied health professionals.[3]

Social Determinants of Health in Surgery. https://doi.org/10.1016/B978-0-443-12366-5.00002-4

The healthcare market has additional aspects that contribute to its financial complexity. Numerous externalities can stem from individual decisions. For example, patients who get vaccinated benefit both themselves and everyone around them by contributing to lower transmission rates (positive externality). Meanwhile, those who choose to smoke harm those around them who are exposed to secondhand smoke (negative externalities). Asymmetric information is another challenge defined in health economics that applies to surgical decision-making. Most patients lack medical training and may have limited insight into how financial costs are balanced against the risks, benefits, and recommendations that impact treatment decision-making, as a patient may not fully understand why an expensive intervention is needed.[4] Physicians too, despite their training, cannot always know exactly what benefit or cost a specific procedure will have for a given patient. Furthermore, insurers have only limited knowledge of their beneficiaries' health risks and behaviors and thus depend on broad rules based on the average patient; this may prevent certain patients from receiving the treatment or intervention that they need.

Healthcare systems today are also marked by mergers that increase consolidation, leading to regional gaps in access to care (e.g., towns and cities with fewer hospitals and insurers), which research shows can reduce competition, raise prices, and negatively impact healthcare delivered. When subspecialty care is limited to a small number of facilities, these healthcare settings have more leverage to charge higher prices. For example, prices at monopoly hospitals have been found to be 12% higher than in markets with >4 hospitals providing the same services.[5] In contrast, mergers may also be an opportunity to improve quality of care by bringing together partnerships of subspecialty expertise and generalists or academic medical center programs into the community.

Insurance also introduces a unique challenge to healthcare economics. When payers primarily pay for healthcare, rather than the individual receiving the healthcare services, purchasing behavior may be altered. This "moral hazard" among insured patients has been well described; if the entire cost is covered by your insurance, there arguably is less reason to be cost-conscious when making healthcare decisions.[6,7] Insurers attempt to mitigate moral hazard through the implementation of copays, deductibles, coinsurance, and preauthorization approval rules. While a detailed discussion of insurance is deferred to a later chapter, insurance is inextricably linked with healthcare finances. As such, certain key definitions are needed to understand the impact of finances on surgical patients as an SDH. In the United States, many patients are covered by insurance plans that require individuals to pay a portion of their healthcare costs directly via so-called "cost sharing." Common forms of cost sharing include copayments (a flat fee charged for drug prescriptions, office visits, or procedures), coinsurance (a fee equaling a percentage of total spend on drugs, visits, or procedures), and/or deductibles (a set amount that the enrollee has to pay out-of-pocket (OOP) before insurance contributions begin).[2] High-deductible plans are defined by the IRS as an individual deductible > $1400 and family deductible >$2800.[8]

Due to this extensive system of cost sharing, even insured patients in the United States are often *underinsured* and have significant direct spending costs. Research shows that underinsurance impacts patients up to 400%–600% above the federal poverty line (defined as $30,000/year for a family of 4 in 2023); this population has been shown to have increased rates of OOP spending.[9] In 2023, the IRS defined in-network OOP maximum spending, including deductibles, as $9100 for individuals and $18,200 for a family.[8] These costs can be prohibitively expensive for patients. Despite recent national efforts to expand insurance coverage through Medicaid expansion and passage of the Affordable Care Act (2010), individuals who remain uninsured face even greater challenges with health-related finances. Recent predictions find that more than 30 million people in the United States still lack health insurance, which was exacerbated by the COVID-19 global pandemic.[10] The confluence of both uninsurance and underinsurance contributes to the complexity of healthcare costs in the United States, both at a national and individual level, and shows how finances impact patient outcomes as an SDH.

Healthcare Finances—a Ballooning Cost in the United States

To fully understand finances as an SDH in surgery, it is important to acknowledge the significant societal costs of healthcare in the United States. Since 1970, total healthcare costs as part of gross domestic product (GDP) have tripled to 18.3% (Fig. 5.1) and totaled $4.3 trillion USD. Contemporary healthcare expenditures include direct spending on healthcare services and related activities such as public health initiatives and medical research.[11] The primary driver of cost increases has been the development of new therapeutics, combined with an aging population, growing prevalence of chronic diseases, and expanded access to insurance.[12,13]

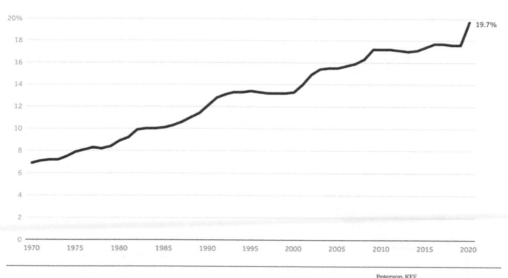

Peterson-KFF
Health System Tracker

FIG. 5.1 Total national health expenditures as a percent of gross domestic product, 1970–2020. (KFF analysis of National Health Expenditure (NHE) data.)

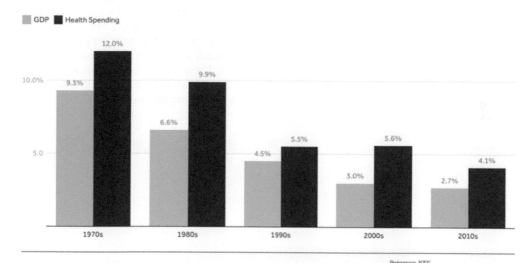

Peterson-KFF
Health System Tracker

FIG. 5.2 Average annual growth rate of GDP per capita and total national health spending per capita, 1970–2020. (KFF analysis of National Health Expenditure (NHE) data.)

Spending on hospitals, physicians, and prescription drugs currently represents 60% of total US healthcare expenditures with growth rates exceeding that of overall GDP (Fig. 5.2).[11,14] Increases in healthcare spending are due to some combination of increases in price and the quantity and "intensity" of health-related products (i.e., use of drug-eluting stents vs. bare metal). A 2021 national spending breakdown by the Centers for Medicare and Medicaid Services (CMS) delineated that the 10% growth in personal healthcare spending was not due to price increase but was instead overwhelmingly driven by the quantity and intensity of services. Most healthcare is funded by the US federal government (34%), with the remainder supported by households (27%), businesses (17%), and state and local governments (15%).[11] Total US healthcare spending includes several interrelated sectors, which all contribute to finances; hospital-based care accounts for the plurality of US health expenditures, followed by physicians and clinics, and prescription drugs (Fig. 5.3).[14]

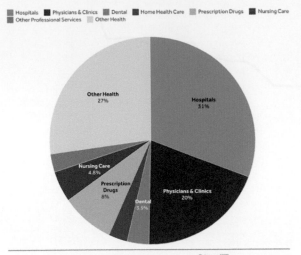

Hospitals   Physicians & Clinics   Dental   Home Health Care   Prescription Drugs   Nursing Care
Other Professional Services   Other Health

Peterson-KFF
Health System Tracker

FIG. 5.3 Relative contributions to total national health expenditures, 2020. (Note: "Other health" includes spending on durable and nondurable products; residential and personal care; administration; health insurance; and other state, private, and federal expenditures. "Other professional services" includes spending for services provided by chiropractors, optometrists, physical, occupational, and speech therapists, podiatrists, private-duty nurses, and others. Nursing care represents expenditures for nursing care facilities and continuing care retirement communities. KFF analysis of National Health Expenditure (NHE) data.)

Compared with peer-industrialized countries, the United States spends approximately twice as much on healthcare without improvements in health as measured by outcomes and quality (e.g., life expectancy, infant mortality).[15,16] While wealthier countries tend to spend more on healthcare compared with poorer countries, the United States is an outlier even when adjusting for its greater wealth (Fig. 5.4). Higher spending may reflect unmeasured differences in quality, such as higher rates of subspecialty visits or greater use of novel technology; whether such quality improvements are commensurate with higher costs—that is, whether they provide real value—is a more complex question than simply knowing a country's healthcare expenditures. An additional major driver of cost differences between the United States and peer nations is the lack of a centralized single payer reimbursement; specifics of different insurance structures will be discussed in a later chapter.

As detailed earlier, it is clear that rising healthcare spending in the United States remains a major societal challenge due to (1) disproportionate spending on treatment vs. prevention; (2) loss of funds to potentially beneficial social spending; (3) risk of growing tax burdens to fund public insurance programs like Medicare and Medicaid; and (4) increased costs to patients and families.[17] These trade-offs illustrate the importance of ensuring high value for every healthcare dollar spent, a goal we continue to work toward.

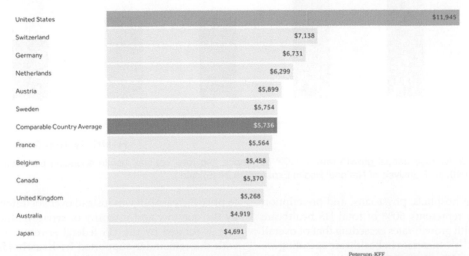

Peterson-KFF
Health System Tracker

FIG. 5.4 Health consumption expenditures per capita, US dollars, PPP adjusted, 2020 or nearest year. (Note: US value obtained from National Health Expenditure data. Data from Australia, Belgium, Canada, Japan, and Switzerland are from 2019. Data for Australia, France, and Japan are estimated. Data for Austria, Canada, Germany, Netherlands, and Sweden are provisional. Health consumption does not include investments in structures, equipment, or research. KFF analysis of National Health Expenditure (NHE) and OECD data.)

THE PATIENT IMPACT: FINANCIAL TOXICITY

The extraordinary rise in healthcare expenditures have increasingly been impacting patients and their families. Average cost statistics mask substantial variation in spending for Americans, which vary widely over the course of an individual lifetime[18]; existing data show that a disproportionate amount of spending each year is generated by a small proportion of the population. In 2019, 5% of the population with the highest healthcare spending accounted for nearly half of medical expenditures, at an average of $61,000 per person.[18] The opposite end of the distribution shows similar results; Americans with health-related spending below the 50th percentile accounted for only 3% of total spending, averaging $374 per person. Not surprisingly, higher healthcare costs are associated with advanced age and serious or chronic health conditions.

As the cost of medical care has continued to rise, the financial burden on patients has gained new attention. In 1999, the Institute of Medicine (IOM) charged the US Healthcare system with "Ensuring Quality Cancer Care" and highlighted the ability to afford care as a key component of quality.[19] Cost sharing via deductibles, copayments, and coinsurance has led to high healthcare costs being offloaded to patients and their families, resulting in often unaffordable individual cost burden. Not only have direct OOP payments increased for patients receiving care, but the indirect costs of care (e.g., employment disruption, lost wages, and need for transportation) also contribute to the financial burden of patients and their families. Notably, this burden of healthcare has been shown to impact treatment adherence and decision-making.[2] In 2007, the American Society of Clinical Oncology (ASCO) created the Task Force on the Cost of Cancer Care in response to rapid increases in the cost of cancer care and the vulnerability of patients to this cost increase. The Task Force's guidance statement, published in 2009, highlighted significant financial burdens faced by cancer patients and specifically recommended that (1) physicians communicate with their patients about their cost of care; (2) clinical support tools be created to help oncologists discuss costs with patients; (3) patients be given resources regarding cost of treatment; and (4) conversations about greater healthcare reform should focus on "high-quality, cost-effective care for all members of society."[20]

These national efforts prompted research regarding the impact of finances on patients and their decision-making. In 2013, the term "financial toxicity" (FT) was introduced into the literature by Dr. Zafar et al., describing the mental and emotional stress related to the increasing burden of unaffordable cancer care.[21] Although financial toxicity has been described on a global scale, this phenomenon is particularly pronounced in the United States due to lack of universal insurance coverage and frequent high OOP payments for commercially or federally insured patients.[22,23] Real-time patient-reported outcome (PRO) tools have been developed to allow for early identification of patients who may suffer from FT with hopes to intervene and help alleviate the burden of care.[24] Acknowledging the variation in individual patients' insurance coverage, salary, resources, and family support, use of such a PRO including the Comprehensive Score for Financial Toxicity (COST) tool developed by de Souza et al. at the University of Chicago allows for an objective and generalizable evaluation of patient risk of financial toxicity.[25] This tool, a freely available and validated 11 question survey, allows for an efficient and thorough evaluation of patients' risk of treatment-related financial hardship without requiring granular knowledge of each specific patient's baseline financial status.[25,26] Tools such as COST have been used to describe the impact of healthcare costs on individuals as an adjunct to specific spending data.

Financial toxicity was initially studied in the oncology setting due to the high costs of complex oncology care, which often include a combination of surgery, radiation, chemotherapy, and newer immunotherapy and targeted therapy regimens.[27] In 2020, 18.1 million cancer survivors in the United States were estimated to contribute to $157.77 billion spent nationally.[28] Medicare beneficiaries with a new cancer diagnosis have been found to spend an average of 23.7% of their income on OOP healthcare costs.[29] Cost considerations have been shown to influence surgical decision-making in 28% of breast cancer patients; those making less than $45,000 per year prioritized treatment costs over considerations of appearance or breast preservation.[30] Advanced cancer stage and poor financial status at time of breast cancer diagnosis have also been linked with worse financial toxicity.[31] Patients with gynecologic malignancies have been shown to delay or avoid care due to finances,[32] with increased rates of FT in patients with cervical cancer, younger age, and non-White race.[33]

The burden of financial toxicity has been described across surgical disciplines. Patients undergoing coronary artery bypass graft surgery face significant variation in cost of surgery, with prices ranging from $44,000 to $448,000,[34,35] and out-of-network emergency room visits or out-of-network perioperative team members (e.g., radiology, anesthesia, assistants) further contribute to OOP cost differences for unknowing patients.[36] Data from the National Health Interview Survey (2008–2018) found that 55% of patients who had undergone surgery within the prior year reported financial toxicity; surgical patients between 50% and 400% of the federal poverty level were at a twofold greater risk of holding medical debt when compared with participants with higher incomes.[37] Patients with chronic medical conditions are also more likely to have both medical and nonmedical debt, low credit scores, or recent bankruptcy, with higher rates of all financial burdens with additional conditions.[38] Furthermore, recent assessment of insurance cost sharing found that many Americans do not have liquid assets to pay their deductibles. In 2021, average deductibles for single coverage ranged from $1397 to $2379 based on employer size; 45% of surveyed single-person nonelderly households did not have $2000 in liquid assets.

LONG-TERM FINANCIAL IMPACTS: EMPLOYMENT DISRUPTION AND BANKRUPTCY

In addition to direct costs as described earlier, the financial burden of care includes lost productivity due to employment disruption and the resulting lost wages and longer-term impact on job security, promotion, and income growth trajectory. A national survey of women with metastatic breast cancer found that 62% of women stopped work completely related to their diagnosis. Women of color were more likely to stop working, reduce work hours, take paid and unpaid leave, or change jobs, whereas white women were more likely to retire.[39] Women with breast cancer report significant short- and long-term career repercussions including the need to use sick time and vacation for treatment and follow-up appointments, as well as position elimination and being passed over for professional growth opportunities.[40] Similar employment disruptions have been seen in patients with endometrial cancer, a disease often curable with up-front surgery. A study of women with employer-subsidized health insurance and newly diagnosed endometrial cancer found that 21.7% of women had a change in employment after treatment; this was 34% more likely in patients who had chemoradiation in addition to surgery.[41] Employment disruptions are seen even when cancer care is less involved. Among thyroid cancer patients largely treated with surgery and/or radioactive iodine (only 2.7% of the study cohort received chemotherapy), 18.1% of patients reported unemployment for >6 months, while 59.6% reported decreased productivity and 42.5% had lost income.[42]

Despite financial toxicity initially being described in the oncology setting, similar employment disruptions have been demonstrated in other surgical patients. Among individuals undergoing pelvic reconstruction surgery, only 42% of previously employed patients returned to work 1 month postoperatively; of those working prior to surgery, 9% had quit and 11% reported continued reduced work productivity 3 months after surgery.[43] Failure to return to work postoperatively is also not uncommon among individuals undergoing total (18%) or unicompartmental (5%) knee replacement; notably, 12% of these patients reported ultimately permanently leaving jobs due to persistent problems with their operated-on knee.[44] Collectively, these findings highlight the risk of employment disruption or job loss after surgery. Further research is needed to better understand the impact of surgery on employment and target interventions that optimize medical leave and disability policies for professional protection.

In its most extreme form, healthcare-related financial toxicity can result in bankruptcy for patients and families receiving comprehensive medical care. A 2019 analysis of medically induced bankruptcy estimated approximately 530,000 medical bankruptcies annually, even after passage of the Affordable Care Act.[45] Medical-related bankruptcy is the named cause of 62% of individual filings for bankruptcy, and more than 75% of these filers were insured at time of their contributing medical bill.[46] Patients with cancer have been shown to have rates of bankruptcy 2.65 times those of patients without cancer[47]; insured breast surgery patients were more likely to file for bankruptcy if younger and of non-White race.[48] The risk of bankruptcy exists across all cancer stages and is correlated with overall and disease-specific survival. Patients with breast cancer who underwent bankruptcy had a 50% greater risk of death compared with propensity-matched controls.[49] Uninsured patients admitted for trauma have been shown to have significant risk of catastrophic health expenditure risk (defined as inpatient charges ≥40% of annual postsubsistence income); 70% of these individuals were at risk of catastrophic health expenditure, which increased to 82% when individuals were severely injured.[50] Additional work is needed to further understand the rates of bankruptcy among patients undergoing elective or nonemergent surgery.

WHAT IS HIGH-VALUE SURGICAL CARE AND WHY DOES IT MATTER?

Healthcare spending in the United States has increased at both the national and individual patient levels without associated demonstrable improved health outcomes. Compared with peer nations, the United States has the lowest life expectancy, an average of 79.1 years for women and 73.2 for men, compared with peer nations' averages of 84.7 and 80, respectively.[51] In the 1980s, US life expectancy previously mirrored peer nations but has rapidly diverged despite outspending other countries at nearly double the rate. Other healthcare quality metrics show further divides between the United States and peer nations. The maternal mortality rate in the United States was 17.4 deaths per 100,000 live births in 2018, double that of other high-income countries.[52] The United States also has the highest infant mortality rate of developed nations and higher rates of chronic disease and adverse outcomes for ischemic heart disease and diabetes.[53] Given this clear discrepancy with unsustainable medical care without improvements in health outcomes, the development of high-value care models has become a priority.

To better understand high-value surgical care, several key definitions are needed. Value, a concept first proposed by Porter and Teisberg, is a uniquely global metric for defining healthcare quality because it refers to the end result of combined practices.[54] Value is defined as quality divided by cost, or patient health outcomes achieved per healthcare dollars spent. Quality and cost can differ significantly based on measurement challenges and definitions of appropriate metrics as well as prioritization of quality versus cost. A University of Utah survey of 700 surgeons, 5000 patients, and 540 employers highlighted these differences; 88% of surgeons felt that quality was the most important aspect of value and only 5% considered cost, whereas 62% of patients prioritized quality and 26% prioritized cost.[55]

Establishing "good value care" is challenging when considering the diverse perspectives and stakeholders within surgical care. The National Academy of Medicine defines quality as "the degree to which health services for individuals and populations increase the likelihood of desired health outcomes and are consistent with current professional knowledge."[56] The WHO adds that health services should be effective, safe, people-centered, timely, equitable, integrated, and efficient.[57] Said simply, quality care is providing the right treatment for each patient at the right time, done effectively and safely.

For nearly 100 years, the American College of Surgeons (ACS) has developed focused programs to improve overall healthcare and attain excellence in surgical quality. In 1994, in response to Congressional mandated reporting of surgical outcomes, the Department of Veteran Affairs (VA) developed the National Surgical Quality Improvement Program (NSQIP). NSQIP established dedicated reviewers at each of the 133 major VA surgical centers to measure and record for all major surgeries: (1) patients' preoperative status, (2) intraoperative outcomes, and (3) postoperative outcomes.[58] Reports focused on observed/expected ratios for 30-day mortality and postoperative morbidity, self-assessment tools, and advisory site visits were added to continue to improve quality of surgical care throughout the system.

Within 10 years of NSQIP implementation, VA surgical patient mortality had decreased by 37% and morbidity by 42%, despite similar severity of illness in patient populations across time periods.[58] NSQIP was then expanded to 14 academic medical centers across the United States through the Patient Safety in Surgery Study, a prospective cohort study.[59] A study examining 118 institutions between 2006 and 2007 showed improvement in both morbidity (82%) and mortality rates (66%) at all hospitals implanting ASC-NSQIP, and implementation of the program continued nationwide in search of improving surgical quality.[60] As of 2022, 708 hospitals are participating in ASC-NSQIP.

Measuring surgical quality is key to ensuring that quality of care remains high and is comparable across centers. Several metrics for quality assessment exist, including the National Quality Forum, which provides reliable, feasible, and useable metrics to address performance gaps.[61] Billing and claims data, as well as databases and clinical registries, are also widely used with attempts to evaluate the quality of care, despite the generally poor sensitivity and high false positive rates associated with administrative data when compared with clinical data.[62] Calculating value also depends on defining cost. As detailed earlier in the chapter, healthcare costs have ballooned in the United States and now significantly exceed those of peer nations. Cost is multifactorial and includes cost to the hospital, reimbursement from third-party payers, charge billed to the insurance company, price (including OOP costs and deductibles) paid by the patient, as well as harder-to-measure costs—distress, physical and emotional suffering, lost income, and impact on quality of life resulting.

BUILDING HIGH-VALUE SURGERY

One intervention to prioritize high-value care has been implementation of bundled care payments, which have predetermined total allowable acute and/or postacute expenditures (target price) for an episode of care.[63,64] Participating providers share in any losses or savings that result from the difference between this target price and actual costs to incentivize more judicious use of resources. Medicare has led the charge on incorporation of bundled payments with mixed success. The initial Bundled Payments for Care Improvement (BPCI) program had significant losses, but a reworked program known as BPCI Advanced—which incorporates prospective pricing, risk adjustment at beneficiary and provider levels, and annual rebasing of target prices, among other changes—is currently being trialed.[65] It remains to be seen how bundled payments can be rolled out successfully in the United States but offers potential to reward high-value care across the healthcare continuum, including in surgery.

Within surgery, several subspecialty organizations have prioritized high-value surgical care by choosing the appropriate patients in which to deescalate care through initiatives such as Choosing Wisely. The Choosing Wisely Campaign, originally created in 2012 by the American Board of Internal Medication Foundation in partnership with multiple specialty organizations, identifies low-value medical care and encourages its subspecialists to avoid these procedures/ interventions.[66] One such campaign has centered on Breast Surgical Oncology; the ACS, Society of Surgical Oncology, and American Society for Breast Surgeons identified four low-value breast cancer surgery as outlined in the following, which are now discouraged.[67]

1. Axillary lymph node dissection for limited nodal disease in patients getting lumpectomy and radiation
2. Lumpectomy reexcision for close but negative margins for invasive cancer
3. Contralateral prophylactic mastectomy (CPM) in average-risk women with unilateral cancer
4. Sentinel lymph node biopsy in women >70 years old with hormone positive disease and clinical node negative status

Of note, compliance with these surgical Choosing Wisely Campaigns in breast has varied significantly. While axillary lymph node dissections and lumpectomy reoperation rates have decreased significantly, rates of CPM in average-risk women and SLNB for older women have risen since 2004.[67] Additional work is needed to ensure that providers use existing guidelines to avoid low-value care and prioritize high-value, patient-centered surgical decision-making. Similar interventions across other surgical subspecialties may be an important first step in prioritizing high-value surgical care and continuing to reduce the financial burden on our patients.

THE FUTURE OF VALUE-BASED SURGICAL CARE

As the cost of surgical care continues to rise, the potential barrier to equitable care for our patients becomes even more significant. In addition to previous efforts to improve the value of care, thereby eliminating extraneous costs for low-benefit interventions, the ACS began a collaboration with Harvard Business School to better measure cost and quality of care to identify areas of low-valued care.[68] The new initiative, called ACS THRIVE (Transforming Healthcare Resources to Increase Value and Efficiency), is working to increase production cost transparency for surgical procedures to better understand the cost of care delivery. Allowing institutions to understand their production costs of certain surgical procedures empowers them to identify ways to improve value-based care models. Initial work has focused on colon, bariatric, and breast cancer surgery with input from both the Harvard Business School on the cost analysis piece and the ACS on the quality standards aspect of value.[68] To calculate production costs, a specific methodology known as Time-Driven Activity-Based Costing (TDABC) is being used to identify three major components of cost:

1. Determine the care process: Identify what activities are performed for each condition, who performs them, and how long each takes.
2. Calculate cost rates: Identify cost per unit of time
3. Account for consumables: Identify what materials, supplies, and drugs are used during the care cycle.

The goal of THRIVE is to create a patient-centric episode of care with a defined production cost to help institutions and providers understand the cost of providing surgical care and move toward a value-based model of care. Collaborative projects such as these demonstrate the ongoing commitment to improve the delivery of value-based care to minimize the effects cost has on our health outcomes. This project, among others, represents a way to continue to narrow the gap in access for patients and to decrease the potentially disastrous financial consequences of surgical care to our patients, in both the immediate and delayed postoperative setting.

CONCLUSIONS

The cost of healthcare in the United States continues to rapidly grow, and the impact of this on both the overall market and individual patient finances is profound. Increasing cost across the healthcare spectrum remain concerning as it relates to health equity and access to care for our patients; resource allocation and waste; continued focus on the treatment of late-stage disease instead of upstream prevention; and financial sustainability of federal insurance. Existing work has shown that a patient's socioeconomic status, which is largely driven by finances, is an independent risk factor for perioperative complications, length of stay, and 30-

day mortality for patients undergoing elective cardiac surgery.[69] In many surgical specialties, the ability of a patient to access reliable preventative healthcare and cancer screening allows for earlier detection of disease and better outcomes. In addition, a patient's financial ability to obtain Medicaid insurance and, thus, have access to care has been linked to improved surgical outcomes.[70] Even when patients are able to access appropriate, warranted healthcare, the long-term financial implications cannot be ignored. As programs such as NSQIP, Choosing Wisely, and THRIVE continue to be utilized across the country, the focus on promoting high-value care while reducing extraneous or low-benefit surgical interventions remains a critical component of decreasing the financial burden of healthcare costs on our patients. Additional work to allow for individual monetary support, early identification of financial distress, and prevention of job loss and bankruptcy through targeted interventions is also needed, especially when protecting generational financial security and social mobility. Lastly, reducing the burden of cost sharing from insurance will further reduce the disparities that currently exist when considering finances as an SDH.

Highlights

- The cost of surgical care is complex and multifaceted and is particularly elevated in the United States, in parallel with higher rising costs of healthcare compared with other industrialized nations.
- The rising cost of healthcare has led to increased rates of patient hardship and "financial toxicity," first described in cancer patients but since seen throughout healthcare including across surgical disciplines.
- Surgery, including pre- and post-op care, has been linked to longer-term financial impacts outside of the immediate treatment setting. It is important to consider impact of surgical care on employment and bankruptcy when counseling patients about their options.
- Efforts to identify high-value surgical care balance the cost of care with the quality of care provided.
- Guidelines such as ASC-NSQIP, Choosing Wisely, and ACS-THRIVE are measures taken by surgeons on a national scale to identify and promote high-value surgical care and minimize cost and complications on the individual level.

REFERENCES

1. *Addressing Social Determinants of Health: Examples of Successful Evidence-Based Strategies and Current Federal Efforts.* Department of Health and Human Services, Office of the Assistant Secretary for Planning and Evaluation; 2022. https://aspe.hhs.gov/reports/sdoh-evidence-review.
2. Politi MC, Housten AJ, Forcino RC, Jansen J, Elwyn G. Discussing cost and value in patient decision aids and shared decision making: a call to action. *MDM Policy Pract.* Jan-Jun 2023;8(1):23814683221148651. https://doi.org/10.1177/23814683221148651.
3. Arrow KJ. Uncertainty and the welfare economics of medical care. *Am Econ Rev.* 1963;53(5):941–973.
4. Finkelstein A, McGarry K. Multiple dimensions of private information: evidence from the long-term care insurance market. *Am Econ Rev.* 2006;96(4):938–958. https://doi.org/10.1257/aer.96.4.938.
5. Cooper Z, Craig SV, Gaynor M, Van Reenen J. The price AIN'T right? Hospital prices and health spending on the privately insured. *Q J Econ.* February 2019;134(1):51–107. https://doi.org/10.1093/qje/qjy020.
6. Pauly MV. The economics of moral hazard: comment. *Am Econ Rev.* 1968;58(3):531–537.
7. Chernew ME, Fendrick AM. Improving benefit design to promote effective, efficient, and affordable care. *JAMA.* 2016;316(16):1651–1652. https://doi.org/10.1001/jama.2016.13637.
8. Healthcare.gov Glossary. US Centers for Medicare and Medicaid Services, Department of Health and Human Services. https://www.healthcare.gov/glossary/out-of-pocket-maximum-limit/ Accessed March 2023.
9. Glied S, Zhu B. *Catastrophic Out-of-Pocket Health Care Costs: A Problem Mainly for Middle-Income Americans with Employer Coverage;* 2020. https://www.commonwealthfund.org/publications/issue-briefs/2020/apr/catastrophic-out-of-pocket-costs-problem-middle-income.
10. Cohen R, Cha A. *Health Insurance Coverage: Early Release of Quarterly Estimates from the National Health Interview Survey, January 2021–March 2022;* 2022. https://www.cdc.gov/nchs/data/nhis/earlyrelease/quarterly_estimates_2022_q11.pdf.
11. Martin AB, Hartman M, Benson J, Catlin A, Team TNHEA. National health care spending in 2021: decline in federal spending outweighs greater use of health care. *Health Aff.* 2022. https://doi.org/10.1377/hlthaff.2022.01397.
12. Thorpe KE. The rise in health care spending and what to do about it. *Health Aff.* 2005;24(6):1436–1445. https://doi.org/10.1377/hlthaff.24.6.1436.
13. Finkelstein A. The aggregate effects of health insurance: evidence from the introduction of Medicare. *Q J Econ.* 2007;122(1):1–37. https://doi.org/10.1162/qjec.122.1.1.
14. Kurani N, Ortazila J, Wager E, Fox L, Amin K. How has U.S. Spending on Healthcare Changed over Time? Peterson-KFF Health System Tracker. Updated February 25, 2022.

https://www.healthsystemtracker.org/chart-collection/u-s-spending-healthcare-changed-time/#Total%20national%20health%20expenditures,%20US%20$%20Billions,%201970-2020.

15. Wager E, Ortazila J, Cox C. How Does Health Spending in the U.S. Compare to Other Countries? Peterson-KFF Health System Tracker. Updated January 21, 2022. https://www.healthsystemtracker.org/chart-collection/health-spending-u-s-compare-countries-2/#GDP%20per%20capita%20and%20health%20consumption%20spending%20per%20capita,%202020%20(U.S.%20dollars,%20PPP%20adjusted).

16. Baicker K, Chandra A. Do we spend too much on health care? *N Engl J Med*. August 13, 2020;383(7):605−608. https://doi.org/10.1056/NEJMp2006099.

17. Baicker K, Chandra A. The health care jobs fallacy. *N Engl J Med*. June 28, 2012;366(26):2433−2435. https://doi.org/10.1056/NEJMp1204891.

18. Ortazila J, McGough M, Wgaer E, Claxton G, Amin K. How Do Health Expenditures Vary across the Population? Peterson-KFF Health System Tracker. Updated November 12, 2021. https://www.healthsystemtracker.org/chart-collection/health-expenditures-vary-across-population/#Proportion%20of%20individuals%20by%20health%20status,%202019.

19. Board IoMUaNRCUNCP. Ensuring quality cancer care. In: Hewitt M, Simone JV, eds. *Ensuring Quality Cancer Care*. 1999.

20. Meropol NJ, Schrag D, Smith TJ, et al. American Society of Clinical Oncology guidance statement: the cost of cancer care. *J Clin Oncol*. August 10, 2009;27(23):3868−3874. https://doi.org/10.1200/JCO.2009.23.1183.

21. Zafar SY, Abernethy AP. Financial toxicity, Part I: a new name for a growing problem. *Oncology*. February 2013;27(2):80−81, 149.

22. Carroll A. *What's Wrong with Health Insurance? Deductibles are Ridiculous, for Starters*. The New York Times; 2022. The New York Times Company.

23. Schoen C, Osborn R, Squires D, Doty MM. Access, affordability, and insurance complexity are often worse in the United States compared to ten other countries. *Health Aff*. December 2013;32(12):2205−2215. https://doi.org/10.1377/hlthaff.2013.0879.

24. Zafar SY, Abernethy AP. Financial toxicity, Part II: how can we help with the burden of treatment-related costs? *Oncology*. April 2013;27(4):253−254, 256.

25. de Souza JA, Yap BJ, Hlubocky FJ, et al. The development of a financial toxicity patient-reported outcome in cancer: the COST measure. *Cancer*. October 15, 2014;120(20):3245−3253. https://doi.org/10.1002/cncr.28814.

26. De Souza JA, Aschebrook-Kilfoy B, Grogan R, Yap BJ, Daugherty C, Cella D. Grading financial toxicity based upon its impact on health-related quality of life (HRQol). *J Clin Oncol*. 2016;34(3_suppl l). https://doi.org/10.1200/jco.2016.34.3_suppl.16, 16-16.

27. Tran G, Zafar SY. Financial toxicity and implications for cancer care in the era of molecular and immune therapies. *Ann Transl Med*. May 2018;6(9):166. https://doi.org/10.21037/atm.2018.03.28.

28. Mariotto AB, Yabroff KR, Shao Y, Feuer EJ, Brown ML. Projections of the cost of cancer care in the United States: 2010-2020. *J Natl Cancer Inst*. January 19, 2011;103(2):117−128. https://doi.org/10.1093/jnci/djq495.

29. Narang AK, Nicholas LH. Out-of-Pocket spending and financial burden among Medicare beneficiaries with cancer. *JAMA Oncol*. June 1, 2017;3(6):757−765. https://doi.org/10.1001/jamaoncol.2016.4865.

30. Greenup RA, Rushing C, Fish L, et al. Financial costs and burden related to decisions for breast cancer surgery. *J Oncol Pract*. August 2019;15(8):e666−e676. https://doi.org/10.1200/jop.18.00796.

31. Offodile 2nd AC, Asaad M, Boukovalas S, et al. Financial toxicity following surgical treatment for breast cancer: a cross-sectional pilot study. *Ann Surg Oncol*. May 2021;28(5):2451−2462. https://doi.org/10.1245/s10434-020-09216-9.

32. Bouberhan S, Shea M, Kennedy A, et al. Financial toxicity in gynecologic oncology. *Gynecol Oncol*. July 2019;154(1):8−12. https://doi.org/10.1016/j.ygyno.2019.04.003.

33. Aviki EM, Manning-Geist BL, Sokolowski SS, et al. Risk factors for financial toxicity in patients with gynecologic cancer. *Am J Obstet Gynecol*. June 2022;226(6):817 e1−e817 e9. https://doi.org/10.1016/j.ajog.2021.12.012.

34. Slavin SD, Khera R, Zafar SY, Nasir K, Warraich HJ. Financial burden, distress, and toxicity in cardiovascular disease. *Am Heart J*. August 2021;238:75−84. https://doi.org/10.1016/j.ahj.2021.04.011.

35. Giacomino BD, Cram P, Vaughan-Sarrazin M, Zhou Y, Girotra S. Association of hospital prices for coronary artery bypass grafting with hospital quality and reimbursement. *Am J Cardiol*. April 1, 2016;117(7):1101−1106. https://doi.org/10.1016/j.amjcard.2016.01.004.

36. Chhabra KR, Sheetz KH, Nuliyalu U, Dekhne MS, Ryan AM, Dimick JB. Out-of-Network bills for privately insured patients undergoing elective surgery with in-network primary surgeons and facilities. *JAMA*. February 11, 2020;323(6):538−547. https://doi.org/10.1001/jama.2019.21463.

37. Taylor KK, Neiman PU, Liu C, Sheetz K, Sinco B, Scott JW. Financial toxicity among surgical patients varies by income and insurance: a cross-sectional analysis of the national health Interview survey. *Ann Surg*. July 1, 2022;276(1):e56−e58. https://doi.org/10.1097/SLA.0000000000005382.

38. Becker NV, Scott JW, Moniz MH, Carlton EF, Ayanian JZ. Association of chronic disease with patient financial outcomes among commercially insured adults. *JAMA Intern Med*. October 1, 2022;182(10):1044−1051. https://doi.org/10.1001/jamainternmed.2022.3687.

39. Samuel CA, Spencer JC, Rosenstein DL, et al. Racial differences in employment and cost-management behaviors in patients with metastatic breast cancer. *Breast Cancer Res Treat.* January 2020;179(1):207–215. https://doi.org/10.1007/s10549-019-05449-9.

40. Oshima SM, Tait SD, Rushing C, et al. Patient perspectives on the financial costs and burdens of breast cancer surgery. *JCO Oncol Pract.* June 2021;17(6):e872–e881. https://doi.org/10.1200/OP.20.00780.

41. Nitecki R, Fu S, Lefkowits C, et al. Employment disruption following the diagnosis of endometrial cancer. *Gynecol Oncol.* January 2021;160(1):199–205. https://doi.org/10.1016/j.ygyno.2020.10.041.

42. Mongelli MN, Giri S, Peipert BJ, Helenowski IB, Yount SE, Sturgeon C. Financial burden and quality of life among thyroid cancer survivors. *Surgery.* March 2020;167(3):631–637. https://doi.org/10.1016/j.surg.2019.11.014.

43. Wang R, Sappenfield EC. Return to work following pelvic reconstructive surgery: secondary analysis of operations and pelvic muscle training in the management of apical support loss trial. *Am J Obstet Gynecol.* 2022;227(2). https://doi.org/10.1016/j.ajog.2022.05.037, 322-322.

44. Zaballa E, Ntani G, Harris EC, Arden NK, Cooper C, Walker-Bone K. Return to work and employment retention after uni-compartmental and total knee replacement: findings from the Clinical Outcomes in Arthroplasty study. *Knee.* January 2023;40:245–255. https://doi.org/10.1016/j.knee.2022.11.022.

45. Himmelstein DU, Lawless RM, Thorne D, Foohey P, Woolhandler S. Medical bankruptcy: still common despite the affordable care act. *Am J Publ Health.* March 2019;109(3):431–433. https://doi.org/10.2105/ajph.2018.304901.

46. Shrime MG, Weinstein MC, Hammitt JK, Cohen JL, Salomon JA. Trading bankruptcy for health: a discrete-choice experiment. *Value Health.* January 2018;21(1):95–104. https://doi.org/10.1016/j.jval.2017.07.006.

47. Ramsey S, Blough D, Kirchhoff A, et al. Washington state cancer patients found to be at greater risk for bankruptcy than people without a cancer diagnosis. *Health Aff.* June 2013;32(6):1143–1152. https://doi.org/10.1377/hlthaff.2012.1263.

48. Obeng-Gyasi S, Timsina LR, Bhattacharyya O, Fisher CS, Haggstrom DA. Bankruptcy among insured surgical patients with breast cancer: who is at risk? *Cancer.* June 15, 2021;127(12):2083–2090. https://doi.org/10.1002/cncr.33468.

49. Ramsey SD, Bansal A, Fedorenko CR, et al. Financial insolvency as a risk factor for early mortality among patients with cancer. *J Clin Oncol.* March 20, 2016;34(9):980–986. https://doi.org/10.1200/JCO.2015.64.6620.

50. Scott JW, Raykar NP, Rose JA, et al. Cured into destitution: catastrophic health expenditure risk among uninsured trauma patients in the United States. *Ann Surg.* June 2018;267(6):1093–1099. https://doi.org/10.1097/sla.0000000000002254.

51. Rakshit S, McGough M, Amin K, Cox C. How Does U.S. Life Expectancy Compare to Other Countries? Peterson-KFF Health System Tracker. https://www.healthsystemtracker.org/chart-collection/u-s-life-expectancy-compare-countries/#Life%20expectancy%20at%20birth%20in%20years,%201980-2021.

52. O'Neil S, Platt I, Vohra D, et al. *The High Costs of Maternal Morbidity Show Why We Need Greater Investment in Maternal Health*; 2021. https://www.commonwealthfund.org/publications/issue-briefs/2021/nov/high-costs-maternal-morbidity-need-investment-maternal-health.

53. Squires D, Anderson C. *U.S. Health Care from a Global Perspective*; 2015. https://www.commonwealthfund.org/publications/issue-briefs/2015/oct/us-health-care-global-perspective.

54. Porter M, Teisberg E. *Redefining Health Care: Creating Value-Based Competition on Results.* Harvard Business School Press; 2006.

55. FORUM UV. BEST QUALITY? YES AND NO. University of Utah Health. https://uofuhealth.utah.edu/value/best-quality.

56. Medicine Io. *Envisioning the National Health Care Quality Report.* The National Academies Press; 2001:256.

57. *Quality Health Services Fact Sheet*; 2020. https://www.who.int/news-room/fact-sheets/detail/quality-health-services.

58. Khuri SF. The NSQIP: a new frontier in surgery. *Surgery.* November 2005;138(5):837–843. https://doi.org/10.1016/j.surg.2005.08.016.

59. Khuri SF, Henderson WG, Daley J, et al. The patient safety in surgery study: background, study design, and patient populations. *J Am Coll Surg.* June 2007;204(6):1089–1102. https://doi.org/10.1016/j.jamcollsurg.2007.03.028.

60. Hall BL, Hamilton BH, Richards K, Bilimoria KY, Cohen ME, Ko CY. Does surgical quality improve in the American College of surgeons national surgical quality improvement program: an evaluation of all participating hospitals. *Ann Surg.* September 2009;250(3):363–376. https://doi.org/10.1097/SLA.0b013e3181b4148f.

61. *NQF-endorsed Measures for Surgical Procedures Technical Report.* 2015.

62. Lawson EH, Louie R, Zingmond DS, et al. A comparison of clinical registry versus administrative claims data for reporting of 30-day surgical complications. *Ann Surg.* December 2012;256(6):973–981. https://doi.org/10.1097/SLA.0b013e31826b4c4f.

63. Agarwal R, Liao JM, Gupta A, Navathe AS. The impact of bundled payment on health care spending, utilization, and quality: a systematic review. *Health Aff.* January 2020;39(1):50–57. https://doi.org/10.1377/hlthaff.2019.00784.

64. What is value-based healthcare? *NEJM Catalyst.* 2017;3(1). https://doi.org/10.1056/CAT.17.0558.

65. Services CfMM. Bundled Payments for Care Improvement Advanced General Frequently Asked Questions (FAQs). https://innovation.cms.gov/files/x/bpci-advanced-faqs.pdf.

66. Mafi JN, Reid RO, Baseman LH, et al. Trends in low-value health service use and spending in the US Medicare fee-for-

service program, 2014-2018. *JAMA Netw Open*. February 1, 2021;4(2):e2037328. https://doi.org/10.1001/jamanetwo rkopen.2020.37328.

67. Wang T, Bredbeck BC, Sinco B, et al. Variations in persistent use of low-value breast cancer surgery. *JAMA Surg*. April 1, 2021;156(4):353−362. https://doi.org/10.1001/jamasurg.2020.6942.

68. About ACS THRIVE. American College of Surgeons. https://www.facs.org/quality-programs/standards-and-sta ging/acs-thrive/.

69. Jerath A, Austin PC, Ko DT, et al. Socioeconomic status and days alive and out of hospital after major elective noncardiac surgery: a population-based cohort study. *Anesthesiology*. April 2020;132(4):713−722. https://doi.org/10.1097/aln.0 000000000003123.

70. Hoehn RS, Rieser CJ, Phelos H, et al. Association between Medicaid expansion and diagnosis and management of colon cancer. *J Am Coll Surg*. February 2021;232(2):146−156. https://doi.org/10.1016/j.jamcollsurg.2020.10.021.

CHAPTER 6

Neighborhood as a Social Determinant of Health in Surgery

ADRIAN DIAZ, MD, MPH • ANDREW M. IBRAHIM, MD, MSC

INTRODUCTION

Social determinants of health (SDOH) defined broadly are the nonclinical factors that impact a person's health.[1-3] According to the World Health Organization, SDOH consist of the conditions in which people are born, grow, learn, work, and age.[4] Alongside schools and workplaces, neighborhoods represent one of the major contexts in which people lead a considerable portion of their lives. Place and location can determine the quality of schools, access to services, job, transportation, as well as exposure to pollution crime, noise, and other environmental features. It follows that residential location can exert a decisive influence on variations in a person's health.

Attempts to link residential location to health outcomes long predate modern medicine. As earlier as the 5h century BCE, Hippocrates' treatise On Airs, Waters, and Places laid the foundation for one of the earliest understandings of the relationships between places, health, and disease. It is Jon Snow (a surgeon!), however, who is frequently cited as an early pioneer who literally drew the connection between neighborhoods and health by means of a map in the 19th century. By developing a precise dot map of cases of and deaths from cholera in 1854, Snow pinpointed the source of cholera to the now infamous Broad Street pump in the Soho neighborhood of London.

Today the study of "contextual effects" has exploded in large part due to the ease with which neighborhood variables as proxied by various census measures could be attached to existing individual-level data. As a result, this is forcing us to clearly articulate why and how context might be important and, more generally why multilevel thinking (and multilevel analysis) is critical not only to fully understand causation but also to identify promising polices to improve health.

COMMONLY USED MEASURES OF NEIGHBORHOODS

The term "neighborhood" generally refers to the place where a group of people live. This, of course, can be defined at several scales starting with an individual building all the way up to regional delivery region. Given the increasing body of literature about neighborhoods, it seems reasonable to assume a consensus definition has been proposed. However, this is far from the case. Although there have been many proposed definitions of what constitutes a neighborhood, the focus of how these neighborhoods can be operationalized in research design has not received a formal or exhaustive assessment. In other words, how to meaningfully delineate boundaries to assess features contained within them and the implications of their features for health of individuals who live, work, and play within these areas remains much to the researcher's discretion. Here, we provide an overview and describe some commonly used examples in public health research. Neighborhood measures are herein organized in ascending order from small geographic area to largest.

Census block group—Developed and used by the US Census Bureau, census block group is a subdivision of a census tract. Census block groupings are the smallest geographic unit for which the US Census Bureau publishes sample data. Typically, census block groups have a population of 600 to 3000 people.

Census tract—Developed and used by the US Census Bureau, census tracts have an average of approximately 4000 people and are designated to be a homogenous spatial units with respect to population characteristics, economic status, and living conditions.

ZIP code and ZCTAs—A zone improvement plan code or "ZIP code" is one of the more commonly used geographic level exposures in research. The ZIP code is classically used by the United States Postal Service and crudely defines geographic areas into a five-digit code. Each ZIP code may include upward of 30,000 people. Alternatively, *ZIP Code Tabulation Areas (ZCTAs)* were created by the US Census Bureau based on census blocks and for the most part coincide with ZIP codes. The ZIP+4 code is a basic five-digit code with four digits added as an extra identifier. It helps to identify a geographic segment within the five-digit delivery area, such as a city block or a group of apartments.

County—Administrative or political subdivision of the state in which their boundaries are drawn. Today, 3142 counties and county equivalents carve up the United States, ranging in number from 3 for Delaware to 254 for Texas.

For the purposes of research, there are trade-offs with each of these scales. While census block groups have the most granularity, most datasets have privacy provisions that prevent that level of granularity. Moreover, at that scale, there may not be enough surgical patients to acquire adequate statistical power. On the other end, county is widely available in several datasets and carries far more people. County-level measures may oversimplify the differences that may exist within a county. As such, ZIP code, ZCTAs, and census tract are the most used scales that manage these granularity and scale trade-offs.

NEIGHBORHOOD DESIGNATIONS SPECIFIC TO HEALTHCARE

Given the growing attention toward health and neighborhoods, there are also health-specific designations for neighborhoods. Examples are summarized here.

Building designations—Perhaps the most important aspect of where a patient lives in the actual building or their home. While this scale can be difficult to measure in large datasets, it has important policy relevance as several housing efforts explicitly try to improve health. For example, the Low-Income Housing Tax Credit provides government subsidies to housing in low-income communities that meets specific health criteria. Similarly, Fannie Mae provides preferable home mortgage rates to housing developments that meet health-promoting design features. Together, these building-level exposures provide on level by which we can measure the built environment where patients may live.

Hospital service area (HSA)—The HSA designation was created by the Dartmouth Atlas. Based on Medicare Claims Data, it aggregates the ZIP codes around a hospital reflect the catchment of its patients. There are approximately 3436 HSAs in the United States.

Hospital referral region (HRR)—HRRs are a designation also created by the Dartmouth Atlas. In aggregate, these boundaries are meant to reflect the broader referral regions for specialty care. The United States contains 306 HRRs.

Health professional shortage areas (HPSAs)—The HPSA designation is created by Health Resources and Services Administration of the US government. These designations are designed to identify communities that lack an appropriate number of healthcare providers. These designations are subsequently used for targeted policy interventions to help improve healthcare access. For example, the Affordable Care Act provided surgeons a 10% payment bonus for procedures provided at hospitals located within an HPSA.

COMMON INDEXES TO MEASURES NEIGHBORHOODS

Given the increased attention to understand neighborhoods, several indexes have been developed. Three most common and widely are summarized in the following.

Area deprivation index (ADI)—Allows for rankings of neighborhoods by socioeconomic disadvantage in a region of interest (e.g., at the state or national level). It includes factors for the theoretical domains of income, education, employment, and housing quality. It is updated every 5 years based on US Census Bureau American Community Survey 5-year estimates. Geographic areas are ranked by national percentile rankings: ranks 1–100 at the block group level and in deciles from 1 to 10 for each state. A ranking of 1 indicates the lowest level of disadvantage within the nation and a ranking of 100 indicates the highest level of disadvantage. All data are generated at the block group level. However, there are two linkage options: the Census block group or 9-digit ZIP codes. The data are publicly available from https://www.neighborhoodatlas.medicine.wisc.edu.

Social vulnerability index (SVI)—Developed by the Centers for Disease Control to identify communities that need support throughout natural disasters or human-made hazardous events in a region of interest (e.g., at the state or national level). The SVI includes factors for the domains of socioeconomic status, household composition and disability, minority status and language, and housing type and transportation. The data are updated every 2 years based on US Census Bureau American Community Survey data releases. Geographic areas are ranked based on percentile rank: ranks from 0 to 1, with higher values indicating greater vulnerability. Data are generated at the census tract or the county level. The data are publicly available from https://www.atsdr.cdc.gov/

Distressed community index (DCI)—A tool for measuring the comparative economic well-being of US communities and helps illuminate ground-level disparities across the country. The DCI is derived from the US Census Bureau's Business Patterns and American Community Survey 5-Year Estimates for 2016—20 and sorts zip codes into quintiles of well-being: prosperous, comfortable, midtier, at risk, and distressed. The seven components of the index are as follows: no high school diploma, housing vacancy rate, adults not working, poverty rate, median income ration, change in employment, and change in establishments. The data are not publicly available but can be purchased through the Economic Innovation Group.

Given the broad proliferation of these indexes, it is important to thoughtfully choose the index based on the underlying hypothesis and the intent of the index. In Table 6.1, we summarize how we conceptualize application of each index.

HOW MIGHT NEIGHBORHOODS INFLUENCE SURGICAL OUTCOMES?

Surgical quality has for a long time focused on the hospital where patients received care. More recently, however, this has been increasing attention to where patients spend their time outside of the hospital and how that influences their care. Specifically, the neighborhoods where they live and their ability to access surgical care and their outcomes afterward. How might this occur?

The following is our conceptual model attempting to understand how the neighborhood where someone lives may ultimately impact their outcomes after surgery (Fig. 6.1).

NEIGHBORHOODS AND SURGICAL OUTCOMES

Putting all these together, we provide the following three examples of how we have started to think about neighborhoods and outcomes after surgery.

Example 1. Historic Housing Policy and Modern-Day Surgical Outcomes

In 1933, the United States Government Home Owners Loan Corporation (HOLC) used racial composition of neighborhoods to determine creditworthiness and labeled them "Best," "Still Desirable," "Definitely Declining," and "Hazardous." Although efforts have been made to reverse these racist policies that structurally disadvantage those living in exposed

TABLE 6.1

Potential Application of Common Neighborhood Indexes to Evaluate Surgical Care

Index	Creator	Original Intent	Potential Applications in Surgery
Area deprivation index	Center for Health Disparities Research, University of Wisconsin School of Medicine and Public Health	A publicly available metric that is applicable to a wide variety of research and health policy efforts, including research into fundamental sociobiologic mechanisms of disease and initiatives to better align resources with needs	To evaluate surgical outcomes such as postoperative complications, mortality, or readmissions
Social vulnerability index	Centers for Disease Control	To identify communities that are most vulnerable after unforeseen emergency natural disasters such as hurricanes or tornados to guide resiliency planning	To evaluate surgical patients with "unforeseen emergencies" such as bowel perforation or ruptured aneurysms
Distressed communities index	The Economic Innovation Group	To measure the comparative economic well-being of US communities	To evaluate surgical patients resource utilization across communities

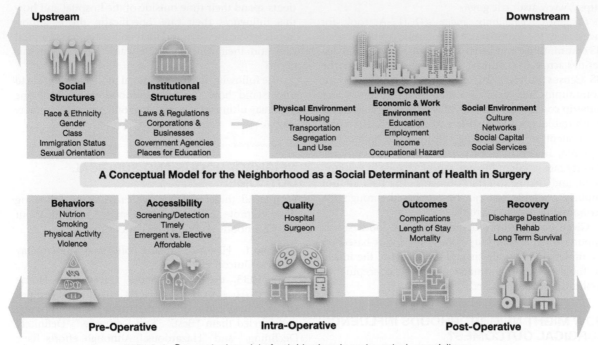

FIG. 6.1 Conceptual model of neighborhoods and surgical care delivery.

neighborhoods, the lasting legacy on modern-day healthcare outcomes is uncertain.

In effort to understand how these polices are associated with surgical outcomes, the authors performed a cross-sectional retrospective review of 212,179 Medicare beneficiaries' living in 171,930 unique neighborhoods historically labeled by the HOLC who underwent one of five of common surgical procedures—coronary artery bypass, appendectomy, colectomy, cholecystectomy, and hernia repair—between 2012 and 2018. The authors compared 30-day mortality, complications, and readmissions across HOLC grade and area deprivation index (ADI) of each neighborhood.

The study noted that 212,179 Medicare beneficiaries resided in 171,930 unique neighborhoods historically graded by the HOLC. Outcomes worsened in a stepwise fashion across HOLC neighborhoods (Fig. 6.2). Overall, 30-day postoperative mortality was 5.4% in "Best" neighborhoods, 5.8% in "Still Desirable," 6.1% in "Definitely Declining," and 6.4% in "Hazardous" (Best vs. Hazardous odds ratio [OR]: 1.23, 95% CI: 1.13–1.24, $P < .001$). The same stepwise pattern was seen from "Best" to "Hazardous" neighborhoods for complications (30.5% vs. 32.2%; OR: 1.12 [95% CI: 1.07–1.17]; $P < .001$) and readmissions (16.3% vs. 17.1%; OR: 1.06 [95% CI: 1.01–1.11]; $P = .023$).[5]

The study had three principal findings that improve our understanding of discriminatory housing policies and modern-day healthcare outcomes. After adjusting for known patient-level factors, patients residing in neighborhoods previously redlined or labeled "Hazardous" were more likely to experience death within 30 days of surgery, a postoperative complication after surgery, and a readmission within 30 days of discharge compared patients residing in neighborhoods previously labeled "Best." In addition, the rise in adverse postoperative outcomes occurred in stepwise fashion across worsening neighborhoods strengthening the correlation of discriminatory housing policy and adverse health outcomes. Even after adjusting for modern-day measures of neighborhood disadvantage, these findings persisted.

Example 2. Neighborhood Segregation and Surgical Outcomes

Recently, the US Senate identified healthcare segregation, the concentration of racial and ethnic groups within specific hospitals, as a key barrier to achieving health equity in medical care. Research has also demonstrated that racial and ethnic minority patients are more likely to undergo surgery at low-volume, low-quality hospitals compared with White patients, contributing

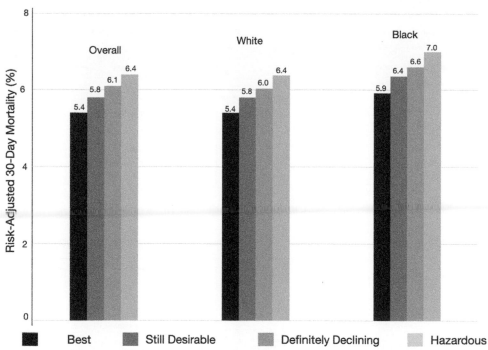

FIG. 6.2 Mortality after surgery by race and historic neighborhood designation. (Authors' analysis of 100% MedPar fee-for-service claims for beneficiaries who underwent selected operative procedures from January 1, 2012 to December 31, 2018. Note. Risk-adjusted rates were derived from marginal means in logistic regression models. All models adjusted for patient age, sex, and 27 Elixhauser comorbidities, type of admission (i.e., elective, nonelective), overall time trends, and hospital characteristics.)

to persistent racial and ethnic disparities in surgical outcomes. However, to date, the extent and effect of hospital-level segregation in US surgical care is unknown. As such, authors utilized 100% Medicare fee-for-service claims to assess hospital-level racial and ethnic segregation among beneficiaries who underwent appendectomy, colectomy, hernia repair, or cholecystectomy.

Of 1,580,359 patients (mean [SD] age, 75.3 [7.3] years), 0.5% were American Indian/Native American; 1.5%, Asian; 2.3%, Hispanic; 8.2%, non-Hispanic Black; and 85.9%, non-Hispanic White. Of all hospitals, 12.6%, 19.0%, 18.6%, and 25.9% performed 90% of surgeries for American Indian/Native American, Asian and Pacific Islander, Hispanic, and non-Hispanic Black beneficiaries, respectively (Fig. 6.3). Compared with hospitals serving lower volumes of minority patients, the top 10% of hospitals serving the largest volumes of minority patients had higher rates of 30-day mortality (6.64% vs. 6.07%; OR, 1.08; 95% CI, 1.08−1.08; $P < .001$), complications (30.30% vs. 28.06%; OR, 1.14; 95% CI, 1.14−1.14; $P < .001$), serious complications (15.96% vs. 14.49%; OR, 1.13; 95% CI, 1.13−1.13; $P < .001$), and 30-day

readmissions (14.90% vs. 14.49%; OR, 1.03; 95% CI, 1.03−1.03; $P < .001$).[6]

These findings demonstrate that a small percentage of hospitals provided a disproportionate amount of surgical care to racial and ethnic minority Medicare beneficiaries with inferior surgical outcomes, suggesting that ongoing concentration of racial and ethnic minorities within certain hospitals may contribute to surgical disparities. The results further suggest that resource allocation for quality improvement, community−hospital partnerships, and delivery model innovation to hospitals that disproportionately provide surgical care to racial and ethnic minority groups is important to mitigate disparities.

Example 3. Neighborhood Depravation and Surgical Outcomes

Rates of death following inpatient surgery vary widely across both the hospitals at which patients receive care and the neighborhoods in which they live. Widespread and resource-intensive efforts to reduce variation in surgical mortality have primarily focused on hospital quality improvement. Because most of

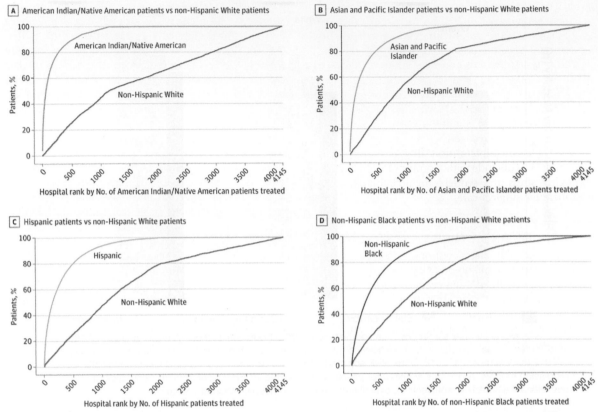

FIG. 6.3 Racial and ethnic distribution of Medicare beneficiaries undergoing common surgeries across US hospitals from 2014 to 2018.

these large-scale efforts have not been able to reduce variation in mortality and surgery-related spending now accounts for more than half of CMS's annual budget, there is increasing interest from surgeons, health systems, and health insurers to understand and intervene on factors outside the hospital, including the neighborhood living conditions of people undergoing surgery. In that context, authors evaluate the relative association of surgical outcomes with neighborhood deprivation and hospital quality using a large national cohort of Medicare beneficiaries who had undergone common inpatient surgical procedures.

A risk matrix across hospital quality and neighborhood deprivation was created to determine the relative contribution of each to mortality after surgery. A total of 1,898,829 Medicare beneficiaries were included in analyses. Patients from all neighborhood deprivation group quintiles sought care at hospitals across hospital quality levels. Thirty-day risk-adjusted mortality varied across high- and low-quality hospitals (4.3% vs. 7.2%;

adjusted odds ratio [aOR], 1.78; 95% CI, 1.66–1.92) and across the least and most deprived neighborhoods (4.5% vs. 6.8%; aOR, 1.58; 95% CI, 1.53–1.64). When combined, comparing patients from the least deprived neighborhoods going to high-quality hospitals versus patients from the most deprived neighborhoods going to low-quality hospitals (Fig. 6.4), the variation increased further (3.8% vs. 8.1%).[7]

The study had three principal findings that improve understanding of variation in postoperative surgical mortality. Despite longstanding efforts in mitigating variation in surgical mortality across hospitals, significant variation persists. There was significant variation in surgical mortality among patients from across neighborhoods at each level of hospital quality. Neighborhood deprivation and hospital quality may also have an additive association with postoperative mortality. Specifically, beneficiaries from the neighborhoods with the highest deprivation who underwent surgery at the lowest-quality hospitals had 2.8-fold greater

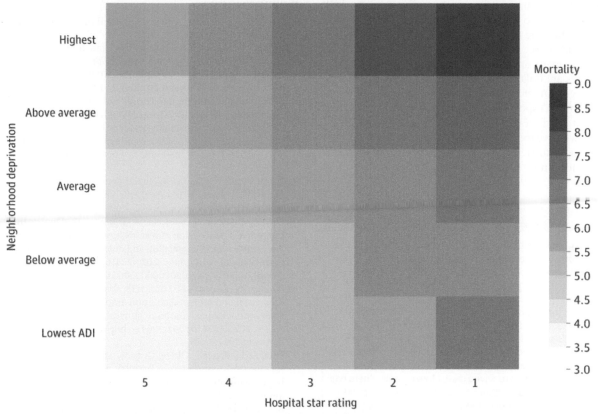

FIG. 6.4 Risk Matrix of Surgical Mortality by Hospital Quality and Neighborhood Deprivation.   (Risk-adjusted rates were derived from marginal means in logistic regression models. All models were adjusted for patient age, sex, and 27 Elixhauser comorbidities, type of admission (i.e., elective, nonelective), overall time trends, hospital characteristics, and patient's area deprivation index. The area deprivation index rankings range from 1 to 100, with least disadvantaged neighborhood conditions designated by lower scores and most disadvantaged by higher scores. Examples of neighborhood-level factors incorporated within the area deprivation index include education, employment, housing quality, and poverty measures.)

odds of postoperative mortality compared with their counterparts from the neighborhoods with the lowest deprivation undergoing surgery at the highest-quality hospitals. Taken together, these findings suggest that the neighborhoods people come from and the hospitals they go are both associated with risk of death after commonly performed inpatient surgical procedures.

DEVELOPING AREAS OF NEIGHBORHOODS AND SURGICAL OUTCOMES

The aforementioned examples, including the indexes and their application to administrative claims data, have been relatively recent advances in surgical research. Moving forward, we anticipate this space improving in three specific ways.

Intentional index selection—As alluded to earlier, there are several indexes now and even more that continue to emerge. Research must resist the urge to choose arbitrarily, but instead be guided by a hypothesis and conceptual model to specify why a specific index was chosen.

Identifying underlying mechanisms—A significant challenge in this space is attempting to disentangle the underlying mechanisms associating neighborhoods and surgical outcomes. It is possible that many of our neighborhood measures may simply be measures of other risk variables that are driving surgical outcomes. Application of more sophisticated analytic techniques, such as causal inference and exploiting natural experiments, will be needed to specific isolate and elucidate specific underlying mechanisms.

Linking findings to interventions—While readers will likely be able to identify a lifetime work of research understanding the relationship of neighborhoods to surgical outcomes, focus must be kept on ultimately improvement. Specifically, as different neighborhood exposures are linked to worse surgical outcomes, we then must go further and test whether a dedicated intervention to that exposure will improve surgical outcomes.

For much of our recent quality improvement in surgery, we have focused on the hospital you go to for care. We ought to step back and appreciate again what surgeon Jon Snow identified; where you come from matters as well.

Highlights

- There have been many proposed definitions of what constitutes a neighborhood, the focus of how these neighborhoods can be operationalized in research design has not received a formal or exhaustive assessment.
- Neighborhood designations specific to healthcare include building designations, HSAs, HRRs, and HPSAs, while common indexes to measure neighborhoods include ADI, SVI, and DCI.
- Surgical quality has long focused on the hospital where patients received care. More recently, there has been increasing attention to where patients spend their time outside of the hospital and how that influences their care.
- Housing policies, neighborhood segregation, and deprivation can each have an important effect on access to care and healthcare outcomes.

REFERENCES

1. Hahn RA, Truman BI, Williams DR. Civil rights as determinants of public health and racial and ethnic health equity: health care, education, employment, and housing in the United States. *SSM - Population Health*. 2018;4:17−24. https://doi.org/10.1016/j.ssmph.2017.10.006.
2. Artiga S, Hinton E. Beyond Health Care: The Role of Social Determinants in Promoting Health and Health Equity. 13.
3. Thornton RLJ, Glover CM, Cené CW, Glik DC, Henderson JA, Williams DR. Evaluating strategies for reducing health disparities by addressing the social determinants of health. *Health Aff*. 2016;35(8):1416−1423. https://doi.org/10.1377/hlthaff.2015.1357.
4. World Health Organization. Social determinants of health. Accessed March 17, 2021. https://www.who.int/westernpacific/health-topics/social-determinants-of-health.
5. Diaz A, O'Reggio R, Norman M, Thumma JR, Dimick JB, Ibrahim AM. Association of historic housing policy, modern day neighborhood deprivation and outcomes after inpatient hospitalization. *Ann Surg*. 2021;274(6):985−991. https://doi.org/10.1097/SLA.0000000000005195.
6. Bonner SN, Kunnath N, Dimick JB, Ibrahim AM. Hospital-level racial and ethnic segregation among Medicare beneficiaries undergoing common surgical procedures. *JAMA Surg*. 2022;157(10):961−964. https://doi.org/10.1001/jamasurg.2022.3135.
7. Diaz A, Lindau ST, Obeng-Gyasi S, Dimick JB, Scott JW, Ibrahim AM. Association of hospital quality and neighborhood deprivation with mortality after inpatient surgery among Medicare beneficiaries. *JAMA Netw Open*. 2023;6(1):e2253620. https://doi.org/10.1001/jamanetworkopen.2022.53620.

CHAPTER 7

Addressing the Social Determinants of Health to Enhance Clinical Trial Participation

J.L. CAMPBELL, MD • JOHN H. STEWART IV, MD, MBA

INTRODUCTION

Notwithstanding the evident advances in cancer screening, detection of disease, and treatment options, health disparities in cancer care and treatment remain the leading cause of life-years lost in the United States.[1] This trend continues to plague minority populations at an inequitable rate compared with their counterparts.[1] Overcoming these iniquities will not be easy but can be obtained by approaching clinical trials through a lens committed to the social determinants of health. Achieving this goal will require that interventions are implemented consistently and equitably across all populations of persons.

The clinical trial mechanism for evaluating patients with similar stages and patterns of disease is the most powerful approach available for evaluating the efficacy of novel therapies.[1] Clinical trials are foundational pillars for enhancing cancer care and treatment worldwide. In addition, clinical trials afford the ability to discover optimal interventions and treatment plans for the population. However, such interventions and treatment plans are only effective if all races and ethnicities are represented.

A British Medical Journal commentary once stated, "Good surgeons know how to operate, better ones when to operate and the best when not to operate."[2] The requisite platform for clinical trials in the surgical field inculcates the prior quote. One surgeon at The Ohio State University College of Medicine asked a single question of every medical school who entered the operating room: Whom does this patient live with/who is in the home with them? It was a question that frustrated even the most astute medical student who had spent the entire evening studying the branches of the internal iliac artery but failed to look at their social demographics in the patient's chart. Shifting our singular focus from pathology and physiology to a holistic approach illuminating the importance of the social determinants of health will be critical in achieving health equity and bridging the gap in health disparities.[3]

In 1993, Congress enacted the National Institutes of Health (NIH) Revision Act to ensure the appropriate inclusion of women and members of racial and ethnic minority groups in all NIH-funded clinical research. The primary goal of this mandate was to ensure that research findings could be generalizable to the entire population. With a growing minority and ethnic population in the United States, this has increased relevance.[4] Since 1993, the appropriated funds for clinical trials have increased over the past decades, although an increase in minority participation has not.[4] As part of the Revitalization Act, prominent cancer support and funding organizations such as the American Cancer Society and Susan G. Komen for the Cure aggressively advocate for augmented outreach to minority communities for clinical trial participation.[4] Inclusive clinical trials are the only proven strategy to date, proving the safety of new cancer treatments to improve standards of care. However, less than 5% of all eligible adult patients enroll in oncology clinical trials. Furthermore, of those enrolled persons, only approximately 14% are members of minority populations.[5] According to Unger et al., from 1956 to 2016, in the Southwest Oncology Group Research Network, 12,361 patients were enrolled in 23 trials.[5] The study estimated a 3.34 million life-years (95% CL, 2.39–4.15 million) were gained from the 23 trials through 2015.[5] The fundamental elements of clinical trial design—standardized delivery of care and follow-up for novel treatments—are essential to make meaningful advances in the fields of surgery and medicine.

Social Determinants of Health in Surgery. https://doi.org/10.1016/B978-0-443-12366-5.00004-8

CURRENT DATA AND LITERATURE ON CLINICAL TRIAL PARTICIPATION

Advani et al.[6] conducted a study with 218 patients with malignant disease (72 African Americans and 146 white patients) who were interviewed with a standardized survey. Results demonstrated a willingness to participate in a clinical trial depending on clinical site and race.[6] 45% of White patients, compared with 31% of African American patients, were willing to participate in a clinical trial.[6] There was no difference in percentages between the White and African American patients regarding patients who had heard of a clinical trial, knew what a clinical trial was, or had been asked to participate in a clinical trial. Overall, 40% noted they were willing to participate in a clinical trial, 22% were unwilling, and 39% were undecided.[6] It is positive to see such a discrepancy between those willing and those unwilling to participate. However, undecided persons are where the focus of researchers, patient navigators, and recruiters needs to place their attention.

Recognizing the low numbers of racial and ethnic minority clinical trial involvement despite national efforts, Fayanju et al. performed a case–control study examining disparities in clinical trial participation among breast surgical oncology patients.[7] The American College of Surgeons Oncology Group (ACOSOG) is a surgically based clinical trials cooperative group funded by the National Cancer Institute of the National Institutes of Health.[8] The enrollment of African American and Latino patients from the ACOSOG clinical trials was congruent with the burden of cancer in these populations. Women with breast cancer enrolled in National Cancer Institute-sponsored, cooperative-group trials from 2000 to 2012, and who underwent oncologic surgery (n = 17,125) were compared with trial-eligible women in the National Cancer Database diagnosed in 2000–12 (n = 792, 719).[8] Results demonstrated that from 2000 to 2003, Asian-Pacific Islander, Hispanic, and White patients from the highest-income groups had greater participation than their lower-income counterparts. From 2008 to 2012, only high-income White patients participated more than their lower-income counterparts. Blacks and Latino patients were much less likely to participate than Whites. However, high-income Black patients were 50% less likely to participate than White patients demonstrating statistically significant area-based patient income associated with clinical trial participation.

The accrual of African American participants was 7.4%.[8] When evaluated by site, participation rates for African American patients were 5.7% for thoracic studies, 8.6% for breast studies, and 11.6% for colorectal studies. The accrual of non-White Latino/a patients was 2.2% (0.6%—thoracic, 3.7%—breast, 5.8% —colorectal).[8]

Fayanju et al. recently evaluated zip code–level data from patients included in the CTEP Surgical Oncology Trial Database to identify population-level determinants of participation in breast surgery trials.[7] Patients from the highest area-based income bracket (>$63 000) were less likely to participate than those from the lowest-income bracket (<$38 000: OR = 0.63, 95% CI = 0.59–0.68). Furthermore, the likelihood of enrollment declined with increasing income ($P < .001$). The impact of underrepresentation on clinical trials is critical for two reasons. First, if the sample size of participants is small, the results cannot be generalized to the entire population. Second, per the National Cancer Institute, the severity of cancer among minorities is prevalent. Definitive data and novel treatments are needed to improve cancer survival rates and reduce treatment side effects. This will only be accomplished if the understood barriers are overcome.

BARRIERS TO PARTICIPATION IN CLINICAL TRIALS UNDERLYING THE SOCIAL DETERMINANTS OF HEALTH

There have been substantial barriers to minority participation in clinical trials. Murthy et al. summarize them as follows: minorities are more likely to express concerns regarding exploitation, dishonesty, and mistrust surrounding the motivation of the researchers, minorities are less likely to be offered clinical participation compared with their white counterparts, and disproportionately low-income facing potential minority participants can hinder appropriate and timely follow-up.[1] In 2019, 116th Congress and Representative Elijah Cummings approved Bill H.R. 1966—Henrietta Lacks Enhancing Cancer Research Act of 2019.[9] This act directed the Comptroller General of the United States to complete a study on barriers to participation in federally funded cancer clinical trials by populations traditionally underrepresented in such trials. For over 20 years, the advances made possible by Henrietta Lacks' cells, who died in 1951 from cervical cancer, were made possible without her or her family's consent. The generous revenues were not shared with or made known to her family. In conjunction with the Tuskegee Study of Untreated Syphilis in the Negro Male," there is a legacy of mistrust and doubt surrounding researchers and clinical trials among minority communities.[10]

From 1996 to 2002, approximately 3.1% of trial participants were Hispanic, 85.6% were White, 9.2% were Asian/Pacific Islanders, and 0.3% were American Indians/Alaskan Natives.[2] This lack of participation from minority groups evidences the known litany of barriers to patient participation in clinical trials. Addressing the social determinants of health (SDH)—the environments where people are born, live, learn, work, play, worship, and age—may reduce such barriers. Creating a society where most persons are considered healthy and may successfully navigate cancer, and other chronic illnesses necessitate clinical trials (discoverable interventions and treatments) representative of the general population. This will require the further analysis of several areas of health policy as it pertains to barriers to clinical trial participation: decreasing food deserts in urban areas, augmenting the quality of free education, safeguarding persons from toxic exposure, providing equitable access to healthcare regardless of transportation option or the lack thereof. Education and income are the two main factors more detrimental to one's health than any other determinants.[4] Furthermore, being poor, unemployed, or socially stigmatized may eliminate potential trial participants in studies pivotal to the population they represent. African Americans and Hispanic Americans are overrepresented among the impoverished and underinsured resulting in less likelihood they will have access to private/university/academic centers where clinical trials are more commonly offered. Most AA and HA patients often receive their healthcare at safety-net institutions.[11]

Literature shows that even in randomized clinical trials, patients with Medicaid or no insurance may not contrive the same benefits associated with experimental therapies as patients with private insurance.[11] If underinsured patients are unequal in the survival benefit from experimental therapies, a refocus on the social determinants of the patients is required. Inspection of their caregivers, communities, treatment teams, and health access before and after interventions might address the observed discrepancy.[12,13] The Delaware Cancer Consortium (established 2002) focused on the reduction

of disparities within colorectal cancer outcomes statewide have implemented a nurse navigator system, screening reimbursement for low-income patients, cost coverage for uninsured patients who receive a positive diagnosis, and targeted community interventions to address disparities among the African American subpopulation.[14]

Low participation in cancer clinical trials has become more common.[1] This may be attributable to the rising cost of cancer care, a lack of transparency from insurance companies, and the perceived institutional impediments to patient financial support.[1,3,10,11,13] Moreover, the participation of diverse patients is tantamount to the discovery and implementation of therapies and interventions. Hindering such achievement has been found in the socioeconomic status of persons and other factors underlying the social determinants of health. Educational barriers among clinicians and patients also open the chasm between a heterogenous and exclusively homogenous population. Financial toxicity is another factor that has been studied and found to disallow patients from enrolling or continuing with participation in a clinical trial.[15]

Implicit bias—associations outside conscious awareness that lead to a negative evaluation of a person based on irrelevant characteristics—displayed by a healthcare provider may significantly impact clinician–patient interaction.[22] Fitzgerald and Hurst performed a systematic review of 42 articles demonstrating that physicians display similar bias to the broader population. Furthermore, a significant positive relationship was found between the level of implicit bias and lower quality of care.[22] Addressing implicit bias among providers is requisite for creating an equitable environment. Implicit biases often disadvantage those already vulnerable—minority populations, immigrants, the poor, low health-literacy individuals, children, the mentally ill, and the elderly.[22]

The consortium for Enhancing Minority Participation in Clinical Trials (EmPaCT), established in 2009 at five national cancer institutions, was designed to systematically address the limited enrollment of minorities in cancer clinical trials.[16–18] From a series of reviewed and analyzed questions, five themes were found: (1) interactions with potential minority participants viewed as challenging, (2) potential minority candidates perceived to be nonideal study candidates, (3) clinic-based barriers in conjunction with negative perceptions of minority study participants by investigators led to providers withholding clinical trial opportunities from potential minority candidates. (4) when clinical trial recruitment practices were tailored to minority patients, addressing misconceptions to build trust was a common strategy, and for some providers, race was viewed as irrelevant when screening and recruiting for clinical trials.[19–22]

Effective pathways can only be discovered and reproduced if the problem is understood or acknowledged. Naranjan et al. concluded that despite best intentions to provide equal clinical trial access to all patients' disparities in clinical trials persisted and may lead to increased morbidity and mortality for individuals underrepresented in the trials.[23]

PATHWAYS AND MECHANISMS THROUGH THE SOCIAL DETERMINANTS OF HEALTH FOR AUGMENTING RECRUITMENT AND RETENTION IN CLINICAL TRIAL PARTICIPATION

Successful recruitment of minority patients, despite historical atrocities such as the "Tuskegee Study of Untreated Syphilis in the Negro Male," will require education and behavior modification at the physician–provider and patient levels.[9] Patients deserve to be educated to understand that enrollment in a clinical trial can serve as a safeguard to ensure the delivery of well-monitored and standardized care that is free of physician/provider bias and discriminatory practices.[9]

Historically, biomedical research has focused on the physiologic pathways and processes that affect health. Recent literature combined with augmented social awareness has illuminated how the social determinants of health are a significant factor that deserves deliberate focus. Successful mechanisms for recruiting and retaining minorities for clinical trials necessitate biological and behavioral mechanisms in a social context to identify the factors affecting specific populations more appropriately (age, gender, race, ethnicity).

Community Engagement

Engagement, requiring trust, respect, and cultural humility, is distinct from recruitment and retention.[24] Yet, engagement enhances recruitment and retention—enrollment and keeping participants in the study until completion, respectively. The NIH All of US program desires to recruit 1,000,000 patients from diverse backgrounds to enhance biomedical research and improve health.[24] Engaging participants, communities, healthcare providers, and stakeholders in a unique manner.

Renaming participants as partners should make the research more relevant to the involved communities and increase the translation rate of discoveries into clinical practice. The program opened in May 2018 and enrolls patients 18 years of age or older from a network of more than 340 recruitment sites.[24] The core values for the All of US initiative are as follows:
- Participation is open to all.
- Participants reflect the rich diversity of the United States.
- Participants are partners.
- Trust will be earned through transparency.
- Participants will have access to their information.
- Data will be accessed broadly for research purposes.
- Security and privacy will be of the highest importance.
- The program will be a catalyst for positive change in research.

Participants in All of Us will have access to their data and most of the results of the research testing. This proves pivotal to creating transparency, a prerequisite for recruiting and retaining minority participants. In addition, patient navigators have become crucial in providing education and confidence in participants from their shared backgrounds and cultural upbringings. Finally, this program shares some of the same challenges facing clinical trial principal investigators: reaching persons in rural areas far from recruitment sites may require alternative strategies for success.

Clinical Trials Navigation

On Jun 29, 2005, President Bush signed into law the Patient Navigator Outreach and Chronic Disease Prevention Act of 2005.[24] Dr. Harold P. Freeman first introduced this concept. Dr. Freeman witnessed a disproportionate number of patients with late-stage cancers leading him to ponder how he could practice the best medicine if he saw patients when the disease process was too far along. It also led him to question what was causing the delay in these patients seeking medical care earlier. In 1990, Dr. Freeman launched his first patient navigation program focused on getting people for medical care earlier. He knew that for this to be successful, it had to come from community members, themselves, whom he trained.[24]

Patient navigators bridge the patient and the healthcare system by providing enhanced education and facilitative services to the patient. As such, patient navigator training is relatively extensive and includes education and training on topics ranging from cancer care to cultural competency and ethics. Clinical trial navigators serve to increase clinical participation through clinic-based education about clinical trials; thus, they require additional training in the principles of cancer clinical trial design, human subjects research policies, and the risks and benefits of trial participation. These strategies have succeeded in small studies reporting clinical trial enrollment between 61% and 86% among study-eligible minority patients. Investigators of the Increasing Minority Participation in Clinical Trials (IMPACT) reported a 74.5% trial retention and completion rate for patients who received clinical navigation compared with 37.5% for those who did not receive navigation support ($P < .001$).[25,26]

Advocacy

The Henrietta Lacks Enhancing Cancer Research Act of 2019, per Representative Elijah E. Cummings, has significantly addressed clinical trial participation barriers.[27] This legislation ensures that all patients, especially those from communities of color, are proportionately represented in clinical trials and ultimately receive the treatments they deserve. This law requires that the Government Accountability Office (GAO) complete a study that reviews what actions Federal agencies have taken to help to address barriers to participation in federally funded cancer clinical trials.[27] This law also requires the GAO to identify additional actions that Federal agencies can take to address barriers to participation in federally funded cancer clinical trials. Finally, the GAO must submit a report to Congress on the results of such a study, including recommendations on potential changes in practices and policies to improve participation in such trials by such populations.

August 1, 2020, would have been Henrietta Lacks' 100th birthday. Mrs. Lacks was an African American woman whose cervical cancer cells, later known as HeLa cells were preserved without the consent of Lacks or her family. Theses HeLa cell lines have played an extraordinary role in biomedical research enabling medical advances for polio, cancer, Ebola virus disease, sickle cell disease, and many other medical conditions and disease processes.[28]

CONCLUSION

Addressing the social determinants of the health of individual participants will augment the recruitment and retention for clinical trial participation. Acknowledging the barriers to successful participation and directly combatting such hindrances is necessary for the future of clinical trials. The need for participation. This will only come to fruition through community engagement, patient navigators, and the eradication of physician−provider bias concomitant with patient education and connection.[29]

Highlights

- Less than 5% of all eligible adult patients enroll in oncology clinical trials, and among those enrolled persons, only approximately 14% are members of minority populations.
- In 1993, Congress enacted the National Institutes of Health (NIH) Revision Act to ensure the appropriate inclusion of women and members of racial and ethnic minority groups in all NIH-funded clinical research.
- Minorities are less likely to be offered clinical participation, and when offered, minorities are more likely to express concerns regarding exploitation, dishonesty, and mistrust surrounding the motivation of the researchers.
- Engagement, requiring trust, respect, and cultural humility, is distinct from recruitment and retention.
- The Henrietta Lacks Enhancing Cancer Research Act of 2019 addressed clinical trial participation barriers by ensuring that all patients, especially those from communities of color, are proportionately represented in clinical trials.

REFERENCES

1. Murthy VH, Krumholz HM, Gross CP. Participation in cancer clinical trials: race-, sex-, and age-based disparities. *JAMA.* 2004;291(22):2720−2726. https://doi.org/10.1001/jama.291.22.2720.
2. BMJ 1999; 318 doi: https://doi.org/10.1136/bmj.318.7180.0a (Published 06 February 1999).
3. Snyder RA, Chang GJ. Insurance status as a surrogate for social determinants of health in cancer clinical trials. *JAMA Netw Open.* 2020;3(4):e203890. https://doi.org/10.1001/jamanetworkopen.2020.3890.
4. *NIH Revitalization Act. Subtitle B. 131-133.* 1993.
5. Unger JM, Blanke CD, LeBlanc M, et al. Association of patient demographic characteristics and insurance status with survival in cancer randomized clinical trials with positive findings. *JAMA Netw Open.* 2020;3(4):e203842. https://doi.org/10.1001/jamanetworkopen.2020.3842.
6. Advani AS, Atkeson B, Brown CL, et al. Barriers to the participation of African-American patients with cancer in clinical trials. *Cancer.* 2003;97:1499−1506. https://doi.org/10.1002/cncr.11213.
7. Fayanju OM, Ren Y, Thomas SM, et al. A case-control study examining disparities in clinical trial participation among breast surgical oncology patients. *JNCI Cancer Spectr.* December 16, 2019;4(2):pkz103. https://doi.org/10.1093/jncics/pkz103. PMID: 32211583; PMCID: PMC7083236.

8. Diehl KM, Green EM, Weinberg A, et al. Features associated with successful recruitment of diverse patients onto cancer clinical trials: report from the American College of Surgeons Oncology Group. *Ann Surg Oncol*. December 2011;18(13):3544−3550. https://doi.org/10.1245/s1043 4-011-1818-9. Epub 2011 Jun 17. PMID: 21681382; PMCID: PMC5773065.

9. Brawley OW. The study of untreated syphilis in the Negro male. *Int J Radiat Oncol Biol Phys*. 1998;40(1):5−8.

10. Garrett BE, Dube SR, Babb S, McAfee T. Addressing the social determinants of health to reduce tobacco-related disparities. *Nicotine Tob Res*. August 2015;17(8):892−897. https://doi.org/10.1093/ntr/ntu266. Epub 2014 Dec 16. PMID: 25516538; PMCID: PMC5104348.

11. Halpern MT, Bian J, Ward EM, Schrag NM, Chen AY. Insurance status and stage of cancer at diagnosis among women with breast cancer. *Cancer*. 2007;110(2):403−411. https://doi.org/10.1002/cncr.22786.

12. Roberson NL. Clinical trial participation: viewpoints from racial/ethnic groups. *Cancer*. 1994;74:2687−2691. https://doi.org/10.1002/1097-0142(19941101)74:9+<2687:: AID-CNCR2820741817>3.0.CO;2-B.

13. Wendler D, Kington R, Madans J, et al. Are racial and ethnic minorities less willing to participate in health research? *PLoS Med*. February 2006;3(2):e19. https://doi.org/10.1371/journal.pmed.0030019. Epub 2005 Dec 6. PMID: 16318411; PMCID: PMC1298944.

14. Felder TM, Pena GD, Chapital BF. Disparities in cancer clinical trials: an analysis of comprehensive cancer control plans. *Prev Chronic Dis*. October 2009;6(4):A116. Epub 2009 Sep 15. PMID: 19754992; PMCID: PMC2774630.

15. Ayanian JZ, Kohler BA, Abe T, Epstein AM. The relation between health insurance coverage and clinical outcomes among women with breast cancer. *N Engl J Med*. 1993;329(5):326−331. https://doi.org/10.1056/NEJM199307293 290507.

16. Chen Jr MS, Lara PN, Dang JH, Paterniti DA, Kelly K. Twenty years post-NIH Revitalization Act: enhancing minority participation in clinical trials (EMPaCT): laying the groundwork for improving minority clinical trial accrual: renewing the case for enhancing minority participation in cancer clinical trials. *Cancer*. April 1, 2014; 120(Suppl 7(0 7)):1091−1096. https://doi.org/10.1002/cncr.28575. PMID: 24643646; PMCID: PMC3980490.

17. Vickers SM, Fouad MN. An overview of EMPaCT and fundamental issues affecting minority participation in cancer clinical trials: enhancing minority participation in clinical trials (EMPaCT): laying the groundwork for improving minority clinical trial accrual. *Cancer*. April 1, 2014; 120(Suppl 7(0 7)):1087−1090. https://doi.org/10.1002/cncr.28569. PMID: 24643645; PMCID: PMC4133979.

18. Durant RW, Wenzel JA, Scarinci IC, et al. Perspectives on barriers and facilitators to minority recruitment for clinical trials among cancer center leaders, investigators, research staff, and referring clinicians: enhancing minority participation in clinical trials (EMPaCT). *Cancer*. April 1, 2014; 120:1097−1105. https://doi.org/10.1002/cncr.28574. PMID: 24643647; PMCID: PMC4395557.

19. Gehan EA, Schneiderman MA. Historical and methodological developments in clinical trials at the National Cancer Institute. discussion 903-6 *Stat Med*. August 1990;9(8):871−880. https://doi.org/10.1002/sim.4780090803. PMID: 2218190.

20. Hernandez ND, Durant R, Lisovicz N, et al. African American cancer survivors' perspectives on cancer clinical trial participation in a safety-net hospital: considering the role of the social determinants of health. Epub 2021 Mar 16 *J Cancer Educ*. December 2022;37(6):1589−1597. https://doi.org/10.1007/s13187-021-01994-4. PMID: 33728872; PMCID: PMC8443686.

21. Byrne MM, Tannenbaum SL, Glück S, Hurley J, Antoni M. Participation in cancer clinical trials: why are patients not participating?. Epub 2013 Jul 29 *Med Decis Making*. January 2014;34(1):116−126. https://doi.org/10.1177/0272989X13497264. PMID: 23897588.

22. FitzGerald C, Hurst S. Implicit bias in healthcare professionals: a systematic review. *BMC Med Ethics*. 2017;18:19. https://doi.org/10.1186/s12910-017-0179-8.

23. Niranjan SJ, Martin MY, Fouad MN, et al. Bias and stereotyping among research and clinical professionals: perspectives on minority recruitment for oncology clinical trials. Epub 2020 Mar 9 *Cancer*. January 1, 2020;126(9):1958−1968. https://doi.org/10.1002/cncr.32755. PMID: 32147815.

24. Freeman HP, Rodriguez RL. History and principles of patient navigation. *Cancer*. 2011;117:3537−3540. https://doi.org/10.1002/cncr.26262.

25. Fouad MN, Acemgil A, Bae S, et al. Patient navigation as a model to increase participation of African Americans in cancer clinical trials. Epub 2016 May 17 *J Oncol Pract*. June 2016; 12(6):556−563. https://doi.org/10.1200/JOP.2015.008946. PMID: 27189356; PMCID: PMC4957258.

26. Cronin RM, Jerome RN, Mapes B, et al. Vanderbilt university medical center pilot team, and the participant provided information committee. Development of the initial surveys for the All of US research program. *Epidemiology*. July 2019;30(4):597−608. https://doi.org/10.1097/EDE.0000000000001028. PMID: 31045611; PMCID: PMC6548672.

27. Henrietta Lacks Enhancing Cancer Research Act of 2019.

28. Wolinetz CD, Collins FS. Recognition of research participants' need for autonomy: remembering the legacy of Henrietta lacks. *JAMA*. 2020;324(11):1027−1028. https://doi.org/10.1001/jama.2020.15936.

29. Fouad MN, Johnson RE, Nagy MC, et al. Adherence and retention in clinical trials: a community-based approach. *Cancervol*. 2014;120:1106−1112. https://doi.org/10.1002/cncr.28572.

FURTHER READING

1. Unger JM, LeBlanc M, Blanke CD. The effect of positive SWOG treatment trials on survival of patients with cancer in the US population. *JAMA Oncol*. October 1, 2017; 3(10):1345–1351. https://doi.org/10.1001/jamaoncol.2017.0762. PMID: 28586789; PMCID: PMC5710507.

2. Martin LW, Wigle DA. Thoracic surgery trials network. Clinical trials in thoracic surgery: a report from Ginsberg day 2017 and early risers at STS 2017. *Ann Thorac Surg*. August 2017;104(2):712–713. https://doi.org/10.1016/j.athoracsur.2017.04.029. PMID: 28734410.

CHAPTER 8

Race, Ancestry, and Social Determinants of Health in Surgery

MELISSA B. DAVIS, PHD • LISA NEWMAN (ANN), MD, MPH, FACS, FASCO, FSSO

OVERVIEW

Health inequities related to racial/ethnic identity are associated with a substantial economic burden in the United States. A recent analysis of data from the Medical Expenditure Panel Survey, the Behavioral Risk Factor Surveillance System, the National Vital Statistics System, and the American Community Survey estimated these costs at $421−451 billion.[1] Most of this economic burden was attributable to the poorer health of the Black population, but the burden attributable to the Hispanic/Latino, American Indian, Alaska Native, and Native Hawaiian communities was also disproportionately high.

Surgeons are arguably most intensely aware of the complex relationship between social determinants of health (SDOH) and the ancestral components of race with regard to a cancer diagnosis. Well-documented variation exists in the burden of cancer between different population subsets defined by race−ethnicity, and the majority of solid organ malignancies continue to require operative intervention as a component of multidisciplinary care. This chapter will therefore focus on race, ancestry, and SDOH in surgical oncology.

In the United States, the most commonly used race/ethnicities categorize individuals as belonging to broad, heterogenous, and inconsistently labeled groups such as those with White/European ancestry (hereafter White); Black/African ancestry (hereafter Black); Hispanic/Latino (hereafter Hispanic); American Indian/Alaska Native (AI/AN); Asian; American Indian or Alaska Native (hereafter AI/AN); Asian/Pacific Islander (hereafter API); or Asian American and Native Hawaiian/Other Pacific Islander (hereafter AA/NHOPI) backgrounds. Much more research is necessary in defining the details of cancer burden related to the disaggregated subsets of these populations, but existing patterns of progress versus persistent challenges in understanding

and managing these differences are documented in the American Association of Cancer Research "AACR Cancer Disparities Progress Report 2022"[2] and the American Cancer Society's "Cancer Statistics for African American/Black People 2022"[3]; a few of these cancer variations are summarized in the following in comparison with White Americans:

- Overall cancer incidence is 6% higher and mortality is 19% higher in Black compared with White men.
- Overall cancer incidence is 8% lower yet mortality is 12% higher in Black compared with White women.
- Endometrial cancer mortality rates are twice as high in Black compared with White women.
- Breast cancer mortality rates are 41% higher in Black compared with White women.
- Breast cancer incidence rates are approximately 50% higher in Black men compared with White men.
- Gastric cancer incidence rates are approximately twofold higher, and mortality rates are more than twofold higher in Blacks compared with Whites.
- Asians have the lowest overall cancer incidence rates compared to other race/ethnic groups, but a disproportionately higher burden of cancers caused by infectious agents, such as liver cancer secondary to chronic hepatitis B virus.
- Compared with Whites, mortality from nasopharyngeal cancer is nearly 10 times higher in individuals with Chinese background, nearly 4 times higher in those with Filipino background, and more than 5 times higher in those with AA/NHOPI background.
- Compared with Whites, incidence of liver cancer is more than twofold higher in AI/AN and API individuals.
- Compared with Whites, mortality from liver cancer is more than twofold higher in AI/AN and API individuals.

Social Determinants of Health in Surgery. https://doi.org/10.1016/B978-0-443-12366-5.00018-8

- Compared with Whites, incidence of gastric cancer is nearly twofold higher in API individuals.
- Compared with Whites, mortality from gastric cancer is more than twofold higher in API individuals.
- Compared with Whites, mortality from gastric cancer is 2–4 times higher in Korean, Japanese, and NHOPI individuals.
- Compared with White women who have never smoked, incidence of lung cancer is more than twofold higher in Chinese American women that have never smoked.
- Compared with White men, mortality rates from gastric cancer are more than twofold higher in Chinese American men, but less than half for South Asian men.
- Compared with Whites, incidence of liver cancer is more than twofold higher in Hispanic individuals.
- Compared with Whites, mortality from liver cancer is more than twofold higher in Hispanic individuals.
- Compared with Whites, incidence of gastric cancer is nearly twofold higher in Hispanic individuals.
- Compared with Whites, mortality from gastric cancer is nearly twofold higher in Hispanic individuals.

The aforementioned patterns summarize cancer disparities relevant to surgeons with regard to multiple different population subsets. However, the unique and horrific experience of slavery in the history of individuals with African ancestry in America has resulted in the long-lasting legacy of systemic racism that exerts a particularly strong adverse effect on the health of Blacks in the United States today. Contemporary manifestations of systemic racism include residential racial segregation, disproportionately high rates of poverty, unemployment, and uninsurance in the Black community, all of which undoubtedly contribute to healthcare access barriers.[4] The disproportionately greater severity of various comorbidities (e.g., hypertension, cardiovascular disease, asthma, and most recently COVID-19) as well as cancer mortality that is documented in Black compared with White Americans is clearly related to the impact of SDOH. African ancestry is also associated with germline genetic factors that can affect cancer burden, and advances in technologies that can quantify geographically defined ancestry have accelerated the pace of research regarding the genetics of cancer disparities. This chapter will therefore also feature an emphasis on the influence of genetic African ancestry on cancer risk. Breast cancer will dominate in the review of correlations between the ancestral germline genetic aspects of race and SDOH because the large-

magnitude disparity in breast cancer burden between populations with African ancestry compared with those with European ancestry has generated the most extensive research.

DISPARITIES IN SURGICAL MANAGEMENT OF CANCER RELATED TO RACE AND SDOH

Most solid organ malignancies require surgical intervention for diagnostic, therapeutic, and/or palliative aspects of management. It is a tragic reality that implicit biases related to a provider's preconceived opinions regarding a patient's understanding of the diagnosis, ability to complete treatment, and/or level of interest in various treatment options will influence the content of that provider's clinical discussion. This is true in surgical oncology as well as in other specialties. The physical appearance of a patient and the provider's perception of their race (which is closely tied to their ancestral background) therefore plays an important role in the delivery of surgical oncology care.

Examples of race-related disparities in delivery of surgical care to cancer patients have been well documented in multiple cancer types. A review of National Cancer Data Base (NCDB) records reveals that Black women experience longer delays in breast cancer surgery[5] and a study from the M.D. Anderson Cancer Center[6] showed that Black mastectomy patients were less likely to be referred to plastic surgeons and less likely to be triaged for reconstruction when seen by the plastic surgeon. The NCDB also reveals disproportionately prolonged surgical treatment delays in AA/PI patients with melanoma,[7] and in Black patients with colon cancer.[8]

Advances in cancer are made possible through the conduct of clinical trials, and the generalizability of clinical research results requires a patient participant population that is comparable with the general population.[9] While the National Institutes of Health Revitalization Act of 1993 mandated inclusion of women and minorities in all federally funded research, underreporting of accrual demographics and underrepresentation of minorities based upon reported data are both persistent problems.[10,11]

The history of abuse in medical research has definitely led to patient fears and mistrust, especially among Black patients because of atrocities such as the Tuskegee experiments of untreated syphilis in Black men.[12] The Tuskegee research misconduct has furthermore been shown to contribute to mistrust among White as well as Black patients.[13] Nonetheless, it has also been demonstrated that substantial barriers to accruing patients from minority race/ethnicities onto clinical trials are related to implicit biases and failure of the clinician to offer clinical trial opportunities.[14,15] Eggly et al.[16] have documented that oncologists spend less time with their Black patients compared with their White patients, and in particular, they spend less time discussing clinical trial opportunities.

While many biases may be completely subconscious, others are actually well recognized by the providers themselves. The consortium for Enhancing Minority Participation in Clinical Trials (EMPaCT) was established in 2009 at five National Cancer Institute—designated comprehensive cancer centers (the University of Minnesota; the University of Alabama at Birmingham; Johns Hopkins University; the University of Texas M.D. Anderson cancer Center; and the University of California at Davis).[17-19] Survey studies emanating from EMPaCT research revealed important discriminatory practices contributing to underrepresentation of minorities onto cancer clinical trials. Niranjan et al.[18] documented several comments made by providers indicating that they did not feel that patients from communities of color (Black, Hispanic) would be interested in clinical trial participation or that they would not have the financial resources to support commitment to clinical trial participation. Many of these providers therefore did not want to invest time into presenting and explaining clinical trial opportunities to these patients. One of the respondent principal investigators commented that "African Americans I think have less knowledge"; and a referring clinician stated "... I think in the end people sort of say it's almost easier just to ignore that group and just give them standard stuff ..." The EMPaCT investigators also documented the importance of educating all staff involved with the continuum of outreach, recruitment, and retention of clinical trial participants and that this training must prioritize an understanding of accrual diversity.[19]

The lack of diversity in the general surgery and surgical oncology workforce likely contributes to and perpetuates inadequate diversity in our clinical trial patient population. A surgical workforce that does not reflect the diversity of the patient population is problematic for at least two reasons: (1) it creates a disconnect between patients and their providers related to a lack of shared experiences and perspectives and (2) the lack of diversity in the workforce has resulted in a weakened research enterprise related to the loss of creativity and innovation from generations of minds that were excluded from health professions because of systemic racism. Unfortunately, however, the demographics of senior- as well as junior-level surgical oncologists has

demonstrated progressive worsening of this pipeline problem. Blacks represent approximately 13% of the American population, and Hispanics represent approximately 19%,[20] yet they comprise fewer than 10% of physicians in the United States. Abelson et al.[21] utilized publicly available datasets to demonstrate the progressive decline in diversity along the academic continuum of medical student graduates (6% Black; 4% Hispanic); general surgery residents (5% Black; 5% Hispanic); Assistant Professor of Surgery (4% Black; 5% Hispanic); Associate Professor of Surgery (3% Black; 5% Hispanic) to Full Professor of Surgery (2% Black; 4% Hispanic). Collins et al.[22] reviewed 2015 to 2020 data from the American Association of Medical Colleges and Accreditation Council of Medical Education and reported that the proportion of White Complex General Surgery Oncology fellows increased from 54.5% to 69.2%, but the proportion of Black fellows decreased from 5.0% to 2.5% and the proportion of Hispanic fellows remained stable at 4.0%—4.2%.

GERMLINE GENETIC ASPECTS OF RACE RELATED TO ANCESTRY, SDOH, AND BREAST CANCER BURDEN

Population-based breast cancer mortality rates are 40% higher among African American/Black (hereafter Black) compared with White American/European ancestry (hereafter White) women in the United States.[23] The complex, multifactorial etiology of this disparity has been the subject of extensive research and debate regarding the meaning of race as a sociopolitical construct versus a biologically relevant metric of identity. Nearly all breast cancer patients will require some type of surgical care, and most newly diagnosed patients will meet with a surgeon as their initial clinical consultation. A review of the interrelationships between race/ancestry and SDOH is therefore especially relevant to surgeons.

The impact of systemic racism as a long-lasting legacy of slavery and manifested by residential racial segregation, disproportionately high rates of poverty, unemployment, and uninsurance in the Black community undoubtedly contributes to healthcare access barriers. The disproportionately greater severity of various comorbidities (e.g., hypertension, cardiovascular disease, asthma, and most recently COVID-19) as well as cancer mortality that is documented in Black compared with White Americans is clearly related to the impact of SDOH. African ancestry is also associated with germline genetic factors that can affect cancer burden, and advances in technologies that can quantify geographically defined ancestry have accelerated the pace of research regarding the genetics of breast cancer disparities.

Of note, breast cancer outcome disparities did not become apparent until the early 1980s, and prior mortality rates were equal for Black and White women. It is likely that the divergent survival curves are explained by the unmasking of differences in primary breast tumor biology between Black and White women.[24] The subsequent survival difference was largely related to declining death rates in White women but mostly stable death rates in Black women. The advent of endocrine therapy in the late 1970s, with its beneficial effects on outcomes in hormone receptor–positive breast cancer, probably accounted for this disproportionate race-related change. Since the incidence of hormone receptor–negative breast cancer is approximately twofold higher in Black women compared with White women, availability of targeted therapy for hormone receptor–positive breast cancer led to the inadvertent consequence of generating outcome disparities related to race-related variation in tumor phenotype.

Hormone receptor–negative breast cancer is a subset of the biologically aggressive tumors known as triple negative breast cancer (TNBC) differences, representing cancers that are negative for the growth factor protein HER2/*neu* as well as the estrogen receptor and progesterone receptor. Tremendous progress has been made in expanding the armamentarium of systemic therapies that target the hormone receptors as well as HER2/*neu*, but population-based incidence of TNBC is twice as high in Black compared with White women, and this has contributed to a widening of the mortality gap. Another example of targeted therapy for breast cancer is use of PARP inhibitors among patients that carry pathogenic mutations in the BRCA1 or BRCA2 genes. Unfortunately, however, disproportionately low rates of genetic testing performed on Black compared with White patients have led to higher frequency of variants of uncertain significance in Black women,[25,26] thereby leaving them less likely to be eligible for PARP inhibition.

SDOH and disparities in care to be delivered to Black compared with White patients, as well as differences in breast tumor biology, create a cascade of negative influences on the outcomes of Black breast cancer patients. "Oncologic anthropology"[27,28] is a proposed terminology to describe the interdisciplinary research looking at how population migration patterns, ancestral germline genetics, and the societal context of where contemporary population subsets reside impacts on cancer risk as well as cancer disparities. Oncologic anthropology can therefore be described as having three different but related aspects that can influence cancer risk in racial/ethnic population subsets: (1) germline genetics and ancestry informative markers (AIMs) that reflect geographically defined ancestral heritage and evolutionary selection pressure to survive various environmental threats related to infectious disease, food sources, or climate; (2) allostatic load and the cumulative lifetime effects of stress on biological homeostasis; and (3) social epigenetics and the effects of neighborhood characteristics (including poverty) on genetic patterns.

Lee et al.[29] conducted a pan-cancer analysis based upon The Cancer Genome Atlas and found that genetic ancestry correlated with survival disparities in breast, squamous head/neck, renal cell, and cutaneous cancers. Mueller et al.[30] found that genetic ancestry analyses from the Breast Cancer Association Consortium resulted in the identification of candidate genes associated with breast cancer risk.

Newman et al.[31] and Martini et al.[32] have reported on the association between the western sub-Saharan African ancestral germline genetics and risk of TNBC based upon an international database enriched with individuals from west and east Africa. For example, the Duffy null variant is an allele in the Duffy antigen receptor for chemokines/atypical chemokine receptor 1 that is seen almost exclusively in individuals with western sub-Saharan African ancestry, because it was acquired through evolutionary selection pressure to survive malaria that was endemic to the tropical areas in that part of the continent where mosquitoes (the host vector for the malaria parasite) thrived. The higher altitude of many east Africa regions is more hostile to the mosquito life cycle, and the Duffy-null variant is therefore less common among individuals with east African ancestry. The Duffy-null variant accounts for some malaria resistance because it leads to absence of the Duffy protein on erythrocytes, which is the portal of entry for the parasite to cause disease. However, downstream consequences of this Duffy protein absence affect the balance of circulating chemokines,[33] and associated effects on the mammary tissue microenvironment may explain the high frequency of TNBC in west Africa compared with the low TNBC frequency in east Africa.[31,34,35] The trans-Atlantic slave trade has resulted in substantial shared ancestry between contemporary Black Americans and western sub-Saharan Africans (including high frequency of Duffy-null in both population subsets) and may therefore also explain the high incidence of TNBC among Black women in the United States.

Obeng-Gyasi et al.[36–38] have conducted comprehensive studies of allostatic load and breast cancer risk. These investigators have reported on the disruption of biological homeostasis by chronic stress and chronic activation of the hypothalamic–pituitary–adrenal axis stress pathway, thereby resulting in disease initiation. Allostatic load describes how repeated and cumulative life stressors, including exposure to racism, can trigger this adverse cascade and provides a framework for understanding how the experiences of Blacks in America can be associated with adverse breast cancer outcomes.[38] A variety of metabolic markers can be used to estimate allostatic load, and Adams-Campbell et al.[39] have furthermore studied the possibility that an exercise intervention trial reduce these measures of allostatic load in Black women with increased breast cancer risk. Shen et al.[40] reported on elevated allostatic load among breast cancer patients living in socioeconomically disadvantaged neighborhoods, with Black patients being disproportionately represented in these communities.

Social epigenetics represent a variation on the concept of allostatic load, but with a stronger emphasis on the neighborhood-level features of socioeconomic disadvantage. Goel et al. have correlated the Area Deprivation Index with breast cancer outcomes and demonstrated shorter breast cancer–specific survival among women residing in the most disadvantaged neighborhoods, even after controlling for individual level patient features, tumor characteristics, and treatment delivered.[41] In another study,[42] they found that extreme racial/ethnic and economic segregation were associated with lower breast cancer–specific survival. Joshi et al.[43] and Carlos et al.[44] describe how structural racism and residential racial segregation converge to create environments where inhabitants develop epigenetic alterations that influence breast cancer risk.

CONCLUSIONS

Surgeons play an integral role in managing most solid organ malignancies. Cancer outcome disparities related to race/ethnicity and SDOH therefore represent public health challenges where surgeons can play a pivotal role in efforts to achieve health equity.

Highlights

- Patients with cancer from minoritized and marginalized racial and ethnic groups in the United States experience higher cancer burden and poorer oncologic outcomes.
- Ancestry is associated with germline genetic factors that can affect cancer burden.
- Oncologic anthropology describes interdisciplinary research looking at how population migration patterns, ancestral germline genetics, and the societal context of where contemporary population subsets reside impacts cancer risk as well as cancer disparities.
- Allostatic load and social epigenetics provide avenues to understand the biological implications of exposure to adverse socioenvironmental factors in patients with cancer.
- Strategies to improve workforce diversity and address implicit bias can mitigate and reduce disparities in oncologic outcomes.

REFERENCES

1. LaVeist TA, Perez-Stable EJ, Richard P, et al. The economic burden of racial, ethnic, and educational health inequities in the US. *JAMA*. 2023;329(19):1682–1692.
2. *CancerDisparitiesProgressReport.org*. Philadelphia: American Association for Cancer Research; 2022. http://www.CancerDisparitiesProgressReport.org/.
3. Giaquinto AN, Miller KD, Tossas KY, Winn RA, Jemal A, Siegel RL. Cancer statistics for African American/black people. *CA: A Cancer J Clin*. 2022;72:202–229.
4. Newman LA. Cascading consequences of systemic racism on public health. *Ann Surg*. 2021;273(1):10–12.
5. Chen YW, Kim T, Specht MC, et al. Time to surgery: a health equity metric in breast cancer patients. *Am J Surg*. 2023. https://doi.org/10.1016/j.amjsurg.2023.05.024. epub May 25, 2023.
6. Tseng JF, Kronowitz SJ, Sun CC, et al. The effect of ethnicity on immediate reconstruction rates after mastectomy for breast cancer. *Cancer*. 2004;101(7):1514–1523.
7. Fane LS, Wei AH, Tripathi R, Bordeaux JS. Asian American and Pacific Islander patients with melanoma have increased odds of treatment delays: a cross-sectional study. *J Am Acad Dermatol*. 2023. https://doi.org/10.1016/j.jaad.2023.05.028.
8. Greenberg AL, Brand NR, Zambeli-Ljepovic A, et al. Exploring the complexity and spectrum of racial/ethnic disparities in colon cancer management. *Int J Equity Health*. 2023;22(1):68.

9. Newman LA, Schwartz TA, Boermeester M. Practical guide to recruitment of participants for surgical clinical trials. *JAMA Surg.* 2022;157(12):1156–1157.

10. Duma N, Vera Aguilera J, Paludo J, Haddox CL, Gonzalez Velez M, et al. Representation of minorities and women in oncology clinical trials: review of the past 14 years. *J Oncol Pract.* 2018;14(1):e1–e10.

11. Gopishetty S, Kota V, Guddati AK. Age and race distribution in patients in phase III oncology clinical trials. *Am J Tourism Res.* 2020;12(9):5977–5983.

12. Shavers VL, Lynch CF, Burmeister LF. Racial differences in factors that influence the willingness to participate in medical research studies. *Ann Epidemiol.* 2002;12(4):248–256.

13. Shavers VL, Lynch CF, Burmeister LF. Knowledge of the Tuskegee study and its impact on the willingness to participate in medical research studies. *J Natl Med Assoc.* 2000; 92(12):563–572.

14. Simon MS, Du W, Flaherty L, et al. Factors associated with breast cancer clinical trials participation and enrollment at a large academic medical center. *J Clin Oncol.* 2004;22(11): 2046–2052.

15. Acuna-Villaorduna A, Baranda JC, Boehmer J, Fashoyin-Aje L, Gore SD. Equitable access to clinical trials: how do we achieve it? *Am Soc Clin Oncol Educ Book.* 2023;43: e389838.

16. Eggly S, Barton E, Winckles A, Penner LA, Albrecht TL. A disparity of words: racial differences in oncologist-patient communication about clinical trials. *Health Expect.* 2015;18(5):1316–1326.

17. Niranjan SJ, Wenzel JA, Martin MY, et al. Perceived institutional barriers among clinical and research professionals: minority participation in oncology clinical trials. *JCO Oncol Pract.* 2021;17(5):e666–e675.

18. Niranjan SJ, Martin MY, Fouad MN, et al. Bias and stereotyping among research and clinical professionals: perspectives on minority recruitment for oncology clinical trials. *Cancer.* 2020;126(9):1958–1968.

19. Niranjan SJ, Durant RW, Wenzel JA, et al. Training needs of clinical and research professionals to optimize minority recruitment and retention in cancer clinical trials. *J Cancer Educ.* 2019;34(1):26–34.

20. U.S. Census at https://www2.census.gov/programs-surveys/popest/. Accessed June 6, 2023.

21. Abelson JS, Symer MM, Yeo HL, et al. Surgical time out: our counts are still short on racial diversity in academic surgery. *Am J Surg.* 2018;215(4):542–548.

22. Collins RA, Sheriff SA, Yoon C, et al. Assessing the complex general surgical oncology pipeline: trends in race and ethnicity among US medical students, general surgery residents, and complex general surgical oncology trainees. *Ann Surg Oncol.* 2023:1–8.

23. Giaquinto AN, Sung H, Miller KD, et al. Breast cancer statistics. *CA A Cancer J Clin.* 2022;72(6):524–541.

24. Newman LA. Parsing the etiology of breast cancer disparities. *J Clin Oncol.* 2016;34(9):1013–1014.

25. Ndugga-Kabuye MK, Issaka RB. Inequities in multi-gene hereditary cancer testing: lower diagnostic yield and higher VUS rate in individuals who identify as hispanic, African or Asian and Pacific Islander as compared to European. *Fam Cancer.* 2019;18(4):465–469.

26. Jones JC, Golafshar MA, Coston TW, et al. Universal genetic testing vs. Guideline-directed testing for hereditary cancer syndromes among traditionally underrepresented patients in a community oncology program. *Cureus.* 2023;15(4):e37428.

27. Newman LA, Kaljee LM. Health disparities and triple-negative breast cancer in African American women: a review. *JAMA Surg.* 2017;152(5):485–493.

28. Davis MB, Newman LA. Oncologic anthropology: an interdisciplinary approach to understanding the association between genetically defined African ancestry and susceptibility for triple negative breast cancer. *Curr Breast Cancer Rep.* 2021;13:247–258.

29. Lee KK, Rishishwar L, Ban D, et al. Association of genetic ancestry and molecular signatures with cancer survival disparities: a pan-cancer analysis. *Cancer Res.* 2022;82(7): 1222–1233.

30. Mueller SH, Lai AG, Valkovskaya M, et al. Aggregation tests identify new gene associations with breast cancer in populations with diverse ancestry. *Genome Med.* 2023;15(1):7.

31. Newman LA, Jenkins B, Chen Y, et al. Hereditary susceptibility for triple negative breast cancer associated with western sub-saharan African ancestry: results from an international surgical breast cancer collaborative. *Ann Surg.* 2019;270(3):484–492.

32. Martini R, Delpe P, Chu TR, et al. African ancestry-associated gene expression profiles in triple-negative breast cancer underlie altered tumor biology and clinical outcome in women of African descent. *Cancer Discov.* 2022;12(11):2530–2551.

33. Yao S, Hong CC, Ruiz-Narvaez EA, et al. Genetic ancestry and population differences in levels of inflammatory cytokines in women: role for evolutionary selection and environmental factors. *PLoS Genet.* 2018;14(6):e1007368.

34. Jiagge E, Oppong JK, Bensenhaver J, et al. Breast cancer and African ancestry: lessons learned at the 10-year anniversary of the Ghana-Michigan research partnership and international breast registry. *J Glob Oncol.* 2016;2(5):302–310.

35. Jiagge E, Jibril AS, Chitale D, et al. Comparative analysis of breast cancer phenotypes in African American, white American, and west versus east African patients:

correlation between African ancestry and triple-negative breast cancer. *Ann Surg Oncol.* 2016;23(12):3843–3849.

36. Obeng-Gyasi S, Elsaid MI, Lu Y, et al. Association of allostatic load with all-cause mortality in patients with breast cancer. *JAMA Netw Open.* 2023;6(5):e2313989.

37. Obeng-Gyasi E, Tarver W, Obeng-Gyasi S. Allostatic load and breast cancer: a systematic review of the literature. *Curr Breast Cancer Rep.* 2022;14:180–191.

38. Obeng-Gyasi S, Tarver W, Carlos RC, Andersen BL. Allostatic load: a framework to understand breast cancer outcomes in Black women. *NPJ Breast Cancer.* 2021;7(1):100.

39. Adams-Campbell LL, Taylor T, Hicks J, Lu J, Dash C. The effect of a 6-month exercise intervention trial on allostatic load in black women at increased risk for breast cancer: the FIERCE study. *J Racial Ethn Health Disparities.* 2022;9(5):2063–2069.

40. Shen J, Fuemmeler BF, Sheppard VB, et al. Neighborhood disadvantage and biological aging biomarkers among breast cancer patients. *Sci Rep.* 2022;12(1):11006.

41. Goel N, Hernandez A, Thompson C, et al. Neighborhood disadvantage and breast cancer-specific survival. *JAMA Netw Open.* 2023;6(4):e238908.

42. Goel N, Westrick AC, Bailey ZD, et al. Structural racism and breast cancer-specific survival: impact of economic and racial residential segregation. *Ann Surg.* 2022;275(4):776–783.

43. Joshi S, Garlapati C, Aneja R. Epigenetic determinants of racial disparity in breast cancer: looking beyond genetic alterations. *Cancers.* 2022;14(8).

44. Carlos RC, Obeng-Gyasi S, Cole SW, et al. Linking structural racism and discrimination and breast cancer outcomes: a social genomics approach. *J Clin Oncol.* 2022;40(13):1407–1413.

CHAPTER 9

Community Engagement as a Social Determinant of Health in Surgery

KIRSTEN C. LUNG, MD • NICOLE L. SIMONE, MD • ADESEYE ADEKEYE, MD, PHD

IDENTIFICATION OF SOCIAL DETERMINANTS OF HEALTH

Access to healthcare varies across countries, communities, and individuals, oftentimes influenced by health policies as well as social and economic conditions. The interplay of differing factors, such as insurance coverage, low income, transportation costs, geographical barriers, and sociocultural expectations, must be taken into consideration when analyzing healthcare access. Limitations in access to healthcare not only lead to negative ramifications in the use of medical services but also affect treatment efficacy and overall health outcomes and quality of life. As value-based models are increasingly serving as guides for healthcare systems, the social determinants of health (SDOH) have emerged as key elements to consider when constructing healthcare systems. Many different communities play a role in improving or worsening SDOH, and in this section, we will overview what comprises SDOH, with a particular focus on the role the surgical community plays in addressing SDOH.

The World Health Organization (WHO) defines SDOH as "the conditions in which people are born, grow, live, work, and age" that are "shaped by the distribution of money, power, and resources at global, national and local levels."[1] This phenomenon inevitably leads to social stratification that creates health inequities among differing groups of people based on socioeconomics. Due to the complex relationships and feedback loops that characterize SDOH, SDOH are integral in shaping major health epidemics plaguing society today, such as diabetes, cancer, obesity, heart disease, and mental illness. Examples of SDOH include income/economic stability, access to educational opportunities, employment status, racial/ethnic disparities, gender inequity, access to housing and safe drinking water, availability of transportation, neighborhood conditions, and social support/inclusivity.

Several different community factors can positively or negatively affect SDOH, such as healthcare systems, national governments, local neighborhoods, and schools. Within healthcare systems, notable elements that can affect SDOH include physicians and other healthcare providers, nurses, social workers or case managers, and hospital administration. The surgical community is poised to impact SDOH through pre-, peri-, and postoperative screening and monitoring. National governments are also pivotal in influencing SDOH through public policy, healthcare access, funding, and research. On a more local scale, neighborhoods can affect SDOH, particularly through access to safe housing, adequate nutrition, recreation or exercise, reliable transportation, and community support, especially for the elderly. Furthermore, schools can create an early foundation that may impact SDOH through access to technology, supplies, or safe spaces, such as libraries (Fig. 9.1).

The importance of SDOH in healthcare is evidenced in disparities in survival and treatment access seen in certain patient populations. For instance, Haider et al. reported that both race/ethnicity and insurance status were associated with disparate outcomes following trauma, such that uninsured trauma patients are twice as likely to die from their injuries as insured trauma patients, and black trauma patients are 20% more likely to die from their injuries as white patients.[2] Moreover, despite attempts at standardization of trauma care with protocols in place for treatment at urban trauma centers, racial minority patients, specifically African American and Hispanic patients, with severe blunt traumatic brain injury, continue to receive worse initial management of trauma injuries and are 15% less likely to be placed in rehabilitation facilities, even after accounting for insurance status.[3]

However, there are local and national responses in place to address the systematic inequalities in

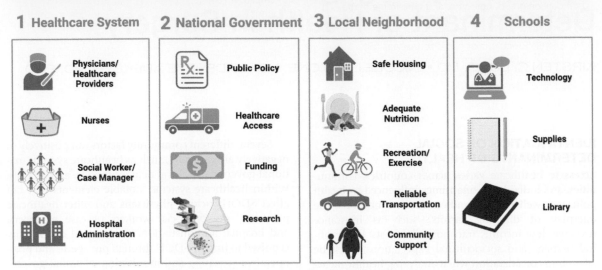

FIG. 9.1 Examples of different communities that can improve or worsen SDOH.

healthcare access to ameliorate the disproportionate impact these inequalities have on long-term functional outcomes and quality of life in patients from certain population groups. Urban safety net hospitals are critical in providing care to underserved populations, but unfortunately face the risk of closure due to various factors. In a retrospective study of all US hospitals with trauma centers in urban regions, Shen et al. found that hospitals in areas with a greater proportion of minorities face a higher risk of trauma center closure (hazard ratio 1.69, $P < .01$).[4] This serves to further exacerbate healthcare access difficulties, thus resulting in worse health outcomes for minorities.

GOVERNMENT RESPONSE TO ADDRESSING SOCIAL DETERMINANTS OF HEALTH

The US annual health expenditures are upward of $3 trillion, but the United States continues to have the lowest life expectancy at birth, highest infant mortality rate, and significant prevalence of chronic diseases in comparison with other countries.[5] Additionally, the United States allots a significantly lower percentage of its gross domestic product toward the maintenance and delivery of social services when compared with other countries with better health outcomes.[5] The Health Resources and Services Administration's Office of Health Equity and the Centers for Medicaid and

Medicare Services (CMS) have recognized SDOH as vital to population health and controlling healthcare costs, as social determinants now represent 40%–50% of the cost structure in Medicare and Medicaid. In response to this and the growing importance of addressing SDOH, the US government introduced the Affordable Care Act (ACA) with the goal of expanding healthcare access in a committed shift toward increasing health equity. Under the ACA, the Prevention and Public Health Fund was established to expand national investments in prevention and public health and to improve health outcomes. Starting in 2016, CMS regulations modernized the Medicaid Managed Care Operations (MCOs) as the "health care only" model has become increasingly antiquated, now empowering states to cover nonmedical interventions and to allot resources at the community level to address activities focused on SDOH and to promote preventative care and population health.[6] A 2016 study by the Yale School of Public Health examined the association between variation in state-level health outcomes and the allocation of state spending between social services and healthcare and found that states with greater allocation of resources toward social services as opposed to medical expenditures demonstrated better health outcomes in various medical conditions, such as obesity, asthma, mental illness, lung cancer, myocardial infarction, and type 2 diabetes mellitus, compared with states that did not.[7] By 2018, approximately 40% of US states had mandated screenings for social services and/or referrals to social services, with the number of additional states with social services screening requirements increasing annually.[8]

IMPORTANCE OF HEALTHCARE PROVIDER SCREENING OF SOCIAL DETERMINANTS OF HEALTH

Although the US government has taken steps to advance the healthcare system to better address SDOH with the goal of improving access to timely, appropriate healthcare, and subsequent patient health outcomes, there is a pervasive and urgent need for activism and engagement at the community and local levels as well. The role of community engagement is critical to increase access to and trust in the healthcare system for racial and ethnic minorities. However, the foundation of community engagement begins with medical providers and the importance of encouraging providers to learn about the population health of the communities within which they serve. The relationship between patients' social needs, such as housing instability, food insecurity, and transportation needs, with health outcomes and associated costs, is now being increasingly recognized by the medical community with studies demonstrating that physician- and hospital-led interventions targeting patients' social needs lead to improvements in health outcomes and reductions in medical expenses.[9] Historically, screening for patients' social needs has not been a traditional component of medical practice despite physicians recognizing the importance of identifying these contributing factors, due, in part, to the often complex nature of social needs coupled with increasing clinical demands. However, social needs screening tools have emerged to enhance the provider's ability to provide holistic care.

In 2013, the National Association of Community Health Centers, Inc., Association of Asian Pacific Community Health Organizations, and Oregon Primary Care Association collaborated together to create the Protocol for Responding to and Assessing Patients' Assets, Risks, and Experiences (PRAPARE), which is a national, standardized, patient-centric SDOH assessment tool and implementation toolkit.[10,11] PRAPARE was the most widely used standardized social risk screening tool among health centers during the COVID-19 pandemic, and the PRAPARE team launched enhanced learning opportunities for PRAPARE users, community partners, and stakeholders to help enable health centers and community-based organizations to address SDOH more effectively and to improve health equity. The implementation of the PRAPARE toolkit nationwide by providers allowed for the gathering of social health data, such as demographics, housing status, socioemotional health, and physical security, which would enable providers to identify their patients' social needs to better address them. Moreover, in 2016, Health Leads created a Social Needs Screening Toolkit that not only had updated languages that would foster more meaningful and effective dialogue between providers and patients, but also a fully translated questionnaire template designed to eliminate access barriers for Spanish-speaking patient populations, and additional questions pertaining to mental health challenges, such as social isolation.[12] This gradual, but marked, increase in utilization of screening tools aimed to identify and address social needs has highlighted the role of the provider in serving as a liaison between patients and critical social services that may contribute greatly to improving patients' quality of life and health outcomes. Hence, it is especially important that healthcare personnel adopt a holistic, patient-centered approach when treating patients.

Screening for SDOH can begin as early as during well-childcare visits. Garg et al. evaluated the effectiveness of a clinic-based screening and referral system entitled Well Child Care, Evaluation, Community Resources, Advocacy, Referral, Education (WE CARE), on the utilization of community-based resources for unmet social needs.[13] The self-reported screening instrument assessed needs for food security, childcare, education, employment, household heating, and housing. Based on the responses, healthcare providers made referrals for social services. It was found that with this screening tool, there was an increase in the number of referrals by providers, family utilization of social support services, employment opportunities for mothers, and childcare resources, as well as a decrease in the number of families with no housing.[13]

Although these screening tools serve as a critical step forward in addressing SDOH, there is the challenge of improving provider access to the questionnaire responses to allow providers to more effectively address unmet social needs. For the surgical community, access to these responses and assuming accountability for appropriate follow-through and referrals for patients with needs are critical in improving surgical outcomes. One solution to this challenge is to allow providers to individually tag electronic medical records to identify patients who may be affected by SDOH, and therefore are at risk for postsurgical complications. However, there currently is no reliable solution to this challenge, and much improvement and research are needed to increase accountability and reliability of access to these screening tools.

ROLE OF THE SURGICAL HEALTHCARE PROVIDER IN COMMUNITY ENGAGEMENT

Surgical patients are particularly poised to be affected by SDOH, as these factors can potentially affect the patient's ability to recover from surgery. Perioperatively, the effects of SDOH are often apparent, as patients of lower socioeconomic status and suffering from chronic conditions that may require surgical treatment frequently lack the support systems necessary for adequate access to healthcare.[14] This inadequate access to preventative healthcare often causes a need for repeat surgeries of an emergent nature, which increases the surgical risk. In a 2010 study conducted by Duke University Medical Center, it was found that a patient's socioeconomic status has a statistically significant effect on operative mortality and that mortality was the greatest among patients with the lowest socioeconomic status.[15] In addition, this study reported a mean decrease in operative mortality risk of 7.1% with a single-level increase in patient socioeconomic status.[15] It therefore becomes imperative that physicians, nurses, and other healthcare personnel involved in the perioperative setting work together to establish trust with patients and to address any SDOH prior to surgery to ensure a successful recovery. Of note, perioperative nurses often encounter the effects of SDOH when patients express concern about surgery scheduling times, transportation, and other support-related issues.[14] Patients living in lower socioeconomic conditions may also be more acutely affected by physiological changes triggered by the chronic stress of their poor living and working conditions, thereby negatively affecting their health and quality of life (Fig. 9.2). This phenomenon stresses the need for collaboration between healthcare communities and patients' own communities to address the SDOH plaguing the residents in their area. In the perioperative period, healthcare providers can establish trust with their patients by acknowledging these concerns, identifying areas of need, and partnering with community-based organizations to find solutions to these needs and to facilitate patient access to community resources, with the intent of reducing patient stress and promoting better postsurgical outcomes.[16] Types of community engagement include connecting patients with social workers or case managers who can assist with basic social needs, including transportation, nutrition, or food access. This becomes critical as patients

may not be willing or able to seek out community resources independently without assistance from a healthcare team member who has a relationship with a community-based organization. Moreover, having interpreter services available in the preoperative area as well as in the operating room is key to ensuring effective and clear communication between patients and healthcare providers.[16] Overall, when developing plans of care, it is imperative that providers recognize the interplay between SDOH and socioeconomic status, which may, in turn, influence the patient's relationship and view toward the healthcare system. This further emphasizes the importance of patient-centered approaches to developing personalized treatment plans for patients.

The term "socially responsible surgery (SRS)" is a field of study and clinical practice that integrates surgery and public health, thereby creating a foundation upon which research, advocacy, community engagement, education, and clinical practice can address the SDOH that negatively affect surgical access and worsen surgical outcomes in underserved populations.[17] SRS aims to provide quality surgical care to underserved patient populations by promoting academic inquiry in rural surgery, urban surgery, and global surgery.[17] Surgeons and trainees in the Department of Surgery at Boston Medical Center (BMC) have developed an SRS initiative to address SDOH among their surgical patients by incorporating various programs including (1) a team of mental health professionals who counsel and advocate for victims of violence, as well as educate trainees about injury prevention and ending cycles of violence; (2) a preventative food pantry that provides access to culturally appropriate nutrition, free of charge, which is critical in ensuring stable postoperative recovery; (3) a medical facility that provides 24/7 medical support for patients without housing; and (4) a medical–legal partnership that provides access to comprehensive legal services to underserved patients with difficulties related to housing, employment, income, or legal status.[17] However, the distinguishing element of the SRS initiatives at BMC is the role of trauma surgeons as consultants to help provide resources and strategies for the prevention of future interpersonal violence and injury. This BMC SRS initiative is unique in its location and access to community resources that will address patients' unmet social needs, and it is this characteristic that allows this SRS initiative to thrive. However, a vast majority of areas affected by SDOH do not have such access to local community resources and programs, which begs the question of what body should be responsible for providing such needed resources to regions with

SDOH on Post-Operative Recovery

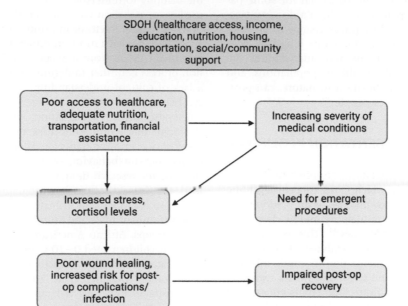

FIG. 9.2 Effects of SDOH on postoperative recovery.

adverse SDOH. In addition to calling upon the national and local governments to provide funding and support for needed resources, it is critical to analyze the role of the healthcare facility and providers, such as surgeons, and how both can share responsibility in addressing SDOH to improve patient outcomes.

SRS initiatives are useful as surgical access varies across regions, which lead to disparities in outcomes of underserved populations in American rural, urban, low-, and middle-income communities. In both rural and urban regions of the United States, underserved populations, traditionally defined as the poor, the uneducated, the uninsured, the homeless, or racial minorities, experience higher rates of traumatic injury, present with cancers at later stages, and receive subpar surgical care.[2,18–22] Surgical access on a global scale is also varied, as approximately 5 billion individuals worldwide lack access to surgical services, with the third of the world's population with the lowest income receiving only 3.5% of the world's surgical procedures.[23–26] The burden of surgical diseases is higher in rural settings compared with urban regions. For instance, rural patients diagnosed with abdominal aortic aneurysms were at greater risk of rupture, more likely to require transfer to another facility for surgical repair, and less likely to undergo definitive repair of the aneurysm.[27] Interestingly, an estimated one-third of all US counties,

of which 95% are considered "nonmetropolitan," had no practicing surgeons in the region, which is a crucial finding, as lack of access to appropriate surgical care correlates to increased morbidity and mortality.[18,20,28] However, surgeons have embraced their integral role in reducing these healthcare disparities and SDOH and have created systems designed to improve patient care and health outcomes. Surgeons practicing in a rural hospital located in central Illinois not only provide perioperative management and surgical treatment of ailments, but they also serve as primary care physicians, reporting a 4% surgical complication rate, which is lower than several urban area facilities.[29] Along a similar vein, while urban communities are often located adjacent to major tertiary and academic medical centers, the urban underserved continue to suffer from poor access to surgical services. Although protocols are instituted to standardize trauma care at urban trauma centers, racial minorities continue to receive subpar initial management and are less likely to be discharged to rehabilitation facilities.[21,22] This brings to light the challenge that faces the surgical community to find ways to preemptively identify patients with known adverse SDOH and to follow up and make appropriate referrals with the goal to address SDOH, to improve postsurgical outcomes, and to serve as patient advocates.

Unfortunately, though efforts by individual providers and health centers are beneficial for some patients, a majority of patients remain at a disadvantage, thus prompting the need for policy change to improve underlying social conditions and create long-term benefits. Community-level input and interventions are necessary to improve the health of populations, and although not specifically medical in nature, can positively impact the health of people.[30]

IMPROVING REPRESENTATION IN CLINICAL TRIALS

Underserved patient populations are often underrepresented in clinical trials, which raises concern regarding the generalizability of study findings, as the predominant population group found in trials are middle-class, well-educated, married white males.[31] This is especially crucial in new drug clinical trials with regard to the safety and efficacy of the new medication in ethnic minority groups.[31] While there is no scientific basis for exclusion of ethnic minority groups from clinical trials, educational programs should be tailored toward clinical trial investigators and funding bodies with the goal to increase awareness of underrepresentation, and to provide guidance for investigators. By educating healthcare professionals on culturally sensitive outreach strategies to successfully interact with ethnic, linguistic, and culturally diverse populations, it will gradually reduce the fear and mistrust of medical professionals. Special advocacy groups or community link workers outside of the medical progression may also play key roles in creating a bridge between underrepresented patient populations and healthcare professionals. However, it is equally as important to examine the review process of clinical trial protocols as more robust reviews of protocols may help to increase minority representation.

There continues to exist significant barriers to minority representation in clinical trials, such as lack of awareness of the importance of representational sampling, the exclusion of women of childbearing age due to ethical considerations, and the exclusion of the elderly based on the assumption of frailty and vulnerability. Hussain-Gambles et al. have identified various factors that hinder equal representation in clinical trials, one of which is cost and the concept that the addition of "extra variables," notably females and ethnic minorities, to conduct subgroup analysis, would require additional subject recruitment, hence driving up costs.[32] The possibility of additional costs incurred from requirements on behalf of the ethics committee, such as translated information sheets or inclusion of an interpreter, is an obstacle to adequate subject recruitment. Similarly, the inability to understand and speak English is often used as an exclusion criterion and therefore poses as a potential barrier to ethnic minority participation as language barrier is seen most prominently when obtaining informed consent from trial subjects. The communication process is further undermined by stereotypes and a lack of cultural understanding.[33] Moreover, prejudicial biases or stereotyping espoused by healthcare providers also affect representation, such as the cultural stereotype that ethnic minorities and individuals with lower socioeconomic status are often difficult to reach, display deviant behavior, or are incapable of understanding the research design.[34-36] Sateren et al. examined the impact of sociodemographics on patient accrual to National Cancer Institute (NCI)—sponsored cancer treatment trials and found that while among minority groups, African American, Asian American, and Hispanic children aged 0—10 years were accrued to trials at rates comparable with their white counterparts, adult cancer patients aged 30—79 years, however, demonstrated lower accrual rates for Asian American and Hispanic men and women compared with their white counterparts.[35] In addition, certain populations' mistrust of healthcare professionals contributes to lower recruitment numbers, and certain historic scientific events, such as the Tuskegee syphilis study, are often cited as key factors in creating mistrust and suspicion of the medical profession by particular minority groups.[36] However, interestingly, this sense of distrust and suspicion may be a key reason why several ethical researchers believe that exclusion of certain population groups from clinical trials is necessary to protect from a repeat of such abuse.[34] Lastly, sociocultural barriers, specifically SDOH, contribute to low ethnic minority accrual to clinical trials as this may be a result of racially constructed socioeconomic factors that cause lower healthcare utilization and subsequent reduced opportunity and exposure to participate in trials[32] (Fig. 9.3). Therefore, we may only see an improvement in the enrollment of underrepresented minorities in clinical trials using a multilevel approach, by targeting changes at an individual level—those responsible for enrollment process, system-based level-hospital infrastructure, and an interpersonal level—a patient's clinical experience.[37]

ROLE OF PATIENT ADVOCACY IN COMMUNITY ENGAGEMENT

As the role of SDOH in determining health outcomes and healthcare access becomes more prominent and widespread on local, national, and global scales, the

Barriers to Minority Participation in Clinical Trials

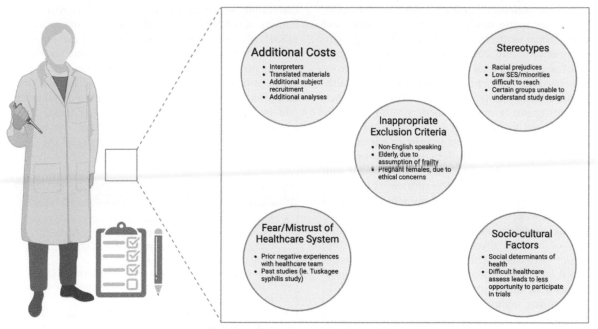

FIG. 9.3 Barriers to minority participation in clinical trials.

importance of community engagement and the need for patient advocacy are more pronounced. Patient advocates are not only vital in assisting vulnerable populations in navigation of the healthcare system but also serve as a bridge between these minority groups and research endeavors as patient advocates are capable of educating clinical trial investigators on outreach strategies that are culturally sensitive. However, the exact role of patient advocates has yet to be clearly defined, although studies have shown support for patient advocates, particularly in instances where patients are unable to advocate for themselves.[38] Healthcare providers have often assumed the role of patient advocate and are often seen sending referral letters to different agencies on behalf of the patient to assist them with unmet basic needs. Several providers have frequently fostered relationships with community organizations and are often able to direct patients to community programs that can assist with child or family care, access to adequate nutrition, and financial assistance.

FUTURE DIRECTIONS

Healthcare providers are increasingly recognizing the importance of reducing health inequity by addressing SDOH through novel integrated care models, community partnerships, and population health assessments, with the goal of improving health outcomes and quality of life for the most vulnerable groups in our communities. Healthcare facilities can help provide underserved patient groups with transportation fare, child care services during appointments or scheduled procedures, interpreter services for those with language barriers, patient navigators, and outreach to local community groups. In addition, the Boston University School of Medicine (BUSM) student Surgical Interest Group has developed an SRS research track designed to support surgeons and trainees committed to addressing social barriers to surgical care.[17] Programs like these are crucial to fostering community around SRS and unifying research, education, and advocacy and creating a community of surgeon researchers, educators, and advocates who are ready to take on the challenge of addressing SDOH.

Furthermore, the randomized controlled trial conducted by Finkelstein et al. investigating the superutilizer intervention created by the Camden Coalition of Healthcare Providers has further supported the importance of randomized trials in identifying ways to adapt existing care delivery models to the needs of its target patient population.[39] The Camden Core Model utilizes real-time data on hospital admissions to identify patients who are superutilizers, with an emphasis on those with chronic conditions and complex medical needs, and to create a care model that engages patients and connects them with appropriate healthcare, government assistance, and community support.[39] The purpose of such a tailored intervention is to improve health outcomes while minimizing unnecessary healthcare utilization. However, challenges remain for superutilizer programs aimed at medically and socially complex populations, and it is possible that current models of connecting patients to existing resources are inadequate for these complex patient groups. For instance, in this study, while patient engagement with the program was high with 95% of patients having at least three encounters with staff documented, sustained engagement was poor as patients failed to consistently reach the predetermined goal of home visit within 5 days of hospital discharge and office visit within 7 days of discharge.[39] This inconsistency reemphasizes the need for future randomized trials as observational evaluations are often subject to transient effects.

Recognizing organizational barriers to overcoming SDOH and incorporating SDOH into novel care model designs are key factors in identifying and addressing patient risk. Predictive models and clinic-based screening tools assessing SDOH are beginnings of standardized approaches to screening for social risk factors during a clinic visit. However, this predicates on the healthcare sector and community sector collaborating as a unit to address SDOH. Provider training on SDOH is imperative.

It is increasingly apparent that to improve population health, health equity and addressing SDOH need to become a priority at the community, national, and global levels and that these measures designed to reduce disparities should be components of future health programs. Policy change is crucial as it has the ability to improve underlying social conditions. However, this process requires community input and investment. Interventions in housing, community outreach, care coordination, and income and nutrition support have led to improvements in health outcomes as well as a decrease in healthcare spending.[40] These findings suggest that future policy changes aimed at these aspects of SDOH may be useful in reducing healthcare costs while improving population health outcomes.

Healthcare leaders have a responsibility to advocate for health equity as a priority in the modern healthcare system construct. Physicians are well positioned to address the disparities that exist in the spectrum of medical care and to lead discussions on the design of care delivery models that would allow for improved

outcomes and medical care access for underserved populations. It is this commitment to health equity, coupled with the investment and engagement by the community sector, that will help society overcome the barriers of SDOH. In the field of surgery, in particular, SDOH play key roles in the postoperative recovery period. Perioperative healthcare personnel are in a unique position to identify and address patients' social needs prior to surgery. The perioperative team is presented with the opportunity to foster trust with patients, and individual efforts to help overcome social challenges, coupled with healthcare initiatives, can have a substantial cumulative effect on improving the outcomes of individuals with SDOH.

Highlights

- Many different communities play a role in improving or worsening social determinants of health (SDOH), including healthcare systems, national governments, local neighborhoods, and schools.
- The surgical community is poised to impact SDOH through pre-, peri-, and postoperative screening and monitoring.
- Although increasing use of SDOH screening tools is a great step forward, there still remains the challenge of improving provider access to these questionnaire responses and creating accountability for appropriate follow-through and referral on behalf of the provider.
- "Socially responsible surgery" (SRS) initiatives are useful in areas with available community resources, but are often challenging to implement in regions with adverse SDOH and scarce funding.
- The challenge remains for the surgical community to find ways to preemptively identify patients with known SDOH and to follow-up and make appropriate referrals to improve postsurgical outcomes and serve as patient advocates.
- Many different factors contribute to the lack of ethnic and racial representation in clinical trials.
- Healthcare providers have a responsibility to advocate for health equity and to work toward minimizing the impact of adverse SDOH on patient health outcomes.

REFERENCES

1. NEJM Catalyst. Social determinants of health (SDOH). In: *NEJM Catalyst Innovations in Care Delivery.* Massachusetts Medical Society; December 1, 2017. https://catalyst.nejm.org/doi/full/10.1056/CAT.17.0312.
2. Haider AH, Weygandt PL, Bentley JM, et al. Disparities in trauma care and outcomes in the United States: a systematic review and meta-analysis. *J Trauma Acute Care Surg.* May 2013;74(5):1195–1205.

3. Shafi S, Marquez de la Plata C, Diaz-Arrastia R, et al. Ethnic disparities exist in trauma care. *J Trauma*. November 2007; 63(5):1138–1142.

4. Shen YC, Hsia RY, Kuzma K. Understanding the risk factors of trauma center closures: do financial pressure and community characteristics matter? *Med Care*. September 2009;47(9):968–978.

5. Bush M. Addressing the root cause: rising health care costs and social determinants of health. *N C Med J*. 2018 Jan-Feb;79(1):26–29.

6. Machledt D. *Addressing the Social Determinants of Health through Medicaid Managed Care*. The Commonwealth Fund; November 2017.

7. Bradley EH, Canavan M, Rogan E, et al. Variation in health outcomes: the role of spending on social services, public health, and health care, 2000-09. *Health Aff*. May 1, 2016;35(5):760–768.

8. Gifford K, Ellis E, Edwards BC, et al. *States Focus on Quality and Outcomes Amid Waiver Changes: Results from a 50-State Medicaid Budget Survey for State Fiscal Years 2018 and 2019*. KFF; October 25, 2018. https://www.kff.org/report-section/states-focus-on-quality-and-outcomes-amid-waiver-changes-managed-care-initiatives/. Accessed February 12, 2023.

9. Solomon LS, Kanter MH. Health care steps up to social determinants of health: current context. *Perm J*. 2018;22: 18–139.

10. Fraze TK, Brewster AL, Lewis VA, et al. Prevalence of screening for food insecurity, housing instability, utility needs, transportation needs, and interpersonal violence by US physician practices and hospitals. *JAMA Netw Open*. 2019;2(9):e1911514.

11. Protocol for Responding to Assessing Patients' Assets, Risks, and Experiences (PREPARE). National Association of Community Health Centers. http://www.nachc.org/research-and-data/prapare/. Accessed February 12, 2023.

12. The Health Leads Screening Toolkit. Health Leads Resource Library. https://healthleadsusa.org/resources/the-health-leads-screening-toolkit/. Accessed February 12, 2023.

13. Garg A, Toy S, Tripodis Y, et al. Addressing social determinants of health at well child care visits: a cluster RCT. *Pediatrics*. 2015;135(2):e296–e304.

14. Spruce L. Back to basics: social determinants of health. *AORN J*. July 2019;110(1):60–69.

15. Bennett KM, Scarborough JE, Pappas TN, et al. Patient socioeconomic status is an independent predictor of operative mortality. *Ann Surg*. 2010;252(3):157–165.

16. Committee on Health Care for Underserved Women. ACOG Committee Opinion No. 729: importance of social determinants of health and cultural awareness in the delivery of reproductive health care. *Obstet Gynecol*. 2018; 131(1):e43–e48.

17. Robinson TD, Oliveira TM, Timmes TR, et al. Socially responsible surgery: building recognition and coalition. *Front Surg*. 2017;4:11.

18. Schecter WP, Charles AG, Cornwell EE, et al. The surgery of poverty. *Curr Probl Surg*. 2011;48(4):228–280.

19. Mackersie RC. For the care of the underserved. *J Trauma Acute Care Surg*. 2014;77(5):653–659.

20. Branas CC, MacKenzie EJ, Williams JC, et al. Access to trauma centers in the United States. *JAMA*. 2005; 293(21):2626–2633.

21. Shafi S, de la Plata CM, Diaz-Arrastia R, et al. Ethnic disparities exist in trauma care. *J Trauma*. 2007;63(5): 1138–1142.

22. Shafi S, Gentilello LM. Ethnic disparities in initial management of trauma patients in a nationwide sample of emergency department visits. *Arch Surg*. 2008;143(11): 1057–1061.

23. Funk LM, Weiser TG, Berry WR, et al. Global operating theatre distribution and pulse oximetry supply: an estimation from reported data. *Lancet*. 2010;376(9746): 1055–1061.

24. Meara JG, Leather AJM, Hagander L, et al. Global Surgery 2030: evidence and solutions for achieving health, welfare, and economic development. *Lancet*. 2015;386(9993): 569–624.

25. Weiser TG, Regenbogen SE, Thompson KD, et al. An estimation of the global volume of surgery: a modelling strategy based on available data. *Lancet*. 2008;372(9633): 139–144.

26. Debas HT, Donkor P, Gawande A, Jamison DT, Kruk ME, Mock CN. *Disease Control Priorities: Volume 1: Essential Surgery*. 3rd ed. Washington, DC: World Bank; 2015.

27. Maybury RS, Chang DC, Freischlag JA. Rural hospitals face a higher burden of ruptured abdominal aortic aneurysm and are more likely to transfer patients for emergent repair. *J Am Coll Surg*. 2011;212(6):1061–1067.

28. Belsky D, Ricketts T, Poley S, Gaul K. Surgical deserts in the U.S.: counties without surgeons. *Bull Am Coll Surg*. 2010; 95(9):32–35.

29. Rossi A, Rossi D, Rossi M, Rossi P. Continuity of care in a rural critical access hospital: surgeons as primary care providers. *Am J Surg*. 2011;201(3):359–362.

30. Health Impact in 5 Years. Centers for Disease Control and Prevention. https://www.cdc.gov/policy/hst/hi5/index.html.

31. Hussain-Gambles M. Ethnic minority under-representation in clinical trials. Whose responsibility is it anyway? *J Health Organisat Manag*. 2003;17(2): 138–143.

32. Hussain-Gambles M, DPhil KA, DPhil BL. Why ethnic minority groups are under-represented in clinical trials: a review of the literature. *Health Soc Care Community*. 2004; 12(5):382–388.

33. Gifford AL, Cunningham WE, Heslin KC, et al. Participation in research and access to experimental treatments by HIV-infected patients. *N Engl J Med*. 2002;346(18): 1373–1382.

34. Swanson GM, Ward AJ. Recruiting minorities into clinical trials: toward a participant-friendly system. *J Natl Cancer Inst*. 1995;87(23):1747–1759.

35. Sateren WB, Trimble EL, Abrams J, et al. How sociodemographics, presence of oncology specialists, and hospital cancer programs affect accrual to cancer treatment trials. *J Clin Oncol*. 2002;20(8):2109–2117.

36. Brawley OW, Freeman HP. Race and outcomes: is this the end of the beginning for minority health research? *J Natl Cancer Inst*. 1999;91(22):1908–1909.

37. Hamel LM, Penner LA, Albrecht TL, et al. Barriers to clinical trial enrollment in racial and ethnic minority patients with cancer. *Cancer Control.* 2016;23(4):327–337.

38. Schwartz L. Is there an advocate in the house? The role of health care professionals in patient advocacy. *J Med Ethics.* 2002;28(1):37–40.

39. Finkelstein A, Zhou A, Taubman S, et al. Health care hot-spotting — a randomized, controlled trial. *N Engl J Med.* 2020;382:152–162.

40. Taylor LA, Tan AX, Coyle C, et al. Leveraging the social determinants of health: what works? *PLoS One.* 2016;11(8): e0160217.

CHAPTER 10

Insurance as a Social Determinant of Health in Surgery

NICOLÁS AJKAY, MD, MBA, FACS

SOCIAL DETERMINANTS OF HEALTH AND INSURANCE STATUS

Social determinants of health (SDOH) are conditions in the environment where people are born, live, learn, work, play, worship, and age, that can affect their health, functioning, and quality-of-life outcomes and risks. According to the Office of Disease Prevention and Health Promotion from the US Department of Health and Human Services (DHHS), SDOH can be grouped into five domains: economic stability, education access and quality, neighborhood and built environment, social and community context, and healthcare access and quality.[1] In this chapter, health insurance is discussed as part of the last domain.

In the United States, many people do not get the healthcare services they need. In fact, 1 out of 10 people in the United States do not have health insurance and lack basic access to healthcare services and medications. A lack of primary care provider (PCP), for example, is a reason to not get recommended healthcare services, such as cancer screenings.[1] Health insurance, or lack of it, can significantly influence healthcare outcomes on surgical diseases and surgical care.

Information from the US Census Bureau demonstrated that in 2017, 67.2% of people had private health insurance, 37.7% had government insurance, and 8.8% of people (28.5 million) did not have health insurance at any point during the year.[2] Most recent numbers from the 2020 Census show that in 2021, 66% of people had private health insurance, 35.7% had government insurance, and 8.3% (27.2 million) were uninsured, a 0.5% decrease from 2017 (Fig. 10.1).[3]

INSURANCE BASICS AND RECENT POLICY ADVANCES

Private insurance (or employer-based health insurance) is defined as a plan provided though an employer or union, or directly purchased by an individual from an insurance company or an exchange. Government insurance plans include federal programs, such as Medicaid, Medicare, Children's Health Insurance Program (CHIP), individual state plans, TRICARE, CHAMPVA (Civilian Health and Medical Program of the Department of Veterans Affairs, DVA), and also care provided by DVA or the military.[2]

Health insurance is a contract between a company and a consumer, in which the company agrees to pay for some or all healthcare costs in exchange for a monthly premium. As explained by healthcare economists Baiker and Chandra: "Insurance, in its simplest form, works by pooling risks: many pay a premium up front, and then those who face a bad outcome (getting sick, being in a car accident, etc.) get paid out of those collected premiums. The premium for health insurance is the expected cost of treatment for the pool. Uncertainty about when we may fall sick and need more health care is the reason to purchase insurance; the more uncertainty there is, the more valuable insurance is." This last point highlights the importance of being insured: "The key insight is that not everyone will fall sick at the same time, so it is possible to pay for the sick even though it costs more than their premiums. This is why it is so important for people to get insured when they are healthy — to protect against the risk of needing extra resources to devote to health care if they fall ill."[4]

Insurance contracts are usually for 1 year and come with two main exceptions, a deductible or out-of-pocket cost the consumer must pay before the company's coverage begins, and a copayment, or the consumer's share of the cost of specific services or procedures. Federal health insurance plans such as Medicare, Medicaid, and CHIP extend coverage to elderly, disabled, or low-income people without access to private or employer-based health insurance.[5] In the next

Social Determinants of Health in Surgery. https://doi.org/10.1016/B978-0-443-12366-5.00009-7

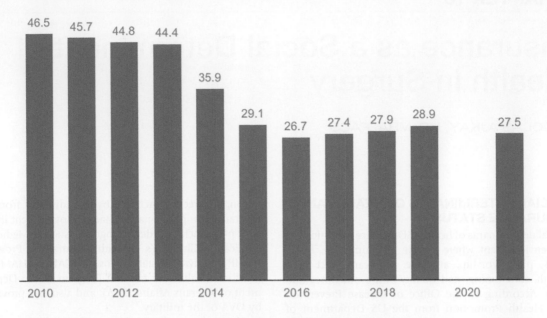

NOTE: Due to disruptions in data collection during the first year of the pandemic, the Census Bureau did not release ACS 1-year estimates in 2020. Includes nonelderly individuals ages 0 to 64
SOURCE: KFF analysis of 2010-2021 American Community Survey, 1-Year Estimates

KFF

FIG. 10.1 Number of nonelderly uninsured, 2010–21.

section, we will discuss the different types of insurances and recent healthcare policy changes in the context of SDOH:

a. Employer-based health insurance: In a 1999 commentary, the economist Uwe Reinhardt discussed the US employer-based healthcare system based on a set of credits and debts it has created.[6] He highlighted four credits or benefits of the system: (1) *Status quo*, the fact that the system exists, as the most effective mechanism of pooling health insurance risk. The tax benefits for employers and employees are significant, since contributions are tax deductible as a business expense, and premiums are paid from pretax wages. (2) *Risk pooling*, where younger and healthier workers subsidize older and/or sicker workers. (3) *Innovation through decentralization* allows the relatively unregulated US employer-based system greater flexibility to experiment and innovate, specifically with physician profiles, multitier pharmaceutical pricing, and home care as an inpatient substitute among other improvements. (4) *Consumer preference*, or the choices of care built into the system, and to some extent, competition as an engine for quality improvement. The author also discusses the system's debits, or the disadvantages of the employer-based system: (1) *Insurance* describes

the fact that the person is only insured while holding a job, so the healthcare protection of the entire family, including children, is tied to being employed. Reinhardt argues that in other industrialized countries, young people know that they have fully portable and permanent health insurance. The US has not been able to offer this benefit to Americans. (2) *Job lock*, a situation caused by healthcare benefits being tied to a particular job. Employees may be induced to hold a job they dislike because it is the only alternative for affordable healthcare. Empirically, it has been shown that a fully portable healthcare insurance, like that afforded to Canadians, facilitates greater labor mobility.[7] (3) *Inequity*, where the tax preferences afforded by the system are inequitable. First, it has not been extended to self-employed and unemployed Americans, and second, it may disproportionally benefit high-income employees more than those in low-income marginal tax brackets. Flexible spending accounts have a similar inequity, as those higher paid employees can fund a flexible spending account for healthcare expenses with pretax dollars and pay much lower after-tax costs than lower income workers unable to fund this accounts (50 cents vs. 85 cents per dollar). (4) *Lack of choice*, as employees are limited by employers to very few healthcare plans. Half of US employees have access to only one plan and about a quarter can only choose between two.[8] This lack of choices stifles competition and may increase cost. (5) *Lack of privacy*, as not only the insurance company, but the employer's personnel departments have access to employees' private health information. (6) *Lack of transparency*, as employees do not exactly know the true total cost of healthcare premiums, or how much of what employers pay is shifted back to them collectively through reductions in take-home pay. Over the long term, the employer-based system, according to the author, is a significant inflationary factor in the cost of healthcare in the United States.

Employer-sponsored wellness programs (ESWP): As cost of healthcare increases, companies are trying to contain cost. ESWPs are designed to make employees healthier by encouraging them to lose weight, stop smoking, participate in health screenings, and modify lifestyle and behavior. There has been an increase in the number of large employers (200 or more employees) that offer these programs, from 70% in 2008 to 84% in 2019.[8] Despite the growing popularity of ESWP, their benefits have been questioned. An opinion piece in the New York Times highlighted a discrepancy between positive findings in observational studies and absence of benefit in randomized trials evaluating the efficacy of ESWP. In other words, once the selection bias of observational studies is eliminated, differences disappear. The author describes the findings from the Illinois Workplace Wellness Study,[9] a large randomized trial based on a wellness program at the University of Illinois at Urbana–Champaign. Out of 5000 employees that volunteered, 1500 were placed in a control group that received no wellness services, and 3300 received a biometric healthcare screening and health risk assessments, and were offered a number of wellness activities with financial incentives for participants, including weight loss, exercise, smoking cessation, and financial wellness programs. After a year of follow-up, the results were disappointing, with no causal effects seen. But when the intervention group was analyzed in an observational fashion, comparing those that took advantage of the program versus those that did not, differences appeared. For example, those who used the program were more likely to go to the gym than those who did not; no difference was seen in the randomized analysis. The observational analysis showed that participants spent less than no

participants in healthcare ($525 vs. $657) and hospital-related costs ($237 vs. $387). The differences in the observation analysis persisted when controlling for several variables, including age, sex, race, salary, and staff versus faculty status. In the randomized trial, no effect was seen when the intervention group was compared with control (healthcare costs, $576 vs. $568, and hospital-related costs $317 vs. $297). There are likely intrinsic unmeasured variables that could predict the benefits of these programs. Most notably, employees' perception of management's culture may influence the program's outcomes. Is there a true interest in workers well-being, or these programs are just part of a company's plan to increase productivity and decrease labor costs?[10]

b. Medicare: It is the federal healthcare insurance program for people 65 and older, regardless of income or health status, or those under 65 who have a long-term disability. It covers up to 60 million people. Medicare Part A coverage eligibility is for patients and their spouses entitled to social security payments. Part A covers inpatient hospital stay, skilled nursing, home health, and hospice. It includes a deductible and requires coinsurance for extended inpatient care. Part B covers outpatient services, including preventative care, and has also deductible and coinsurance requirement. Part C or Medicare Advantage allows beneficiaries to enroll in a private healthcare plan and receive all Medicare-Covered Part A, B, and some Part D benefits. Part D covers prescription drugs though stand-alone prescription drug plans (PDPs) and Medicare Advantage, including high-cost medications. Medicare has benefit gaps, including cost sharing requirements, relatively high deductibles, and no out-of-pocket spending limits, so most beneficiaries have some type of supplemental coverage.[11] In a 2016 survey of Medicare recipients, Medicare supplemental coverage was provided by employer-sponsored insurance to 30%, Medigap (Medicare supplement insurance) to 29% and Medicaid to 22% (low incomes and modest assets). 19% of beneficiaries had no supplemental coverage and were exposed to Medicare's cost sharing requirements and no limit in out-of-pocket spending, unlike beneficiaries enrolled in Medicare Advantage.[12] The same survey showed that in 2016, traditional Medicare beneficiaries spent on average $5460 on out-of-pocket expenses, including premiums, cost sharing, and not covered services, up to 12% of their total income. Although Medicare helps make healthcare more affordable, beneficiaries face high out-of-pocket expenses, particularly for uncovered services, such as long-term care. Beneficiaries who incur the highest out-of-pocket costs include women, those older than 85, in poorer self-reported health, with multiple medical conditions and without supplemental coverage.

c. Medicaid: This program is the largest health insurance in the United States. Data from 2013 showed that the program covered 62 million people, or one in five Americans. It is for those who lack access to the private health insurance system, require long-term skilled nursing care, or need other community-based services and support. It provides core funding for health centers and safety-net hospitals serving low-income or uninsured people, as well as essential community services, as trauma care and neonatal intensive care (Fig. 10.2). It also covers many long-term services that private or other federal insurance, such as Medicare do not, including nonemergency transportation and translation services required to improve access to care. States are responsible for the design and management of their own Medicaid programs, under a broad federal framework. It is publicly financed, but it is not a government-run healthcare system. States pay physicians, hospitals, and other providers for services provided to Medicaid beneficiaries, either on a fee-for-service basis, or through risk-based contracts with managed care plans (either managed care organizations or primary care case management). Medicaid covers one in three children, 40% of all births, millions with severe disabilities, and provides gap coverage to low-income Medicare beneficiaries.[13]

With the passing of the Affordable Care Act, after 2014, Medicaid became a program for people under 65 with income at or below 138% of the federal poverty level ($26,951 for a family of 3), in those states that expanded Medicaid. Only American citizens and some lawfully present immigrants can qualify for Medicaid; undocumented immigrants do not.[13] Data from the 2020 Census show that in 2021, close to 62 million people, or 18.9% of the US population, were covered by Medicaid. This represents a full 1% increase from the previous year (58.8 million, 17.9%), due in part to the COVID 19 pandemic.[3]

The Impact of Medicaid on access to care has been significant. Its coverage of pregnant women and children has improved birth outcomes and child health, with the latter being comparable with privately insured children in core measures of preventative care and primary care.[14] Adult Medicaid beneficiaries, compared with uninsured adults, have increased access to primary and preventive care, reduced out-of-pocket burdens, and are less likely to forgo care. But when compared with adults with private insurance, working age Medicaid adults have greater difficulty obtaining needed medical care.[15] Multiple challenges persist, including provider shortages due to lack of participation, particularly at the specialty level.

The Oregon Health Insurance Experiment: The effects on healthcare outcomes resulting from increasing health coverage to the uninsured have been questioned by some researchers and policymakers, especially because insured individuals tend to be different than the uninsured. Despite attempts to carefully control for differences, uncertainty remains.[16] One of the best attempts to evaluate the effects to increasing healthcare coverage to the uninsured were the results of a study of a lottery that Oregon healthcare officials implemented as part of the state's attempt to increased coverage. After 5 years of budget cuts, in 2008, the state had funds to support 10,000 new enrollees. Predicting a much larger demand, the state used a lottery to select individuals to receive coverage. The application for the lottery had a 30-day window; 90,000 individuals applied and 30,000 of those were selected randomly. Of those, only 60% returned the required forms in time, and half of those were ineligible due to income or other requirements. Around 9000 (30%), were enrolled in Medicaid. As described by journalist Ezra Klein in 2013, "Oregonians who got Medicaid weren't the only winners, though. Early on, a group of eminent health economist realized the lottery offered a chance to conduct a study no one in their discipline had ever managed but everyone had always wanted: a randomized, controlled experiment comparing those who received Medicaid with those who remained uninsured."[17] The 30,000 lottery winners (the treatment group) were then compared with the remainder of the applicants that the lottery excluded (the control group). Researchers collected large amounts of information, including administrative, hospital discharge, mortality, financial and mail survey data for the state, and emergency department visits date for the Portland area (25,000 of treatment and control group).

The first-year data analysis showed key differences between insured and uninsured Oregonians.

MEDICAID'S ROLE IN TRAUMA CARE

AUGUST 2017

Everyone is at risk for a traumatic injury requiring medical attention, such as burns, fractures, or spinal cord or traumatic brain injuries from a car accident, fall or other sudden event.

Medicaid is a safety net for individuals who need trauma care and supports trauma center financing. Over one-third of injuries require ongoing care after the initial hospitalization, and Medicaid is a key provider of long-term care for those with permanently disabling injuries.

Medicaid currently provides federal matching funds with no pre-set limit and enhanced federal funding for states that elect to cover adults who were previously excluded from the program. Medicaid coverage and financing supports states' ability to care for trauma survivors.

Traumatic Injuries are Unexpected and Can Result in Ongoing Health Care Costs

Over 860,000 injuries resulted in an ER visit or hospitalization in 2015.

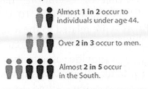

Almost **1 in 2** occur to individuals under age 44.

Over **2 in 3** occur to men.

Almost **2 in 5** occur in the South.

>$25,000

Average outstanding medical bills from injury for people declaring bankruptcy in 2007.

Of the over 860,000 injuries with ER visit or hospitalization in 2015, **7 in 10** involved a fall or car accident.

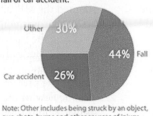

Other 30%

44% Fall

Car accident 26%

Note: Other includes being struck by an object, gun shots, burns and other sources of injury.

Over 40% of injury-related costs result from care after initial hospitalization in 2005.

Average percent of costs for one year following injury:

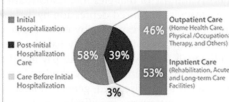

- ■ Initial Hospitalization
- ■ Post-initial Hospitalization Care
- ☐ Care Before Initial Hospitalization

58%   39%

3%

Outpatient Care (Home Health Care, Physical /Occupational Therapy, and Others) 46%

Inpatient Care (Rehabilitation, Acute, and Long-term Care Facilities) 53%

Mean one year costs: $75,210

Medicaid Protects Individuals with Traumatic Injuries from Financial Burdens and Covers Needed Care

The ACA's Medicaid expansion covers people who may lose their income due to an injury and those most at risk of injury such as young men.

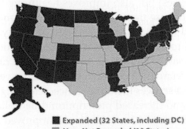

- ■ Expanded (32 States, including DC)
- ☐ Have Not Expanded (19 States)

Half of states offer **optional** Medicaid waiver eligibility and services to people with long-term care needs from **traumatic brain and/or spinal cord injuries**, as of 2013.

Medicaid covers a variety of injury-related care.

All state Medicaid programs cover:
- inpatient and outpatient services
- nursing facilities
- home health care
- prescription drugs
- medical transportation

State Medicaid programs can cover:
- physical therapy and other rehabilitative services
- private duty nursing
- personal care services
- prosthetic devices
- care coordination

Federal Medicaid Financing has Expanded Coverage and Reduced Uncompensated Care Costs

Medicaid covers **22%** of inpatient hospital days at Level I and II Trauma Centers.

Medicaid-covered injury-related hospitalizations have **increased** and **uninsured** stays have **decreased** in Medicaid expansion states compared to non-expansion states.

Median % change between 4th Q 2012 and 2014:

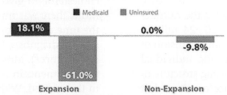

- ■ Medicaid ■ Uninsured

18.1%   0.0%

-9.8%

-61.0%

Expansion   Non-Expansion

Medicaid financing has **increased coverage** of individuals with traumatic injuries for acute and post-acute care, and **protects against unexpected medical bills.**

Sources for this document are available at: http://kff.org/infographic/medicaids-role-in-trauma-care.
The Henry J. Kaiser Family Foundation Headquarters: 2400 Sand Hill Road, Menlo Park, CA 94025 | Phone 650-854-9400
Washington Offices and Barbara Jordan Conference Center: 1330 G Street, NW, Washington, DC 20005 | Phone 202-347-5270
www.kff.org | Email Alerts: kff.org/email | facebook.com/KaiserFamilyFoundation | twitter.com/KaiserFamFound
Filling the need for trusted information on national health issues, the Kaiser Family Foundation is a nonprofit organization based in Menlo Park, California.

FIG. 10.2 Medicaid's role in trauma care.

Medicaid enrollment increased the likelihood of being admitted to the hospital by 30%, outpatient care by 35%, and prescription drug use by 15%. Self-reported outcomes were even more impressive, with 92% of Medicaid recipients reporting receiving all necessary care compared to 68% of the control group. Despite the increase in healthcare utilization, the impacts of health outcomes were less clear. Medicaid had no significant effect on the typical markers of health, including blood pressure, cholesterol, glycosylated hemoglobin, depression, or Framingham cardiovascular risk scores. Glucose control did not improve despite increased diabetes diagnosis and use of diabetes medications after the lottery. Insurance reduced depression by 30% and catastrophic medical expenses by 4.5%. From a financial standpoint, it reduced by half the number of individuals borrowing money to pay healthcare bills, or having unpaid nonmedical bills.[18]

The study, as Klein discussed, generated large amounts of controversy, specifically due to being underpowered to detect changes in health, and questioning the increased expense of a Medicaid expansion (ME). It did unequivocally show that Medicaid provided the basic functions of health insurance, which are providing access to healthcare and protecting from catastrophic expenses. He then quotes Oregon's Governor Johh Kitzhaber, a former emergency room physician, discussing the question of how much healthier did Medicare make these new beneficiaries? "Medicaid is a financing tool. Once people get on Medicaid, they are bought into the same hyperinflationary, inefficient, backloaded medical system as everyone else."[17]

d. Affordable Care Act[19]: This landmark piece of legislation, known as the ACA or Obamacare, and enacted in 2010, is the most significant overhaul and expansion in coverage of the US healthcare system since the introduction of Medicare and Medicaid in 1965. Its major provisions were effective in 2014, and by some estimates, roughly halved the number of uninsured Americans in 2016 to 20–24 million (Fig. 10.1). These effects were due to an expansion of Medicaid eligibility and changes to the individual insurance market. It retained the existing structure of government and employer insurance coverage, but the individual insurance market was changed. Insurers were mandated to accept all applicants regardless of preexisting conditions, and cover a list of essential health benefits, and individuals were obligated to buy insurance or pay a fine (individual mandate), to avoid adverse selection (less healthy

will buy insurance, with their care being more expensive than their premiums, while the healthy do not buy it, decreasing the benefit of risk pooling). The ACA has faced fierce political opposition and calls for repeal and major legal challenges. In a 2012 Supreme Court ruling, states were given the freedom to choose not to participate in the Law's ME, while upholding the law. The Tax Cuts and Jobs Act of 2017 set the individual mandate at $0, starting in 2019, and raised questions about the constitutionality of the ACA. In 2021, the ACA was upheld for a third time by the Supreme Court. At the time of this writing, 40 states, including the District of Columbia, have adopted the ME, and 11 states have not (Fig. 10.3).[20] Many concerns with the ACA are related to the ME, including the increased cost to states and the argument that Medicaid does not provide value to its beneficiaries.[21,22] The evidence, though, points toward some proven benefits to being insured. In a 2017 review of the existing evidence, specially focusing on the results of the ACA, Sommers, Gawande, and Baicker[23] discussed how being insured does not only provide a benefit with regard to the beneficiary's finances (decrease in medical bills sent to collection and elimination of catastrophic out-of-pocket expenses) but also improves healthcare utilization, disease treatment and outcomes, and self-reported health and may decrease mortality. With regard to access to healthcare and utilization, the authors saw increasing rates of outpatient care utilization, retaining a personal physician, preventative visits and services including cancer screening and lab testing, and increased prescription drug utilization and adherence. The evidence on improved utilization of emergency department was mixed thought. They saw improvement in chronic condition diagnosis and treatment rates, specifically in depression. As the Oregon Experiment showed, there were no significant changes in blood pressure, cholesterol, or glycosylated hemoglobin. Furthermore, there was mixed evidence on cancer staging at the time of diagnosis (no change on breast cancer stage at diagnosis, but improvements in cervical and colon cancer). Most notably, many studies show improvements in self-reported health and well-being in the insured. With regard to mortality, the results were less clear. The authors acknowledge that the observational studies have mixed results, and the only randomized study lacked the sample size and subject follow-up time, to give a more definitive answer. Quasi-experimental studies, the authors suggest, show that mortality can be improved by

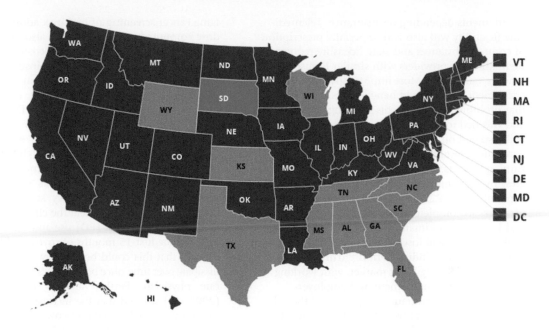

■ Adopted and Implemented   ■ Adopted but Not Implemented   ■ Not Adopted

SOURCE: Kaiser Family Foundation, kff.org

FIG. 10.3 Status of state action on the medicaid expansion decision.

insurance when looking at "healthcare-amenable" conditions such as heart disease, infections, and cancer.

A systematic review of 77 published studies evaluating the effects of the ME under the ACA had similar findings, including increases in access to care, driven by increases in insurance coverage and use of health services. These improvements were seen in non-ACA MEs that preceded the law, in Massachusetts, Oregon, and New York. Gaining access to care resulted in improvements in health, with reduction in chronic condition healthcare spending, improved work productivity, and better quality of life. With regard to quality of care, improvements were seen in at least half of the studies (despite few studies in this area), including preventive care, chronic care management, and postoperative morbidity. A small number of studies looking at healthcare spending showed the increases were almost entirely due to increased federal spending.[24]

e. COVID 19: The coronavirus disease (COVID-19), the infectious disease caused by the SARS-CoV-2 virus, created a worldwide pandemic at the beginning of 2020. The US federal government put in place an emergency declaration early that year to combat the health crisis. It provided the government with flexibility to waive or modify certain requirements in a range of areas, including Medicaid, Medicare, and CHIP programs, as well as in private health insurances. This constituted another major overhaul of health insurance coverage, this time in response to a nationwide catastrophic health event.

The public health emergency will expire at the time of this writing, on May 11, 2023. It will have several implications that will be seen in the years to come. With regard to vaccines, prices will not change for as long as federally purchased supplies last; after that, due to ACA and other provisions, vaccines should continue to be free for insured people. Unfortunately, for the uninsured, the cost of vaccines may become a barrier. At-home or rapid testing cost will increase for those with private insurance, and for those on Medicare, depending on the plan; it will continue to be free for Medicaid beneficiaries and will be costly for the uninsured. COVID treatments, specifically pharmaceuticals, will have cost sharing requirements depending on insurance. Telemedicine flexibility will also end, especially prescription of control substances and state licensure requirement allowing providers with similar licenses to practice remotely.[25] Most importantly, continuous enrollment for Medicaid beneficiaries, a provision that prohibits states from disenrolling beneficiaries and was tied to the public healthcare emergency, will also end on March 31, 2023. Continuous enrollment resulted in record number of people gaining benefits. Medicaid and CHIP enrollment grew by 19.8 million or 27.9%, to 90.9 million in September of 2022. It will take approximately 1 year for states to complete this disenrollment process, and it has been estimated that between 5 and 14 million people will lose Medicaid coverage during the 12-month unwinding period.[26] This effect could be offset by a strong labor market, with working adults regaining employment and employer-sponsored health insurance for them and their dependents. The unemployed, their dependents, the elderly or disabled will likely suffer the negative effects of lack of healthcare access.

Insurance influence in initiation, progression, and outcomes of surgical disease: insurance coverage allows access to healthcare services, including screening for malignancies that require surgical treatment as well as emergent, elective, and specialized surgical care:

a. Cancer screening: The American Cancer Society prevention and early detection guidelines recommend screening tests for the early detection of cancers of the breast, cervix, colon and rectum, endometrium, lung, and prostate, as well as risk reduction strategies including lifestyle changes, smoking cessation, and the use of the papilloma virus vaccine.[27] Lack or lapse of insurance can be responsible for decreased screening rates. In a study of patterns of cancer screening using the US National Health Insurance Survey, researchers found that cervical and breast cancer screening prevalence had decreased in 2015 compared with 2008 and was below DHHS's Healthy People 2020 (HP2020) targets (pap smear 81.5% from 84.5%, target 93%; mammogram 71.7% from 73.7%, target 81.1%). Rates were lower for those without a usual source of healthcare, with public insurance, or uninsured. Conversely, colorectal cancer (CRC) screening increased in both men and women but did not reach HP2020 targets (61.9% and 63.4% respectively, from 52.1%, target 70.5%). CRC screening rates were also lower for those without a usual source of healthcare, with public insurance or uninsured.[28]

Lung cancer screening of high-risk adults with low-dose computed tomography can also be improved by increased access to care, with screening rates being three times higher among the insured than the uninsured.[29] One study shows that turning 65, which allows for universal access to Medicare, increased lung cancer screening rates. From 2017 to 2019, lung cancer screening rates significantly increased in high-risk Medicare eligible men (16.2%), but not significantly in high-risk women (1.6%). Screening rates in high risk men and women below the age of 65 were as low as 5%.[30]

b. Insurance status and emergency surgical care: The Oregon Experiment looked at the effect of the ME in emergency department (ED) use and saw a 40% increase in the first 15 months of coverage. Researchers thought that this could be an early effect that could dissipate over time once beneficiaries found a primary care physician. Further analysis of 2-year data (2007−10) showed that the increase in ED use persisted. Interestingly, Medicaid coverage increased the probability of a person having both an ED and an office visit by 13.2%. PCP office visits may had encouraged ED visits as described by one quoted study participant: "I went to the doctor's office one time and they said, no, you need to go to the ER because your blood sugar is way too high, it's going to take hours to get it down. So you need to go the ER."[31] Acute Cholecystitis is a common surgical condition and can be used to uncover disparities of emergent surgical care related to health insurance status. Researchers from the Massachusetts General Hospital looked at the impact of the 2006 Massachusetts healthcare coverage expansion in the management of acute cholecystitis (cholecystectomy at the time of admission or not), and compared their state to three control states. Prior to the reform, privately insured patients were more likely to receive cholecystectomy during hospital admission than government-insured or self-pay patients (85.9% vs. 76.8%). Adjusted analysis found that compared with the insured, the uninsured had a 6.6% lower probability of cholecystectomy in Massachusetts, and a 9.9% lower probability in the control states prior to the reform, and a 4.3% and 10.3% lower probability postreform, respectively, suggesting a beneficial effect of being insured. The differences were only seen in patients presenting with uncomplicated disease; there were no differences in the rates of presentation, or immediate cholecystectomy for complicated disease.[32] Another study looked at quality of acute cholecystitis care between Medicaid and non-

Medicaid patients and found no differences in rates of laparoscopic cholecystectomy, time to surgery or length of stay. The only difference seen was in hospital readmissions (30.4% vs. 17.9%, $P = .001$), and multivariate analysis could not explain any independent predictors. Researchers point out that one-third of Medicaid patients required an interpreter, potentially complicating postoperative care discharge instructions.[33]

c. Insurance status and elective surgical care: Those surgeries that do not have to be performed emergently are considered elective. The effect of insurance coverage on bariatric or weight loss surgery, due to its proven safety and effectiveness, high cost ($20,000 to $25,000), and potential for life threatening postoperative complications, is a good example to discuss. The American Society of Metabolic and Bariatric Surgery (ASBMS) has recently updated their recommendation for these types of procedures, to include individuals with a body mass index (BMI) of 35 or more regardless of the presence, absence, or severity of obesity-related conditions, and to be considered in people with BMI 30–34.9 with metabolic disease, those with BMI starting at 30 without metabolic disease but unable to achieve substantial or durable weight loss, as well as appropriately selected children and adolescents.[34] Despite increased eligibility criteria for bariatric surgery, insurance coverage is restricted, and some policies do not cover it. Under the ACA, 23 of 50 states require that health insurers selling plans in the marketplace or directly to individuals cover bariatric surgery under the ACA's "essential health benefit" provision. This provision does not apply to employer-sponsored insurance.[35] Uninsured patients must pay out-of-pocket; some bariatric centers will help these patients get a loan. To get coverage, most insurance companies require proof of medical necessity, participation in a physician-supervised diet program for 6 months (with a minimum documentation of no weight gain), a psychological evaluation, and a nutritional evaluation.[36] A study of the effect of presurgical insurance requirements showed that longer diet requirements, PCP letter of necessity, cardiology evaluation, and advanced laboratory testing were independent predictors of not receiving surgery after initial evaluation, despite lack of evidence of improved clinical outcomes with these requirements. During the waiting period, patients experienced significant weight gain.[37]

d. Insurance status and cancer care: Researchers from Georgetown University evaluated the New York State 2001 Pre-ACA ME to nondisabled adults with earnings up to 100% above federal poverty line, and its effect of surgical cancer care. Utilizing the state's Inpatient Database from 1997 to 2006, they found that the proportion of cancer operations paid by Medicaid increased from 8.9% to 15.1% in the 5 years after the expansion, with a precipitous drop of 21.3% in the uninsured rate. The overall all-payer case remained stable though. The authors speculated that when evaluating lifesaving operations, compared with elective surgeries, such as joint replacements, the main effect of expanding insurance coverage is a shift of the financial burden from patients and hospitals to Medicaid, and not an increase in demand.[38]

When looking specifically at the most common cancers in the United States, the effect of the ME shows some interesting insights. In a 2018 study from the University of Louisville, researchers evaluated the effect of the ACA ME in breast cancer care utilizing the Kentucky Cancer Registry (KCR). As expected, after the 2014 ME came into effect, the uninsured rate dropped from 3.7% to 1%, and Medicaid coverage increased from 10.9% to 15%. More importantly, there were significantly increased rates of early-stage breast cancer at presentation (66.7% vs. 64.5%), and breast conservation (48.8% vs. 44%). Despite these improvements, time from diagnosis to first treatment was significantly increased (36 vs. 28 days).[39] A nationwide study in 2017 showed that insurance status could influence local therapy in breast cancer, as well as stage of presentation. Medicaid or uninsured patients were more likely to have large, node-positive tumors. Medicaid insurance was found to be significantly associated with receipt of mastectomy, while both Medicaid and uninsured status were associated with omission of radiotherapy after lumpectomy. The authors concluded that while unable to determine patient's choice, specific insurance status is associated with departure from the standard of care.[40] A 2023 study of breast cancer outcomes, comparing states that expanded Medicaid (Louisiana, Kentucky and Arkansas) to those that did not (Tennessee, Alabama, Mississippi, Texas, and Oklahoma), found a 10% increase in Medicaid patients in the former, with a 1.3% decrease in the latter, and a 2.3% decrease in distant disease diagnosis compared with a 0.5% increase, respectively.[41]

With regard to CRC, researchers from the University of Kentucky, using the KCR, found that after the ME, Medicaid recipients had increases in CRC screening by 230%, incidence of CRC by 6.7%, and early-stage diagnosis by 9.3%. CRC survival was noted to improve also (hazard ration 0.73, $P < .01$).[42] A 2020 National Cancer Database study, comparing ME with non-ME states, found an increase in Medicaid coverage, less distance traveled, and increased likelihood of treatment at integrated network programs in ME states. In these, more early-stage CRC patients were treated within 30 days, more stage IV patients received palliative care, less patients needed urgent surgical intervention, and more patients received minimally invasive procedures.[43]

Ultimately, the goal of early detection via screening and treatment of cancer is to prevent deaths. Researchers from the Harvard School of Public Health compared mortality in ME versus non-ME states in newly diagnosed breast, colorectal, and lung cancers, from the National Cancer Database, from 2012 to 2015. They found that ME was associated with a decreased hazard of mortality, which was largely mediated by earlier stage of diagnosis (mortality improvements were no longer evident after adjusting for cancer stage). After the ME, lung cancer mortality decreased overall but mostly in the ME states, while breast and colorectal cancer mortality was worse overall, but significantly worse in non-ME states. The absolute differences were small but significant at 0.4% (meaning that 250 patients with cancer would need to gain coverage to prevent 1 death, 4 years after cancer diagnosis).[44]

e. Insurance status and organ transplantation: A 2014 article describes the "heartfelt story" of three patients in need for a transplant, who, despite living close to six transplant centers in Chicago, were denied evaluation due to being uninsured. The authors describe how "in theory, the organ allocation system in the US is based on justice and equity (per the National Organ Transplant Act of 1984). Fair allocation of organ transplants is unrealized. The uninsured are systematically denied access to transplant evaluation."[45] Of those insured, outcomes are worse for patients on governmental insurance. A 2020 study of liver transplant outcomes from the US Scientific Registry of Transplant Recipients found a 60:40 private to governmental insurance distribution, with 56% eventually receiving a transplant and 22% dropping off the list. Medicare or Medicaid status was found to be independently associated with lower chance of receiving a transplant and higher posttransplant mortality.[46]

DISCUSSION

Insurance as a SDOH discussions cannot be had without mentioning the increasing cost of care. As discussed by David Goldhill, in his 2009 editorial "How American Health Care Killed My Father", the United States spends 18% of GDP in healthcare. The author questioned if society had a mechanism to determine if healthcare expenditures provide better health than investments in other SDOH, such as cleaner air or water, better nutrition, recreation, or outdoor spaces? His answer: "No, healthcare simply keeps gobbling up national resources, without regard to other societal needs. As new tests and treatments are developed, they are, for the most part, added to our medicare or commercial insurance policies, no matter what they cost."[47]

Value-based insurance design (VBID) is a promising solution to the misallocation of underused high-value care. It selectively reduces or eliminates financial barriers to evidence-based care that improves patient-centered outcomes (such as cardiac and pulmonary rehabilitation, tobacco cessation, and hemoglobin A1 testing) and increases cost sharing for low-value care (such as spinal fusions, vertebroplasty and kyphoplasty, or unnecessary imaging). The incremental expenditures incurred by the increased use of high-value care will be offset by the savings from reduced use of low-value care.[48] It has been suggested that cost containment through high deductible healthcare plans, aimed to discourage unnecessary healthcare utilization, should be replaced by a more nuanced VBID, which aligns patient's out-of-pocket cost with the value of specific services, as in the case of Bariatric surgery discussed before. Surgeons should lobby insurers to make these changes. As suggested in the bariatric surgery example, which applies to many other surgical conditions, it is "time for surgeons to lead the charge."[35]

Highlights

- Insurance allows people to access the healthcare they need and avoid catastrophic healthcare expenses.
- Risk pooling is achieved when both healthy and sick individuals are insured.
- Most working adults and their dependents are covered by employer-based insurance, while Medicare covers the elderly and disabled, and Medicaid covers those with low income, pregnant women, and children.
- The Affordable Care Act (ACA), and especially the Medicaid expansion, has dramatically increased insurance coverage with measurable improvements in surgical care access and surgical outcomes.

> **Highlights—cont'd**
>
> - Despite these gains, Medicaid and uninsured patients are likely to have worse outcomes when compared with privately insured patients for similar surgically treated conditions.

REFERENCES

1. Healthy People 2030, U.S. Department of Health and Human Services, Office of Disease Prevention and Health Promotion. https://health.gov/healthypeople/priority-areas/social-determinants-health.
2. Berchick ER, Hood E, Barnett JC. *Health Insurance Coverage in the United States: 2017*. 2018.
3. Keiser-Starkey K, Bunch LN. *Health Insurance Coverage in the United States: 2021*. US Census; 2022. https://www.census.gov/library/publications/2022/demo/p60-278.html.
4. Baicker K, Chandra A. Myths and misconceptions about U.S. health insurance. *Health Aff*. Nov-Dec 2008;27(6):w533–w543. https://doi.org/10.1377/hlthaff.27.6.w533.
5. Kagan J, Catalano TJ. *Health Insurance: Definition, How it Works*. 2022.
6. Reinhardt UE. Employer-based health insurance: a balance sheet. *Health Aff*. Nov-Dec 1999;18(6):124–132. https://doi.org/10.1377/hlthaff.18.6.124.
7. Gruber J, Hanratty M, Gruber J, National Bureau of Economic R. The labor market effects of introducing national health insurance: evidence from Canada. In: *NBER Working Paper Series No W4589*. National Bureau of Economic Research; 1993.
8. *Kaiser/Commonwealth*. National Survey of Health Insurance; 1997.
9. Jones D, Molitor D, Reif J. What do workplace wellness programs do? Evidence from the Illinois Workplace wellness study. *Q J Econ*. November 2019;134(4):1747–1791. https://doi.org/10.1093/qje/qjz023.
10. Goetzel RZ, Commentary on the Study. What do Workplace wellness programs do? Evidence from the Illinois Workplace wellness study. *Am J Health Promot*. May 2020;34(4):440–444. https://doi.org/10.1177/0890117120906664.
11. Kaiser Family Foundation. *An Overview of Medicare*. KFF; 2019.
12. Kaiser Family Foundation. *Analysis of Center of Medicare and Medicaid Services 2016 Medicare Current Beneficiary Survey*. KFF; 2016.
13. Kaiser Family Foundation. *Medicaid: A Primer*. The Kaiser Commission on Medicaid and the Uninsured; 2013.
14. Services DoHaH. *2012 Annual Report on Quality of Care for Children in Medicaid and CHIP*. December 2012.
15. Office GA. *States Made Multiple Program Changes, and Beneficiaries Generally Reported Access Comparable to Private Insurance*. November 2012.
16. Kolata G. *Study Finds Benefits in Health Insurance for the Poor*. New York Times; July 7, 2011.
17. Klein E. *Is the Future of American Health Care in Oregon?* The Washington Post; May 20, 2013.
18. Finkelstein A, Taubman S, Wright B, et al. The Oregon health insurance experiment: evidence from the first year. *Q J Econ*. August 2012;127(3):1057–1106. https://doi.org/10.1093/qje/qjs020.
19. *Affordable Care Act*. Wikipedia; 2023.
20. Foundation KF. *Status of State Medicaid Expansion Decisions: Interactive Map*. November 09, 2022, 2019.
21. Gottlieb S. *Medicaid Is Worse than No Coverage at All*. Wall Street Journal; March 10, 2011.
22. Sommers BD, Grabowski DC. What is Medicaid? More than meets the eye. *JAMA*. August 22, 2017;318(8):695–696. https://doi.org/10.1001/jama.2017.10304.
23. Sommers BD, Gawande AA, Baicker K. Health insurance coverage and health - what the recent evidence tells Us. *N Engl J Med*. August 10, 2017;377(6):586–593. https://doi.org/10.1056/NEJMsb1706645.
24. Mazurenko O, Balio CP, Agarwal R, Carroll AE, Menachemi N. The effects of Medicaid expansion under the ACA: a systematic review. *Health Aff*. June 2018;37(6):944–950. https://doi.org/10.1377/hlthaff.2017.1491.
25. Cox C. *The End of the COVID-19 Public Health Emergency: Details on Health Coverage and Access*. February 03, 2023.
26. Tolbert J. *10 Things to Know about the Unwinding of the Medicaid Continuous Enrollment Provision*. January 11, 2023.
27. Society AC. American Cancer Society Prevention and Early Detection Guidelines.
28. Hall IJ, Tangka FKL, Sabatino SA, Thompson TD, Graubard BI, Breen N. Patterns and trends in cancer screening in the United States. *Prev Chronic Dis*. July 26, 2018;15:E97. https://doi.org/10.5888/pcd15.170465.
29. Zahnd WE, Eberth JM. Lung cancer screening utilization: a behavioral risk factor surveillance system analysis. *Am J Prev Med*. August 2019;57(2):250–255. https://doi.org/10.1016/j.amepre.2019.03.015.
30. Sun J, Perraillon MC, Myerson R. The impact of Medicare health insurance coverage on lung cancer screening. *Med Care*. January 1, 2022;60(1):29–36. https://doi.org/10.1097/mlr.0000000000001655.
31. Finkelstein AN, Taubman SL, Allen HL, Wright BJ, Baicker K. Effect of Medicaid coverage on ED Use - further evidence from Oregon's experiment. *N Engl J Med*. October 20, 2016;375(16):1505–1507. https://doi.org/10.1056/NEJMp1609533.
32. Loehrer AP, Song Z, Auchincloss HG, Hutter MM. Influence of health insurance expansion on disparities in the treatment of acute cholecystitis. *Ann Surg*. July 2015;262(1):139–145. https://doi.org/10.1097/sla.0000000000000970.
33. Fazzalari A, Pozzi N, Alfego D, et al. Treatment of acute cholecystitis: do Medicaid and non-medicaid enrolled patients receive the same care? *J Gastrointest Surg*. April 2020;24(4):939–948. https://doi.org/10.1007/s11605-019-04471-y.

34. Surgery ASoMaB. *After 30 Years - New Guidelines for Weight-Loss Surgery.* October 21, 2022.

35. Chhabra KR, Dimick JB, Fendrick AM. Value-based insurance coverage for bariatric surgery: time for surgeons to lead the change. *Surg Obes Relat Dis.* January 2019;15(1): 152–154. https://doi.org/10.1016/j.soard.2018.11.012.

36. Davis JL. *Paying for Weight Loss Surgery.* WebMD; 2021.

37. Love KM, Mehaffey JH, Safavian D, et al. Bariatric surgery insurance requirements independently predict surgery dropout. *Surg Obes Relat Dis.* May 2017;13(5):871–876. https://doi.org/10.1016/j.soard.2017.01.022.

38. Al-Refaie WB, Zheng C, Jindal M, et al. Did pre-affordable care act Medicaid expansion increase access to surgical cancer care? *J Am Coll Surg.* April 2017;224(4):662–669. https://doi.org/10.1016/j.jamcollsurg.2016.12.044.

39. Ajkay N, Bhutiani N, Huang B, et al. Early impact of Medicaid expansion and quality of breast cancer care in Kentucky. *J Am Coll Surg.* April 2018;226(4):498–504. https://doi.org/10.1016/j.jamcollsurg.2017.12.041.

40. Churilla TM, Egleston B, Bleicher R, Dong Y, Meyer J, Anderson P. Disparities in the local management of breast cancer in the US according to health insurance status. *Breast J.* March 2017;23(2):169–176. https://doi.org/10.1111/tbj.12705.

41. Laughlin AI, Li T, Yu Q, et al. Impact of Medicaid expansion on breast cancer diagnosis and treatment in southern states. *J Am Coll Surg.* February 1, 2023. https://doi.org/10.1097/xcs.0000000000000550.

42. Gan T, Sinner HF, Walling SC, et al. Impact of the affordable care Act on colorectal cancer screening, incidence, and survival in Kentucky. *J Am Coll Surg.* April 2019;228(4):342–353. https://doi.org/10.1016/j.jamcollsurg.2018.12.035.

43. Hoehn RS, Rieser CJ, Phelos H, et al. Association between Medicaid expansion and diagnosis and management of colon cancer. *J Am Coll Surg.* February 2021;232(2):146–156. https://doi.org/10.1016/j.jamcollsurg.2020.10.021.

44. Lam MB, Phelan J, Orav EJ, Jha AK, Keating NL. Medicaid expansion and mortality among patients with breast lung, and colorectal cancer. *JAMA Netw Open.* November 2, 2020;3(11):e2024366. https://doi.org/10.1001/jamanetworkopen.2020.24366.

45. Ansell D. *When the Only Cure Is A Transplant.* Health Affairs; February 21, 2014.

46. Stepanova M, Al Qahtani S, Mishra A, Younossi I, Venkatesan C, Younossi ZM. Outcomes of liver transplantation by insurance types in the United States. *Am J Manag Care.* April 1, 2020;26(4):e121–e126. https://doi.org/10.37765/ajmc.2020.42839.

47. Godhill D. How American health care killed my father. *Atlantic.* September 2009;304(2):38–55.

48. Michigan Center for Value-Based Insurance Design.

CHAPTER 11

Health Literacy

MIRA L. KATZ, PHD, MPH

The value of using narratives in health has been thoroughly demonstrated; therefore, I begin this chapter with a short story about a patient who taught me the importance of health literacy and the need for clear and effective patient–provider communication.

A 65-year-old female experienced multiple transient ischemic attacks during a 1-week period. A carotid ultrasound examination showed significant bilateral internal carotid artery disease. A surgeon met with the patient and explained the results of the ultrasound examination and recommended the patient have a carotid endarterectomy. As the surgeon left the examination room and the door closed, the patient turned to me and said "I did not understand a word the doctor said. Can you please explain it to me?" I took time with the patient and used plain, everyday language to explain the results of the ultrasound test and the recommended operation.

Before the patient left, I checked her understanding by using the teach-back methodology. Later that day, I told the surgeon that I had clarified everything with the patient because she had not understood his explanation of the ultrasound test or the recommended surgical procedure. The surgeon was genuinely surprised because he thought he had explained everything to her and she had not asked any questions.

This summary of a true story demonstrates that even with good intentions, healthcare professionals often lack awareness of their inability to provide clear medical information to patients. Furthermore, the story highlights two additional important points: first, patients are often unfamiliar with medical information or do not understand the medical terminology, jargon, or acronyms that healthcare professionals use when discussing health-related topics with them, and second, patients may be too uncomfortable or embarrassed to express their lack of understanding. Therefore, clear, direct, and effective communication is essential among patients, surgeons, and members of the surgical team to enable patients to make informed decisions that will result in the best possible surgical outcomes, improve their quality of life, and increase satisfaction with their care.

In this chapter, I provide an overview of health literacy and its relevance to surgical patients, surgeons, and members of the surgical team and the healthcare system. This chapter defines health literacy, reviews health literacy as a social determinant of health, and discusses the prevalence of health literacy among adults in the United States and the importance of health literacy in the practice of surgery. In addition, this chapter describes instruments commonly used to measure health literacy, the estimated cost associated with limited health literacy, potential challenges in and strategies for addressing patients with limited health literacy, and suggestions for future directions.

WHAT IS HEALTH LITERACY?

Several definitions of health literacy have been used during the past decades, and its evolving description highlights the complex role it plays in health. The early definitions of health literacy considered it as an individual-level factor and focused on individuals' skills and deficits. In fact, the American Medical Association Ad Hoc Committee on Health Literacy proposed one of the early definitions in 1999, describing functional health literacy as "a constellation of skills, including the ability to perform basic reading and numerical tasks required to function in the health care environment."[1] Several investigators proposed revised descriptions of the term, including the Institute of Medicine, which defined it as "the degree to which individuals have the capacity to obtain, process, and understand basic health information and services needed to make appropriate health decisions" in its 2004 report, *Health Literacy: A Prescription to End Confusion.*[2]

The national initiative *Healthy People 2030*[3] includes attaining health literacy in one of its foundational principles and in one of its overarching goals and offers an expanded definition that considers health literacy as multidimensional, including both personal and organizational health literacy. This more recent definition of health literacy considers an individual's capabilities as well as their access to resources and the influence of the complex healthcare

Social Determinants of Health in Surgery. https://doi.org/10.1016/B978-0-443-12366-5.00015-2

system on their health and others.[4] It describes personal health literacy as "the degree to which individuals have the ability to find, understand, and use information and services to inform health-related decisions and actions for themselves and others," and organizational health literacy as "the degree to which organizations equitably enable individuals to find, understand, and use information and services to inform health-related decisions and actions for themselves and others."[3,4]

Although there are many dimensions to health literacy, numeracy—often referred to as quantitative literacy—is considered one of its major features and has been defined as "the ability to access, use, interpret, and communicate mathematical information and ideas, to engage in and manage the mathematical demands of a range of situations in adult life."[5] Numeracy has also been described as "how facile people are with mathematical concepts and their applications."[6] In the context of health literacy, health numeracy has been defined as "the degree to which individuals have the capacity to access, process, interpret, communicate, and act on numerical, quantitative, graphical, biostatistical, and probabilistic health information needed to make effective health decisions."[7] An individual's math skills are considered objective numeracy, and their self-assessment of their understanding of mathematical data is characterized as subjective numeracy. A proposed framework has operationalized health numeracy into four functional and overlapping categories: basic (e.g., identifying numbers), computational (e.g., performing simple calculations), analytical (e.g., making sense of information and understanding percentages and basic graphs), and statistical (e.g., understanding probabilities and complex health information).[7] Other investigators have proposed a health numeracy model that includes six main functions (facilitating computation, encouraging more information seeking, improving interpretation of the meaning of provided numbers, facilitating assessment of likelihood and value, increasing or decreasing acceptance of numerical data, and promoting individuals to act and make a behavioral change).[6]

The updated concept of health literacy includes several factors––notably health numeracy (e.g., understanding of risk)––considers the influence of health institutions, provides an ecological perspective of health, and recognizes the complex contextual influences on personal health literacy that enable individuals to access, understand, and use information to navigate the healthcare system. This expanded definition of health literacy is critical for patients, surgeons, and the surgical

team and healthcare organizations in the perioperative period.

HEALTH LITERACY AS A SOCIAL DETERMINANT OF HEALTH

Evaluating the influence of health literacy alone on health outcomes is challenging as it is associated with many other established social determinants of health, including educational, economic, environmental, cultural, and social factors.[8,9] Many of these factors (Fig. 11.1) have been shown to influence individuals' access to care, and their abilities to communicate and apply critical skills to seek, analyze, and use information to address their health. Moreover, having inadequate health literacy is associated with less access to timely and quality care, increased healthcare costs, an extensive range of health-related behaviors and outcomes, including a lack of adherence to prescribed medications, less frequent use of preventive services, poor management of chronic diseases, more use of emergency care and hospitalizations, and higher morbidity and mortality rates.[10,11]

There are two opposing perspectives on health literacy as a social determinant of health.[12] The clinical perspective considers it a *risk factor* and focuses on screening for limited health literacy among patients who interact with healthcare providers and systems. This perspective is goal-oriented and aims to develop health information interventions that improve patient–provider communication to optimize care in complex healthcare environments. The opposing perspective of health literacy considers it an *asset* and is aligned with health promotion and public health. This perspective focuses on developing and implementing interactive and adaptable interventions to improve health outcomes by improving individuals' knowledge and decision-making skills to empower them to take control of their health.[9] Both perspectives are relevant and reflect the importance of health literacy for clinical care and public health as well as its contribution to achieving health equity.[13]

It is also important to recognize that health literacy has three potential causal mechanisms of impacting health: directly as a social determinant of health, as a mediator between other social determinants of health and health, or as a moderator of the effect of other social determinants on health.[13,14] The different potential relationships of health literacy, other social determinants of health, and health outcomes draw attention to this multifaceted concept. To explain the complex causal relationship of health literacy and other factors,

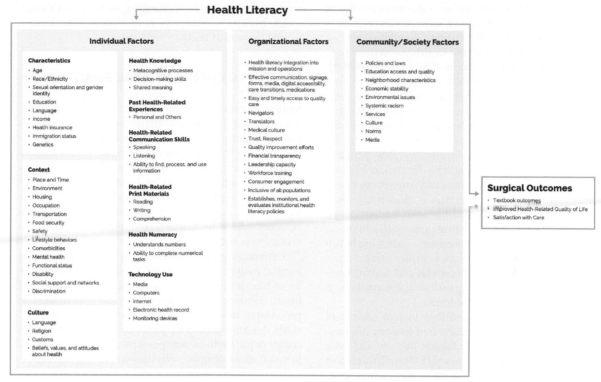

FIG. 11.1 Factors influencing the health literacy of surgical patients.

several frameworks have been proposed to explain the association of health literacy and health outcomes.[15–17]

Social determinants of health are also gaining recognition for the important role they play for surgical patients[18,19]; thus, further research and discussion of health literacy as a social determinant of health is warranted to better understand its impact on how patients navigate the perioperative period.

In addition to personal health literacy, organizational health literacy also impacts the ability of surgical patients to navigate the healthcare system during the perioperative period. In 2012, the Institute of Medicine's Roundtable on Health Literacy published the *Ten Attributes of Health Literate Health Care Organizations*,[20] providing strategies to improve patients' experiences by including health literacy as an organizational value. Surgeons, as healthcare providers and leaders in organizations, can play a significant role in establishing and maintaining strategies to improve organizational literacy to meet the needs of all patients.

The Agency for Healthcare Research and Quality (AHRQ) developed a Health Literacy Universal Precautions Toolkit that includes tools to improve clear communication (oral and print), patient self-management and empowerment, and supportive systems.[21] Although the AHRQ toolkit is designed to provide evidence-based guidance for primary care settings, many of the tools are applicable to and may benefit other types of medical practices, including surgery.

Many factors at the individual, interpersonal, organizational, community, and societal levels may influence an individual's health literacy, which complicates the process of documenting health literacy as an independent social determinant of health. Therefore, a necessary step in understanding the concept of health literacy and the role it may play in the perioperative period is to consider its prevalence in the general adult population and among surgical patients as well as how it measured.

PREVALENCE OF HEALTH LITERACY

The 2003 National Assessment of Adult Literacy (NAAL) assessed more than 19,000 adults (ages 16 and older) in the United States and included 28 health literacy items addressing a range of literacy activities that adults generally face in their everyday life.[22] The health literacy assessment addressed three different domains of healthcare information and services: clinical (e.g., medication instructions), prevention (e.g., how exercise habits decrease the risk for developing serious illness), and navigation of the healthcare system (e.g., what a health insurance plan will or will not pay for). The NAAL results categorized participants into four health literacy levels: *below basic,* indicating the most simple health literacy skills (e.g., locating easily identifiable information in a short text, locating numbers, and performing addition); *basic,* implying health literacy skills needed to perform simple, everyday activities (e.g., reading and understanding information in prose text and simple math); *intermediate,* suggesting health literacy skills needed to perform moderately challenging activities (e.g., reading and understanding moderately dense text and using quantitative information to solve problems); and *proficient,* indicating health literacy skills needed to perform complex literacy activities (e.g., reading complex prose text and making complex inferences and using quantitative information to solve multistep complex problems).

The NAAL findings showed that 14% of adults had below basic health literacy, 22% had basic health literacy, 53% had intermediate health literacy, and only 12% had proficient health literacy.[22] Overall, this report suggests that only 12% of adults in the United States were proficient in the skills needed to manage and navigate the complex healthcare system and that slightly over a third had basic or below basic health literacy skills. Additionally, individuals in the two lowest levels of health literacy tended to be males, Hispanic or Black, and aged 65 and older; have less than a high school education; live below the poverty threshold; have Medicare, Medicaid, or no health insurance; rate their overall health as poor or fair; and not seek information about health-related issues.[22]

Although not specific to health literacy, the Program for the International Assessment of Adult Competencies (PIAAC) conducted in 2012/2014 (combined years) and 2017 offers a more recent measure of literacy, numeracy, and digital problem-solving among adults in the United States.[5] The PIAAC results categorize participants into six proficiency levels for literacy and numeracy and four for digital problem-solving and include those who could not participate due to cognitive or physical inabilities or language barriers. In 2017, 19%, 29%, and 62% of adults in the United States were in the two lowest proficiency levels (below level 1 and level 1) for literacy, numeracy, and digital problem-solving skills, respectively.[5] The findings from these national assessments suggest that more than one-third of adults living in the United States

may find it especially challenging to read and understand health information and/or complete health-related numerical tasks.

HEALTH LITERACY AND THE PRACTICE OF SURGERY

Systematic reviews of health literacy among surgical patients suggest that approximately one-third of patients undergoing surgical procedures have inadequate health literacy.[23,24] The prevalence of limited health literacy among surgical patients is similar to the findings in the general adult population in the United States.[22] Also similar to the general population, surgical patients with limited health literacy tend to be male, older in age, not fluent in English, and have less education and a lower socioeconomic status.[24]

Determining the influence of health literacy among surgical patients is challenging due to the intersectionality of health literacy with other social determinants of health. Furthermore, studies vary by the type of surgical procedure, health literacy measurement instrument, study design, number of patients, and measured outcomes (e.g., length of stay, postoperative complications, hospital readmissions.). But despite the inconsistent results, studies of surgical patients indicate that those with limited health literacy ask fewer questions during office visits,[25] are less adherent to preoperative medication instructions,[26] and have longer hospital stays[27,28] and more postoperative complications.[29,30]

Scoping reviews have also examined health literacy among patients of surgical subspecialities including neurosurgery patients[31] and those undergoing plastic surgery.[32] The findings of these scoping reviews suggest that additional efforts must accommodate surgical patients by assessing their health literacy, using plain language and pictures to develop educational materials aimed at a fifth grade reading level, using teach-back strategies, and developing interventions to improve patients' understanding of their care.

Information about health numeracy among surgical patients is limited. Although numerical information is important in everyday life, the ability to understand and use numbers is an especially valuable skill for patients as it enables them to weigh risks and benefits to make informed decisions in the management of their health. Specifically, surgical patients need good numeracy skills to make informed decisions given the benefits and risks associated with a recommended procedure.[33] In addition, good numeracy skills are important for surgeons, who need to provide patients with accurate information about treatment options, the expected outcomes of a surgical procedure, the risk of potential complications associated with a recommended procedure, and the implications for the patient's quality of life.[33,34]

For surgical patients, health literacy and health numeracy are associated with correctly following preoperative instructions and postoperative discharge instructions as well as understanding the consent process. Although it is impossible to name every factor and behavior associated with a surgical patient's health literacy and health numeracy in the perioperative period, several are listed in Fig. 11.2. Many of these factors may influence a patient's navigation through the complex healthcare system, including their understanding of recommended surgical procedures, keeping scheduled appointments, adherence to medications and other instructions, and communication with healthcare providers about their health. Several of these factors may also influence the frequency of emergency room visits, rehospitalizations, morbidity and mortality rates, and satisfaction with their care.

Furthermore, there is limited information about the assessment of organizational health literacy and the development of targeted interventions to improve health-literate approaches in medical practices, hospitals, and academic health centers. However, a few studies have measured organizational health literacy,[35–37] including one study among surgeons in one department of surgery in an academic medical center.[37] The results of these studies indicate that workforce training in health literacy is one modifiable factor that could improve healthcare practices to assist patients in navigating the complex healthcare system.

Due to the prevalence of limited health literacy and numeracy among adults in the United States, it is important to dedicate time and effort to clearly communicating information so that surgical patients can make informed decisions about their health. This information includes the cause of a patient's health problem, why the surgical procedure is needed, the risks and benefits of the procedure, alternatives to the procedure, the consequences of not having the procedure, and the

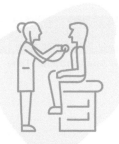

Preoperative

- Understands educational materials and risk
- Navigates and coordinates care
- Keeps appointments
- Follows preoperative instructions including medication (dose and timing) and behavioral changes (e.g., diet)

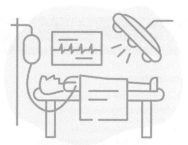

Ambulatory Surgery Center/Hospital

- Organizational literacy
- Consent process
- Forms (e.g., living will)
- Signage
- Stress, Anxiety
- Complications
- Length of stay

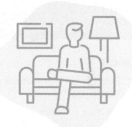

Postoperative

- Follows discharge instructions (written and oral) including medication adherence (e.g., pain control) and behavioral changes (e.g., physical activity restrictions)
- Understands educational materials
- Navigates and coordinates care
- Keeps follow-up appointments
- Monitors and reports signs and symptoms
- Manages: drains, wound care, devices
- Health outcomes: ER visits, rehospitalizations, complications, functional status, mortality
- Satisfaction with care

Cross-cutting Factors

- Patient's demographic characteristics, medical history, health status, health knowledge, and decision-making skills
- Patient-provider communication, medical terminology and jargon
- Challenges: time off work, family care, transportation, psychological (e.g., fear)
- Manages issues associated with health insurance

FIG. 11.2 Factors and behaviors associated with the health literacy of patients in the perioperative period.

importance of correctly following perioperative instructions to achieve the best surgical outcomes.

HEALTH LITERACY INSTRUMENTS

Numerous validated instruments exist to measure different domains of health literacy, numeracy, and organizational literacy for various health disciplines (e.g., vascular surgery, cancer, dentistry), spoken language (e.g., English, Spanish), and patient age groups (e.g., adolescents and adults). The instruments also vary by administration time and method (e.g., self-reported, completed on paper by the patient, administered by an interviewer). In addition, to the wide variety of available instruments, scoring of the different instruments to determine limited health literacy has varied by investigator, making it difficult for providers to decide which instrument and scoring to use in a clinical setting.[38] The Health Literacy Tool Shed offers an online database of more than 200 validated health literacy and numeracy instruments and their psychometric properties (https://healthliteracy.bu.edu/). The following

paragraphs briefly describe some of the instruments that have been used in numerous studies among different populations, including surgical patients and organizations (Table 11.1).

The Test of Functional Health Literacy in Adults (TOFHLA) measures general health literacy in patients with fill-in-the-blank items related to comprehension of prose and numeric calculations.[39] The TOFHLA has been translated into several languages, and a validated shortened format of the TOFHLA[40] reduces the administration time. The Rapid Estimate of Adult Literacy in Medicine (REALM) is a quick screening tool that identifies patients with limited reading skills by measuring medical word recognition and pronunciation.[41] The REALM has also been translated into several languages and has a validated shortened format[42] as well as a validated format for adolescents[50] and, more recently, a validated format for use in virtual environments.[51] The Newest Vital Sign measures patients' functional health literacy (reading comprehension and numerical tasks) through questions about an ice cream nutrition label.[43] Other common instruments used to measure

TABLE 11.1
Instruments That Measure Health Literacy, Numeracy, and Literate Healthcare Organizations

Instrument	Description	Approximate Administration Time (minutes)
Test of Functional Health Literacy in Adults (TOFHLAs)[39]	17 items: numerical ability 3 items: reading comprehension	22
Short form-Test of Functional Health Literacy in Adults (S-TOFHLA)[40]	4 items: numerical ability 2 items: reading comprehension	12
Rapid Estimate of Adult Literacy in Medicine (REALM)[41]	66 words: word recognition and pronunciation	3
Rapid Estimate of Adult Literacy in medicine-Short Form (REALM-SF)[42]	66 words: word recognition and pronunciation 7 words: word recognition and pronunciation	1
Newest Vital Sign (NVS)[43]	6 items: functional health literacy	3
Short Literacy Survey (SLS)[26] Single-Item Literacy screener (SILS)[44]	3 items: inadequate health literacy screening 1 item: limited reading ability	1 1
eHealth Literacy Scale (eHEALS)[45]	8 items: information technology skills	1–2
Numeracy Scale[46]	10 items: objective numeracy and risk	8
Subjective Numeracy Scale (SNS)[47]	8 items: subjective quantitative ability	5
Berlin Numeracy Test[48]	4 items: numeracy and risk	3
Health-Literate Healthcare Organization (HLHO-10)[49]	10 items: attributes of health literate organization	Unknown

health literacy include the Short Literacy Survey[26] and the Single Item Literacy Screener.[44] Finally, the eHealth Literacy Scale is commonly used to measure an individual's knowledge, comfort, and perceived skills in finding, evaluating, and applying electronic information to health problems.[45]

Three instruments are often used to measure numeracy. A numeracy scale focuses on the objective skills needed to complete math tasks.[46] The Subjective Numeracy Scale measures an individual's perceived ability to perform mathematical tasks and preference for math to be presented as numerical values (e.g., percentages) versus prose (e.g., small chance).[47] The third instrument, the Berlin Numeracy Test, assesses math skills and risk literacy (e.g., the ability to interpret risks).[48]

Finally, to measure organizational health literacy, a Health-Literate Healthcare Organization 10-item instrument (HLHO-10) was developed and validated[49,52] based on the 2012 Roundtable on Health Literacy's 10 attributes for organizations.[20] This instrument examines health literacy associated with various attributes of an organization, including its integration into the organization's mission, leadership, communication standards, financial transparency, and workforce training.

LIMITED HEALTH LITERACY COST

It has been difficult to estimate the cost of limited health literacy for patients, healthcare systems, and society in general in the United States given the plethora of affected health outcomes, which may be affected by having less access to timely and quality healthcare; poor adherence to prescribed medications; less frequent use of preventive care; lack of knowledge, ability, and confidence to self-manage acute and chronic disease; and the inadequate skills needed to communicate with healthcare professionals about one's health including physical signs and/or symptoms.[11]

Although the exact dollar amount is unknown, general research findings have demonstrated that limited health literacy (e.g., basic and below basic levels) is associated with significantly increased health care costs.[53-58] For example, one study of over 92,000 veterans who accessed healthcare in the Veterans Health Administration from 2007 to 2009 found that the estimated 3-year cost for veterans with limited health literacy was $143 million more than that for veterans with adequate health literacy.[58] At the national level, based on the 2003 NAAL Health Literacy survey and modeling methods, Vernon and colleagues estimated that limited health literacy costs the US economy between $106 billion and $238 billion annually.[53] A more recent study concluded that individuals categorized as having basic or below basic health literacy have significantly more healthcare costs than individuals categorized as above basic literacy for physicians visits, nonphysician visits, and emergency room visits.[55] With all factors considered, inadequate health literacy is associated with increased healthcare costs, however, studies are needed to fully understand the impact of inadequate health literacy on the healthcare costs and the financial burden among surgical patients during the perioperative period.

POTENTIAL CHALLENGES AND STRATEGIES TO ADDRESS HEALTH LITERACY

Although there may be health-related benefits to screening surgical patients for health literacy, it is important to be cognizant of the potential barriers and risks associated with implementing this activity in clinical practice.

For patients, health literacy screening may cause shame and increased concern about facing stigma.[59,60] Patients who are aware of their limited literacy skills often are embarrassed by this trait and try to conceal it from others, including healthcare providers, by not asking questions, waiting until later to read information or fill out forms, or making up excuses for missing appointments or failing to follow preoperative and discharge instructions.[61]

For surgeons and the surgical team, identifying patients with limited health literacy requires them to devote time and effort to measuring patients' health literacy, improving patient–provider communication, providing additional documentation, and managing care coordination throughout the perioperative period. In addition, providers must decide which health literacy measurement instrument to use in their clinical practice, overcoming any limited resources available to complete this task (e.g., training of staff, time needed for administering, scoring, and documenting results of health literacy instruments), variability in the accuracy and reliability of the different instruments that were often developed for research purposes, and patient unwillingness to answer the questions included in the various validated instruments.

Moreover, even patients with proficient health literacy often face fear, uncertainty, and unfamiliarity with medical terminology and procedures in the context of a surgical procedure.

A shame-free environment where patients can ask questions without fear of being embarrassed or being demeaned is an important feature of a health-literate surgical practice and organization.

Several strategies can be used to accommodate a patient's limited health literacy, such as using plain language in all forms of communication, slowing down during patient–provider discussions, providing limited but key information and repeating it, practicing reflective listening, using visuals, graphics, or small media to explain complex concepts, using active voice verbs and avoiding complex sentence structure in print material, presenting patients with low-literacy consent forms, demonstrating how to complete a task, encouraging questions, and confirming patients' understanding by using the teach-back methodology.[61] It is also important for healthcare providers to frame questions such that patients feel free to admit when they do not understand the medical information or recommendation. For example, instead of asking "Do you have any questions?," a provider can ask, "What are your questions?" Additional ways to create a shame-free environment include engaging a patient's family members in the discussion and encouraging patients to come prepared to medical visits by using the Ask-Me-3 program,[62] which focuses on three questions: "What is my main problem?" "What do I need to do (about the problem)?" and "Why is it important for me to do this?"

CONCLUSIONS AND FUTURE DIRECTIONS

This review of health literacy as a social determinant of health in surgery raises many questions. Approximately one-third of surgical patients have limited health literacy, and many intersecting factors may affect patients' health literacy during the perioperative period. Research using mixed methods to better understand the role of health literacy in the perioperative period is warranted especially since the environment of undergoing a surgical procedure increases stress, which may impact a patient's decision-making, communication skills, and health outcomes. Addressing this specific social determinant of health using quantitative and in-depth qualitative data collection will provide the evidence needed to develop, implement, and evaluate multilevel interventions at the patient, provider, and organizational levels. Bringing awareness of health literacy to surgeons, members of the surgical team, practices, and organizations is an important first of many steps toward improving health equity in surgical outcomes.

Highlights

- A recent and expanded definition of health literacy includes both personal and organizational health literacy.
- At least one-third of surgical patients have limited health literacy, and even patients with a proficient level of health literacy have difficulty understanding medical information and recommended surgical procedures.
- Validated instruments to measure health literacy, numeracy, and organizational literacy are available for use in surgical practices.
- Creating a shame-free, health-literate environment with effective patient–provider communication will improve surgical outcomes, quality of life, and patient satisfaction with their care.
- Future health literacy research should use mixed methods and focus on surgical patients, surgeons and the surgical team, and organizational characteristics to understand how health literacy contributes to surgical outcomes.

REFERENCES

1. Health literacy: report of the council on scientific affairs. Ad Hoc committee on health literacy for the council on scientific affairs, American Medical Association. *JAMA.* 1999; 281(6):552–557.
2. Institute of Medicine Committee on Health Literacy. *Health Literacy: A Prescription to End Confusion.* Washington, DC: The National Academies Press; 2004.
3. United States Department of Health and Human Services, Office of Disease Prevention and Health Promotion. Healthy People 2030. https://health.gov/healthypeople. Accessed February 4, 2023.
4. Santana S, Brach C, Harris L, et al. Updating health literacy for Healthy People 2030: defining its importance for a new decade in public health. *J Publ Health Manag Pract.* 2021; 27(Suppl 6):S258–S264.
5. United States Department of Education. Institute of Education Sciences, National Center for Education Statistics. Program for the International Assessment of Adult Competencies (PIAAC). https://nces.ed.gov/surveys/piaac/index.asp. Accessed February 4, 2023.
6. Lipkus IM, Peters E. Understanding the role of numeracy in health: proposed theoretical framework and practical insights. *Health Educ Behav.* 2009;36(6):1065–1081.
7. Golbeck AL, Ahlers-Schmidt CR, Paschal AM, Dismuke SE. A definition and operational framework for health numeracy. *Am J Prev Med.* 2005;29(4):375–376.
8. Lopez C, Kim B, Saks K. Health Literacy in the United States. Enhancing Assessments and Reducing Disparities. https://milkeninstitute.org/sites/default/files/2022-05/Health_Literacy_United_States_Final_Report.pdf. Published 2022. Accessed October 18, 2022.

9. Nutbeam D, Lloyd JE. Understanding and responding to health literacy as a social determinant of health. *Annu Rev Publ Health*. 2021;42:159–173.

10. Levy H, Janke A. Health literacy and access to care. *J Health Commun*. 2016;21(Suppl):43–50.

11. Berkman ND, Sheridan SL, Donahue KE, Halpern DJ, Crotty K. Low health literacy and health outcomes: an updated systematic review. *Ann Intern Med*. 2011;155(2):97–107.

12. Nutbeam D. The evolving concept of health literacy. *Soc Sci Med*. 2008;67(12):2072–2078.

13. Stormacq C, Van den Broucke S, Wosinski J. Does health literacy mediate the relationship between socioeconomic status and health disparities? Integrative review. *Health Promot Int*. 2019;34(5):e1–e17.

14. Pelikan JM, Ganahl K, Roethlin F. Health literacy as a determinant, mediator and/or moderator of health: empirical models using the European Health Literacy Survey dataset. *Glob Health Promot*. 2018;25(4):57–66, 1757975918788300.

15. Paasche-Orlow MK, Wolf MS. The causal pathways linking health literacy to health outcomes. *Am J Health Behav*. 2007;31(Suppl 1):S19–S26.

16. Squiers L, Peinado S, Berkman N, Boudewyns V, McCormack L. The health literacy skills framework. *J Health Commun*. 2012;17(Suppl 3):30–54.

17. Sorensen K, Levin-Zamir D, Duong TV, Okan O, Brasil VV, Nutbeam D. Building health literacy system capacity: a framework for health literate systems. *Health Promot Int*. 2021;36(Supplement_1):i13–i23.

18. Paro A, Hyer JM, Diaz A, Tsilimigras DI, Pawlik TM. Profiles in social vulnerability: the association of social determinants of health with postoperative surgical outcomes. *Surgery*. 2021;170(6):1777–1784.

19. Diaz A, Hyer JM, Barmash E, Azap R, Paredes AZ, Pawlik TM. County-level social vulnerability is associated with worse surgical outcomes especially among minority patients. *Ann Surg*. 2021;274(6):881–891.

20. Brach C, Keller D, Hernandez LM, et al. *Ten Attributes of Health Literate Health Care Organizations*. Washington, DC: Institute of Medicine; 2012.

21. Brega AG, Barnard J, Mabachi NM, et al. *AHRQ Health Literacy Universal Precautions Toolkit*. AHRQ Publication No. 15-0023-EF. 2nd ed. Rockville, MD: Agency for Healthcare Research and Quality; 2015.

22. Kutner M, Greenberg E, Jin Y, Paulsen C. *The Health Literacy of America's Adults: Results from the 2003 National Assessment of Adult Literacy*. NCES Publication No. 2006-483. Washington, DC: U.S. Department of Education; 2006. Institute of Education Sciences, National Center for Education Statistics.

23. Roy M, Corkum JP, Urbach DR, et al. Health literacy among surgical patients: a systematic review and meta-analysis. *World J Surg*. 2019;43(1):96–106.

24. Chang ME, Baker SJ, Dos Santos Marques IC, et al. Health literacy in surgery. *Health Lit Res Pract*. 2020;4(1):e46–e65.

25. Menendez ME, van Hoorn BT, Mackert M, Donovan EE, Chen NC, Ring D. Patients with limited health literacy ask fewer questions during office visits with hand surgeons. *Clin Orthop Relat Res*. 2017;475(5):1291–1297.

26. Chew LD, Bradley KA, Boyko EJ. Brief questions to identify patients with inadequate health literacy. *Fam Med*. 2004;36(8):588–594.

27. Wright JP, Edwards GC, Goggins K, et al. Association of health literacy with postoperative outcomes in patients undergoing major abdominal surgery. *JAMA Surg*. 2018;153(2):137–142.

28. Rothermel LD, Conley CC, Sarode AL, et al. Health literacy in surgical oncology patients: an observational study at a comprehensive cancer center. *J Natl Compr Cancer Netw*. 2021;19(12):1407–1414.

29. Theiss LM, Wood T, McLeod MC, et al. The association of health literacy and postoperative complications after colorectal surgery: a cohort study. *Am J Surg*. 2022;223(6):1047–1052.

30. Scarpato KR, Kappa SF, Goggins KM, et al. The impact of health literacy on surgical outcomes following radical cystectomy. *J Health Commun*. 2016;21(sup2):99–104.

31. Shlobin NA, Huang J, Lam S. Health literacy in neurosurgery: a scoping review. *World Neurosurg*. 2022;166:71–87.

32. Tiourin E, Barton N, Janis JE. Health literacy in plastic surgery: a scoping review. *Plast Reconstr Surg Glob Open*. 2022;10(4):e4247.

33. Congelosi PD, Carroll MC, Wong SL. Numeracy levels influence shared decision-making and surgical outcomes: a scoping review of the literature. *Am J Surg*. 2023;225(6):967–974.

34. Garcia-Retamero R, Cokely ET, Wicki B, Joeris A. Improving risk literacy in surgeons. *Patient Educ Counsel*. 2016;99(7):1156–1161.

35. Prince LY, Schmidtke C, Beck JK, Hadden KB. An assessment of organizational health literacy practices at an academic health center. *Qual Manag Health Care*. 2018;27(2):93–97.

36. Howe CJ, Adame T, Lewis B, Wagner T. Original research: assessing organizational focus on health literacy in north Texas hospitals. *Am J Nurs*. 2020;120(12):24–33.

37. Park G, Kim DH, Shao C, et al. Organizational assessment of health literacy within an academic medical center. *Am J Surg*. 2023;225(1):129–130.

38. Altin SV, Finke I, Kautz-Freimuth S, Stock S. The evolution of health literacy assessment tools: a systematic review. *BMC Publ Health*. 2014;14:1207–2458.

39. Parker RM, Baker DW, Williams MV, Nurss JR. The test of functional health literacy in adults: a new instrument for measuring patients' literacy skills. *J Gen Intern Med*. 1995;10(10):537–541.

40. Baker DW, Williams MV, Parker RM, Gazmararian JA, Nurss J. Development of a brief test to measure functional health literacy. *Patient Educ Counsel*. 1999;38(1):33–42.

41. Davis TC, Crouch MA, Long SW, et al. Rapid assessment of literacy levels of adult primary care patients. *Fam Med*. 1991;23(6):433–435.

42. Arozullah AM, Yarnold PR, Bennett CL, et al. Development and validation of a short-form, rapid estimate of adult literacy in medicine. *Med Care.* 2007;45(11):1026–1033.

43. Weiss BD, Mays MZ, Martz W, et al. Quick assessment of literacy in primary care: the newest vital sign. *Ann Fam Med.* 2005;3(6):514–522.

44. Morris NS, MacLean CD, Chew LD, Littenberg B. The Single Item Literacy Screener: evaluation of a brief instrument to identify limited reading ability. *BMC Fam Pract.* 2006;7: 21–2296.

45. Norman CD, Skinner HA. eHEALS: the eHealth Literacy Scale. *J Med Internet Res.* 2006;8(4):e27.

46. Lipkus IM, Samsa G, Rimer BK. General performance on a numeracy scale among highly educated samples. *Med Decis Making.* 2001;21(1):37–44.

47. Fagerlin A, Zikmund-Fisher BJ, Ubel PA, Jankovic A, Derry HA, Smith DM. Measuring numeracy without a math test: development of the Subjective Numeracy Scale. *Med Decis Making.* 2007;27(5):672–680.

48. Cokely ET, Galesic M, Schulz E, Ghazal S, Garcia-Teamero R. Measuring risk literacy: the Berlin numeracy test. *Judgment and Decision Making.* 2012;7(1):25–47.

49. Kowalski C, Lee SD, Schmidt A, et al. The health literate health care organization 10 item questionnaire (HLHO-10): development and validation. *BMC Health Serv Res.* 2015;15:47–4015.

50. Davis TC, Wolf MS, Arnold CL, et al. Development and validation of the rapid estimate of adolescent literacy in medicine (REALM-teen): a tool to screen adolescents for below-grade reading in health care settings. *Pediatrics.* 2006;118(6):e1707–e1714.

51. Aker JL, Leonard-Segal A, Christman L, Travis S, Beck M, Newton A. Evaluating health literacy in virtual environments: validation of the REALM and REALM-teen for virtual use. *J Gen Intern Med.* 2022;37(11):2834–2839.

52. Singer D, Howe C, Adame T, Lewis B, Wagner T, Walker D. A psychometric analysis of the health literate health care organization-10 item questionnaire. *Health Lit Res Pract.* 2022;6(2):e137–e141.

53. Vernon JA, Trujillo A, Rosenbaum S, DeBuono B. Low health literacy: Implications for national health policy. https://hsrc.himmelfarb.gwu.edu/cgi/viewcontent.cgi?article=1173&context=sphhs_policy_facpubs   Published 2007. Accessed January 27, 2023.

54. Howard DH, Gazmararian J, Parker RM. The impact of low health literacy on the medical costs of Medicare managed care enrollees. *Am J Med.* 2005;118(4):371–377.

55. Rasu RS, Bawa WA, Suminski R, Snella K, Warady B. Health literacy impact on national healthcare utilization and expenditure. *Int J Health Pol Manag.* 2015;4(11): 747–755.

56. Eichler K, Wieser S, Brugger U. The costs of limited health literacy: a systematic review. *Int J Publ Health.* 2009;54(5): 313–324.

57. Palumbo R. Examining the impacts of health literacy on healthcare costs. An evidence synthesis. *Health Serv Manag Res.* 2017;30(4):197–212.

58. Haun JN, Patel NR, French DD, Campbell RR, Bradham DD, Lapcevic WA. Association between health literacy and medical care costs in an integrated healthcare system: a regional population based study. *BMC Health Serv Res.* 2015;15, 1-1.

59. Parikh NS, Parker RM, Nurss JR, Baker DW, Williams MV. Shame and health literacy: the unspoken connection. *Patient Educ Counsel.* 1996;27(1):33–39.

60. Wolf MS, Williams MV, Parker RM, Parikh NS, Nowlan AW, Baker DW. Patients' shame and attitudes toward discussing the results of literacy screening. *J Health Commun.* 2007;12(8):721–732.

61. Weiss BD. *Health Literacy and Patient Safety: Help Patients Understand. Manual for Clinicians.* 2nd ed. Chicago, Illinois: American Medical Association Foundation and American Medical Association; 2007.

62. Institute for Healthcare Improvement. Ask me 3: Good questions for your good health. https://www.ihi.org/resources/Pages/Tools/Ask-Me-3-Good-Questions-for-Your-Good-Health.aspx Updated 2023. Accessed February 18, 2023.

CHAPTER 12

Psychological Stress and the Surgical Stressor

BARBARA L. ANDERSEN, PHD • KYLIE R. PARK

INTRODUCTION

Perioperative and postoperative morbidity and mortality are seen as correlates of the preoperative condition of the patient, the quality of surgical care provided, and the extent of surgical stress.[1] The latter are of clear importance. Considered here are pre- and postoperative stress responses—psychological, behavioral, biologic—and patients' view of illness, hospitalization, and surgery as stressors. We begin with defining stress and the similarity of physiologic models of surgical stress and psychological stress. We note that stress covaries with negative affect, such as negative mood and anxiety and depressive symptoms. Stress in critical periods in the patients' experience, e.g., awareness of illness/diagnosis, anticipation of surgical treatment, and short- and long-term recovery, is described, and empirical relationships to morbidity and mortality are discussed. We conclude with a prompt to consider psychological stress and sequelae in prehabilitation and postoperative surgical care.

STRESSORS AND STRESS RESPONSES

Stressors and the stress response are conceptually distinct. Though a bit unsatisfying as it is circular, a stressor can be defined as an event in the environment which most people would find stressful. Indeed, data reliably confirm that, on average, people undergoing divorce, bereavement, caregiving, and importantly, surgery, report greater stress than those not experiencing these stressors. What are the characteristics that define a stressor? Several have been offered,[2] including (1) the level of adaptation required to respond to the stressor; (2) the immediacy of harm, the duration, and the degree to which the event is uncontrollable; (3) the demands of the event exceeding one's capacity/resources to respond; and (4) the stressor interrupts one's goals, including those for psychological or

physical well-being. Some characteristics may be more relevant than others in particular situations, but taken together, we can assume that the awareness and anticipation of surgery is a potent stressor and for many, one that does not readily resolve with the occurrence of surgery per se.

Individuals subjectively (psychologically) appraise a stressor, one's capacity to respond to it (behavioral), and physiologic systems are activated (e.g., fight or flight processes) to support behavior to respond. Hypothesized by many (see examples: cardiovascular,[3] diabetes[4]) and tested by some (see example: cancer[5]), biobehavioral elements play a role in adaptation to a health stressor and potentially, downstream disease/illness outcomes.

The principal aspect of psychological stress is cognitive, i.e., perceiving an event as stressful. That is, the individual first appraises the threat and then his or her capacity to respond to it.[6,7] This appraisal process determines the type, direction, and intensity of stress-related emotions (e.g., anxiety, anger, fear, sadness). Individual differences among people also influence appraisals, such as past experience with the stressor, one's perceived ability to cope, and other social determinants (e.g., see associated chapters on financial resources, race, and others). In short, stress responses of individuals vary, even when the precipitating event (e.g., type of surgery) is similar.

In addition to cognitions and negative emotions, stressors prompt behaviors/behavioral change ("flight or fight"). Although there are exceptions, people generally engage in less healthy behaviors when under stress from an event or when perceiving stress. For example, people reporting greater perceived stress are likely to exercise for less time on fewer days, report lower self-efficacy for meeting an exercise goal, or feel less satisfied with their exercise.[8] Stress is also related to sleep difficulties. Stress is not only the leading cause of temporary

Social Determinants of Health in Surgery. https://doi.org/10.1016/B978-0-443-12366-5.00016-4

insomnia, but lack of sleep may also be a source of stress.[9] Stress is associated with increases in health-damaging behaviors. People under stress are likely to increase alcohol intake,[10] smoke more cigarettes,[11] and eat more "fast food," and high calorie foods.[12]

What are the physiologic responses to psychological stress? Essentially, the system wide physiological responses of the surgical stress response are common to physiologic responses to psychological stress.[13] Two major regulatory pathways exist: the hypothalamic–pituitary–adrenocortical (HPA) axis and the sympathetic adrenomedullary (SAM) axis, providing the basis of stress adaptation. In brief, psychologic stressors activate the brain in a top-down fashion; descending information is stored in the hypothalamus and ascending information in the brainstem. The two pathways act in unison, ensured by bidirectional connection between their centers. Both have physiological responses in common and are viewed as innate survival mechanisms designed to reestablish homeostasis as quickly as possible after stress exposure/injury. Repeated demands, however, tax the body's ability to respond and return to normal, producing "wear and tear" or "allostatic load" (see accompanying chapter). Notably, psychological stressors are able to activate the physiologic adaptational systems even without a physiological stimulus.[14]

Stress, Anxiety, and Depression

A 2023 survey revealed more than a quarter (26%) of Americans anticipated that they would experience more stress in the coming year, with over 35% rating their mental health as fair to poor.[15] Among the sources of anxiety for individuals was physical health for virtually half of the sample. Though conceptually and empirically distinct, stress is correlated with negative mood and symptoms of depression and anxiety disorders. Depression is uniquely toxic. Estimated to occur for 7% of the US population, depression is a risk factor for premature death (all-cause mortality) and for all major illnesses and chronic conditions (e.g., cardiovascular,[16] non–small-cell lung cancer[17]). For these reasons, studies which have researched anxiety or depression, along with stress, are reviewed as correlates or predictors of biobehavioral (psychological, behavioral, biologic) responses to and outcomes from surgery.

ILLNESS AS A STRESSOR

Surgery aside, individuals' learning that s/he has a major medical condition (illness) is a stressor for most,

with the added stress from reactions of friends and family members[18] of the news. Patients' perceptions of their illness can function as a guide to the illness that may, in turn, influence psychological, behavioral, and illness outcomes. "Illness perceptions" may be cognitive—pertaining to an individual's thoughts or beliefs—or emotional.[19] Dimensions of cognitive ones[20] are perceptions of the illness *consequences*, the degree to which an individual believes an illness impacts their life, thoughts of the *illness timeline*, or how long an individual believes the illness will last, *personal control* refers to one's belief that the illness can be controlled by oneself, whereas *treatment control* refers to beliefs about the extent to which treatment will help the illness; *identity* reflects the label an individual applies to the illness and the symptoms related to the illness; and *cause* pertains to one's beliefs concerning the illness' etiology. There are *emotional responses*—reflecting negative reactions, such as fear, anger, and distress, in response to an illness.

Data suggest that individuals' negative illness perceptions (IPs) assessed prior to treatment covary with adverse psychological, behavioral, and health outcomes for many conditions, including chronic illnesses.[21] Regarding surgery studies, Juergens et al.[22] reported perceptions of a lengthy timeline and negative preoperative emotions predicted extent of disability at 3 months postcoronary artery graft bypass surgery. Regarding total hip or knee replacement, multiple studies show perceptions of negative consequences have predicted worse knee functioning,[23] pain with daily activity and walking,[24] and disability.[25] These studies suggest that prior to learning one has a need for surgery, patients' perceptions of their illness or condition are relevant to later outcomes.

HOSPITALIZATION AND THE SURGERY STRESSOR

In preface, we note that as long 50 years ago, researchers described anxiety accompanying hospitalization.[26] As studied, the hospital environment was viewed as novel, one of routines and procedures with which individuals are not familiar,[27] with research focused upon identifying characteristics of the surgical patient which covary with risk for any number of undesired outcomes. Some characteristics are well recognized, such as those included in the American College of Surgeons surgical risk calculator, e.g., demographics (age, sex), functional status, frailty,[28] comorbidities and their severity, and others. Additionally, we refer the reader to the accumulating research on social determinant variables[29] and other biologic risk correlates (see Social Determinants of Health in Surgery Overview, Allostatic Load) and related efforts[29] to improve risk prediction.[30]

There is worldwide recognition of surgical patients' having anticipatory stress and anxiety. We begin with a compelling metaanalysis and systematic review of the global prevalence of preoperative anxiety among surgical patients.[31] Reported was a pooled prevalence of anxiety being 48% (95% confidence interval [CI]: 39% −47%; 28 studies; 14,652 patients). This review is consistent with individual studies,[32,33] although some lower estimates can be found (e.g., 33% among patients about to receive low to moderate risk surgery).[33] There are differences that may moderate levels of stress/negativity, such as extent of surgery, e.g., greater distress for patients about to receive segmental mastectomy versus excisional biopsy.[34] There are examples of equivalent high estimates of depressive symptoms, as found in orthognathic surgery patients (42%).[35]

It is relevant to consider the phenomenology of worries and fears grounding patients' high stress and negative emotions. The previously cited metaanalysis identified correlates of anxiety, i.e., fear of complication RR = 3.53 (95% CI: 3.06−4.07), fear of awakening in the middle of surgery RR = 2.58 (95% CI: 2.17−3.06), and fear of medical mistakes RR = 1.93 (95% CI: 1.57−2.36). Sources of preoperative worries of pain, financial instability/loss,[32] disability, and unexpected outcomes of the operation are found among abdominal surgery patients. Though not an exhaustive accounting, the salient summary message is the *commonality of stress, anxiety, and for some, depression, in*

preoperative period. Further, the breadth of fears/concerns makes clear that no single preoperative information session or pamphlet, for example, would be sufficient, but a substantive effort using active stress reduction strategies (see the following discussion). Considering the commonality and severity of preoperative symptoms and concerns, large literature have emerged testing presurgery responses as predictors. Correlational studies such as these cannot establish cause−effect relationships; however, the reliability of the findings across postoperative periods is notable. Summarized here are illustrative metaanalyses and studies of hospital admission/preoperative stress and anxious and depressive responses in relationship to subsequent circumstances and events (see Fig. 12.1).

PREOPERATIVE RESPONSES IN ASSOCIATION WITH OUTCOMES

Postoperative Symptoms. Multiple studies have identified patient characteristics predictive of high levels of stress, distress, and delirium, pain and other physical symptoms, and poor function. The relationship between psychological factors and postoperative pain, both acute and chronic, has been extensively investigated. In a systematic review (48 trials, 23,037 patients),[36] anxiety was a common predictor of postoperative pain, identified in 15 studies. Other factors associated with postoperative pain were preoperative pain, age, and type of surgery.

Chronic postsurgical pain (CPSP) has been described as pain, which (1) develops after surgery or

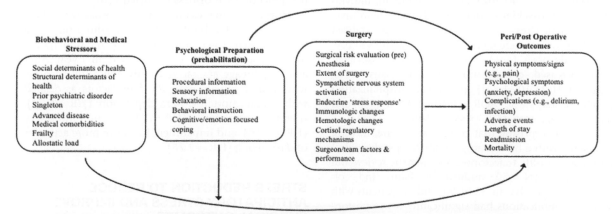

FIG. 12.1 A conceptual framework for preoperative individual differences among patients in stressors and stressful circumstances (biobehavioral and medical stressors), which covary with adverse surgical outcomes (peri/postoperative). Prehabilitation (psychological preparation) is needed for all patients and particularly for those with preoperative risk correlates (stressors) to improve postoperative outcomes and enhance patients' quality of life.

which continues or develops anew after an asymptomatic period; (2) lasts 2 months or longer; (3) is not caused by other factors (e.g., chronic infections being ruled out); and (4) interferes with quality of life.[37] Systematic reviews of psychosocial risk factors for CPSP indicate a high level of evidence (i.e., Grade of Association 1: Association Likely) for the predictive value of presurgical psychological variables. Pooled odds ratios (ORs) for presurgical anxiety (OR = 1.76, 95% CI: 1.07–2.90) and presurgical pain catastrophizing (OR = 2.37, 95% CI: 1.32–4.28) suggest that patients with these responses are approximately twice as likely to go on to develop CPSP.[38]

Complications. Mavos et al.[39] in a systematic review (16 studies, 1473 patients) examined outcomes in the early postoperative months, finding preoperative anxiety significantly related to complications following many surgeries, including cardiac.[40] For example, anxiety has been related to impaired wound healing after inguinal hernia repair.[41] One notable study is that by Myoga et al.[42] testing preoperative stress and health behavior variables in association with adverse events and complications, as defined by the Clavien–Dindo classification of surgical complications.[43] Multivariable analysis revealed that older age ($P = .020$), psychological stress ($P = .041$), and longer anesthesia time ($P < .001$) were significantly associated with adverse events and complications, whereas prior and/or current alcohol usage and smoking dependence was not.

Using nationally representative data from the 2005 to 2008 Nationwide Inpatient Sample, Fox and colleagues[44] identified women aged ≥ 18 years with invasive breast cancer who underwent inpatient mastectomy (N = 40,202), and among them, individuals with a psychiatric diagnosis (major depressive, posttraumatic stress, panic, adjustment, or generalized anxiety disorder) were identified. Analyses showed psychiatric diagnosis (any) to be significantly associated with increased complications (5.9% versus 4.8%; AOR = 1.21 [1.10–1.34]), prolonged hospitalization (8.5% versus 4.8%; AOR = 1.40 [1.32–1.49]), and higher average costs ($9723 vs. $9,108, $P < .001$).

It is not surprising that complications are, in turn, associated with a broad range of adverse psychological and quality-of-life trajectories. A systematic review and metaanalysis (N = 50 studies) by Pinto and colleagues[45] found that in 32 of 50 studies, patients with surgical complications had significantly worse postoperative psychosocial outcomes even after controlling for preoperative psychosocial, clinical, and demographic factors. Further, half of the latter complication studies later found patients reporting continuing anxiety and lower quality of life for 12 months and longer postsurgery. Similar results come from women with breast cancer having arm complications following axillary dissection.[46] Compared with women reporting no arm problems, the adjusted odds ratios of having psychological distress at 3 months for women reporting one to two, three to four, and five to six arm problems were 1.2, 2.3, and 3.1, respectively (chi 2 for trend = 9.5, $P = .002$). The multiple difficult sequelae of esophageal surgery (e.g., eating difficulty, eating in front of others, weight loss) have been found to be significantly worse for those with psychological distress during the two postsurgery years.[47]

Prolonged hospitalization, length of stay (LoS), rehospitalization. Data from the Vascular Events In Noncardiac Surgery Patients Cohort Evaluation (VISION) study[48] (n = 997) found preoperative distress (day of surgery) associated with greater length of stay ($b = 0.01$, 95% CI [0.00–0.02], $R^2 = 0.15$, $f^2 = 0.18$) and increased odds of rehospitalization (AOR = 1.07, 95%CI [1.01–1.13]). Metaanalyses and individual studies have examined predictors of postoperative outcomes, particularly pain, for patients undergoing hip or knee arthroplasty. For example, a metaanalysis (6 studies, 1525 patients) reported poorer 12 month outcomes for patients reporting preoperatively worse mental health, anxiety, and/or depression.[49] Individual studies[50] have found patients (N = 231) preoperative pain-related psychological distress to predict LOS. Another single institution study[51] (N = 863) found 23% of the patients to have significant psychological distress, and controlling for age, education, race/ethnicity, living alone, and smoking, psychological distress predicted LoS.

Mortality. One example is a prospective cohort study[52] supported by the National Institute on Aging that followed 1341 adults over age 65 undergoing high risk surgery, with 17% dying within 1 year. After adjusting for age, sex, race/ethnicity, education, income, wealth, and surgery type, the four factors associated with 1-year mortality were depression (HR = 1.72), cognitive function (HR = 1.10), multimorbidity (HR = 1.16), and impairment in two or more activities of daily living (HR = 2.76).

STRESS REDUCTION TO REDUCE ANTICIPATORY STRESS AND IMPROVE SURGICAL OUTCOMES

Prehabilitation efforts are designed to prepare patients physically and emotionally for surgery stress. Efforts vary, but nutrition, exercise, and psychological elements are the mainstays of multimodal efforts. Collectively, they are used to enhance physiological reserve, improve functional status, and reduce psychological stress and negative affect to reduce surgical morbidities and facilitate recovery and resumption of activities of daily living.[1] Discussed here are psychological efforts to improve patients' emotional states; readers are referred to other resources for review and discussion of nutritional and activity elements.[53–56] It is also the case that psychological interventions can effectively support the latter efforts. Fig. 12.1 provides a framework for considering medical and biobehavioral risk factors, many of them commonly associated with elevated anxiety or depressive disorders,[57] efficacious psychological/behavioral intervention components, and postoperative outcomes.

There is a long history of randomized clinical trials testing interventions to reduce patients' stress prior to surgery[58,59] to improve the outcomes described before. From that early literature, significant, reliable effects were reported for interventions providing procedural information (e.g., exactly what was to happen pre-[e.g., anesthesia] to postoperatively) and, most importantly, sensory information (e.g., type of pain anticipated, location, duration), along with teaching patients progressive muscle relaxation. Decades later, metaanalytic[60] and network analysis[61] results remain in support of psychological preparation for surgery to achieve benefits in reduced emotional distress and less resource use. In particular, relaxation is beneficial for reducing pain, and procedural information, sensory information, and behavioral instruction may be effective in reducing hospital stay.

ERAS is a multimodal perioperative care pathway designed to achieve early recovery for patients undergoing major surgery. The central elements of the ERAS pathways across more than 20 surgeries address key factors (i.e., need for parenteral analgesia, the need for intravenous fluids secondary to gut dysfunction, bed rest caused by lack of mobility) related to extended hospital stay. Within some pathway documents, patient education materials recommended for use are ones mentioning nutrition and physical fitness support. Selected documents (e.g., lung surgery,[62] vascular surgery,[63] gynecologic oncology[64]) provide strong recommendations for counseling in addition to information provision.

In closing, there is an extensive literature regarding psychological preparation for surgery. Even in surgery types with the strongest evidence for improved postoperative outcomes, attention to and adoption of empirically supported psychological interventions (see Fig. 12.1) is modest.[65] Nevertheless, there are actions that can be taken to screen for and document psychological/behavioral risk factors and add psychological components into prehabilitative programs.[66] Examples may include implementing preoperative screening/assessments of anxiety and depressive symptoms and other psychosocial risk factors in routine clinical care (e.g., sociodemographic, financial, allostatic load). Incorporating other risk factors into existing models and surgical risk calculators for risk prediction, as well as integration of mental health professionals within presurgery teams to provide recommendations for interventions, to intervene directly, and/or train nurses and other healthcare professionals to provide timely, preoperative support, and stress reduction and coping interventions should be considered.

Highlights

- Stressors and the stress response are conceptually distinct.
- Individuals subjectively (psychologically) appraise a stressor, one's capacity to respond to it (behavioral), and physiologic systems are activated (e.g., fight or flight processes) to support behavior to respond.
- Though not universal, there is a commonality of stress, anxiety, and for some, depression, in preoperative period.
- Relaxation is beneficial for reducing pain, and procedural information, sensory information, and behavioral instruction may be effective in reducing hospital stay.
- Implementing preoperative screening/assessments of anxiety and depressive symptoms and other psychosocial risk factors in routine clinical care (e.g., sociodemographic, financial, allostatic load) provide significant value added to identifying individuals as risk for poor surgical, functional status, and quality of life outcomes.

REFERENCES

1. Gillis C, Ljungqvist O, Carli F. Prehabilitation, enhanced recovery after surgery, or both? A narrative review. *Br J Anaesth.* 2022;128(3):434–448. https://doi.org/10.1016/j.bja.2021.12.007.
2. Cohen S, Murphy MLM, Prather AA. Ten surprising facts about stressful life events and disease risk. *Annu Rev Psychol.* 2019;70:577–597. https://doi.org/10.1146/annurev-psych-010418-102857.
3. Steptoe A, Kivimaki M. Stress and cardiovascular disease: an update on current knowledge. *Annu Rev Publ Health.* 2013;34:337–354. https://doi.org/10.1146/annurev-publhealth-031912-114452.

4. Subba R, Sandhir R, Singh SP, Mallick BN, Mondal AC. Pathophysiology linking depression and type 2 diabetes: psychotherapy, physical exercise, and fecal microbiome transplantation as damage control. *Eur J Neurosci.* 2021; 53(8):2870—2900.

5. Andersen BL, Kiecolt-Glaser JK, Glaser R. A biobehavioral model of cancer stress and disease course. *Am Psychol.* 1994;49(5):389—404. https://doi.org/10.1037//0003-066x.49.5.389.

6. Lazarus RS, Folkman S. *Stress, Appraisal, and Coping.* Springer Publishing Company; 1984.

7. Folkman S, Lazarus RS, Gruen RJ, DeLongis A. Appraisal, coping, health status, and psychological symptoms. *J Pers Soc Psychol.* 1986;50:571—579. https://doi.org/10.1037/0022-3514.50.3.571.

8. Stults-Kolehmainen MA, Sinha R. The effects of stress on physical activity and exercise. *Sports Med.* 2014;44: 81—121. https://doi.org/10.1007/s40279-013-0090-5.

9. Kalmback DA, Anderson JR, Drake CL. The impact of stress on sleep: pathogenic sleep reactivity as a vulnerability to insomnia and circadian disorders. *J Sleep Res.* 2018; 27(6). https://doi.org/10.1111/jsr.12710.

10. Keyes KM, Hatzenbuehler ML, Grant BF, Hasin DS. Stress and alcohol: epidemiologic evidence. *Alcohol Res.* 2012; 34(4):391—400.

11. Taylor GMJ, Lindson N, Farley A, et al. Smoking cessation for improving mental health. *Cochrance Database Syst Rev.* 2021. https://doi.org/10.1002/14651858.CD013522.

12. Bremner JD, Moazzami K, Wittbrodt MT, et al. Diet, stress, and mental health. *Nutrients.* 2020;12(8):2428. https://doi.org/10.3390/nu12082428.

13. Selye H. The general adaptation syndrome and the diseases of adaptation. *J Clin Endocrinol Metabol.* 1946;6(2): 117—230.

14. Hayley S, Borowski T, Merali Z, Anisman H. Central monoamine activity in genetically distinct strains of mice following a psychogenic stressor: effects of predator exposure. *Brain Res.* 2001;892:293—300. https://doi.org/10.1016/S0006-8993(00)03262-5.

15. Healthy Minds Monthly, Annual Poll. *Americans Anticipate Higher Stress at the Start of 2023 and Grade Their Mental Health Worse;* December 21, 2022. https://www.psychiatry.org/News-room/News-Releases/Americans-Anticipate-Higher-Stress-at-the-Start-of. Accessed May 1, 2023.

16. Meng R, Yu C, Liu N, He M, Jun L. Association between depression and all-cause and cardiovascular mortality in Chinese adults. *JAMA Netw Open.* 2020;3(2). https://doi.org/10.1001/jamanetworkopen.2019.21043.

17. Andersen BL, McElroy JP, Carbone DP, et al. Psychological symptom trajectories and non-small cell lung cancer survival: a joint model analysis. *Psychosom Med.* 2022;84: 215—223.

18. Woolf C, Muscara F, Anderson VA, McCarthy MC. Early traumatic stress responses in parents following a serious illness in their child: a systematic review. *J Clin Psychol Med Settings.* 2016;23:53—66. https://doi.org/10.1007/s10880-015-9430-y.

19. Leventhal EA. Aging and the perception of illness. *Res Aging.* 1984;6(1):119—135.

20. Hagger MS, Orbell S. A meta-analytic review of the common-sense model of illness representations. *Psychol Health.* 2003;18(2):141—184. https://doi.org/10.1080/088704403100081321.

21. Sawyer AT, Harris SL, Koenig HG. Illness perception and high readmission health outcomes. *Health Psychol Open.* 2019;6(1). https://doi.org/10.1177/2055102919844504.

22. Juergens MC, Seekatz B, Moosdorf RG, Petrie KJ, Rief W. Illness beliefs before cardiac surgery predict disability, quality of life, and depression 3 months later. *J Psychosom Res.* 2010;68(6):553—560. https://doi.org/10.1016/j.jpsychores.2009.10.004. Epub 2009 Dec 5. PMID: 20488272.

23. Hanusch BC, O'Connor DB, Ions P, Scott A, Gregg PJ. Effects of psychological distress and perceptions of illness on recovery from total knee replacement. *Bone Joint Lett J.* 2014;96-B(2):2010—2216. https://doi.org/10.1302/0301-620X.96B2.31136.

24. Lindberg MF, Miaskowski C, RustoEn T, Rosseland LA, Cooper BA, Lerdal A. Factors that can predict pain with walking, 12 months after total knee arthroplasty. *Acta Orthop.* 2016;87(6):600—606. https://doi.org/10.1080/17453674.2016.1237440.

25. Magklara E, Morrison V. The associations of illness perceptions and self-efficacy with psychological well-being of patients in preparation for joint replacement surgery. *Psychol Health Med.* 2016;21(6):735—742. https://doi.org/10.1080/13548506.2015.1115109.

26. Lucente FE, Fleck S. A study of hospitalization anxiety in 408 medical and surgical patients. *Psychosom Med.* 1972; 34(4):304—312.

27. Newman S. Anxiety, hospitalization, and surgery. In: Fitzpatrick R, Hinton J, Newman S, Scambler G, Thompson J, eds. The Experience of Illness. Routledge. https://doi.org/10.4324/9781003283966.

28. Evered LA, Vitug S, Scott DA, Silbert B. Preoperative frailty predicts postoperative neurocognitive disorders after total hip joint replacement surgery. *Anesth Analg.* 2020;131(5): 1582—1588. https://doi.org/10.1213/ANE.0000000000004893.

29. Mehaffey JH, Hawkins RB, Charles EJ, et al. Socioeconomic "Distressed Communities Index" improves surgical risk adjustment. *Ann Surg.* 2020;271(3):470—474. https://doi.org/10.1097/SLA.0000000000002997.

30. Charles EJ, Mehaffey JH, Hawkins RB, et al. Socioeconomic Distressed Communities Index predicts risk-adjusted mortality after cardiac surgery. *Ann Thorac Surg.* 2019;107(6): 1706—1712. https://doi.org/10.1016/j.athoracsur.2018.12.022.

31. Abate SM, Chekol YA, Basu B. Global prevalence and determinants of preoperative anxiety among surgical patients: a systematic review and meta-analysis. *Intl J Surgery Open.* 2020;25:6—16. https://doi.org/10.1016/j.ijso.2020.05.010.

32. Williams H, Jajja MR, Baer W, et al. Perioperative anxiety and depression in patients undergoing abdominal surgery

for benign or malignant disease. *J Surg Oncol*. 2019; 120(3):389–396. https://doi.org/10.1002/jso.25584.

33. Kuzminskaite V, Kaklauskaite J, Petkeviciute J. Incidence and features of preoperative anxiety in patients undergoing elective non-cardiac surgery. *Acta Med Litu*. 2019;26(1): 93–100. https://doi.org/10.6001/actamedica.v26i1.3961.

34. Schnur JB, Montgomery GH, Hallquist MN, et al. Anticipatory psychological distress in women scheduled for diagnostic and curative breast cancer surgery. *Int J Behav Med*. 2008;1:21–28. https://doi.org/10.1007/BF03003070.

35. Collins B, Gonzalez D, Gaudilliere DK, Shrestha P, Girod S. Body dysmorphic disorder and psychological distress in orthognathic surgery patients. *J Oral Maxillofac Surg*. 2014;72(8):1553–1550. https://doi.org/10.1016/j.joms.2014.01.011.

36. Ip HYV, Abrishami A, Peng PWH, Wong J, Chung F. Predictors of postoperative pain and analgesic consumption: a qualitative systematic review. *Anesthesiology*. 2009;111(3): 657–677. https://doi.org/10.1097/ALN.0b013e3181aae87a.

37. Weinrib AZ, Azam MA, Birnie KA, Burns LC, Clarke H, Katz J. The psychology of chronic post-surgical pain: new frontiers in risk factor identification, prevention and management. *Br J Pain*. 2017;11:169–177.

38. Theunissen M, Peters ML, Bruce J, et al. Preoperative anxiety and catastrophizing: a systematic review and meta-analysis of the association with chronic postsurgical pain. *Clin J Pain*. 2012;28:819–841.

39. Mavros MN, Athanasiou S, Gkegkes ID, Polyzos KA, Peppas G, Falagas ME. Do psychological variables affect early surgical recovery? *PLoS One*. 2011;6(5):e20306.

40. Stengrevics S, Sirois C, Schwartz CD, Friedman R, Domar AD. The prediction of cardiac surgery outcome based upon preoperative psychological factors. *Psychol Health*. 1996;11:471–477.

41. Broadbent E, Petrie KJ, Alley PG, Booth RJ. Psychological stress impairs early wound repair following surgery. *Psychosom Med*. 2003;65:865–869.

42. Myoga Y, Manabe H, Osaki Y. The effects of preoperative alcohol, tobacco, and psychological stress on postoperative complications: a prospective observational study. *BMC Anesthesiol*. 2021;21:245. https://doi.org/10.1186/s12871-021-01456-w.

43. Dindo D, Demartines N, Clavien PA. Classification of surgical complications: a new proposal with evaluation in a cohort of 6336 patients and results of a survey. *Ann Surg*. 2004;240:205–213.

44. Fox JP, Philip EJ, Gross CP, Desai RA, Killelea B, Desai M. Associations between mental health and surgical outcomes among women undergoing mastectomy for cancer. *Breast J*. 2013:276–288. https://doi.org/10.1111/tbj.12096.

45. Pinto A, Faiz O, Davis R, et al. Surgical complications and their impact on patients' psychosocial well-being: a systematic review and meta-analysis. *BMJ Open*. 2016;6(2): e007224. https://doi.org/10.1136/bmjopen-2014-007224.

46. Maunsell E, Brisson J, Deschenes L. Arm problems and psychological distress after sugery for breast cancer. *Can J Surg*. 1993;36(4):315–320.

47. Liu YJ, Schandl A, Markar A, Johar P, Lagergren P. Psychological distress and health-related quality of life up to 2 years after oesophageal cancer surgery: nationwide population-based study. *BJS Open*. 2021;5(1). https://doi.org/10.1093/bjsopen/zraa038.

48. Sommer JL, Reynolds K, Hebbard P, et al. Healthcare-related correlates of preoperative psychological distress among a mixed surgical and cancer-specific sample. *J Psychosom Res*. 2022;162. https://doi.org/10.1016/j.jpsychores.2022.111036.

49. Sorel JC, Veltman ES, Honig A, Poolman RW. The influence of preoperative psychological distress on pain and function after total knee arthroplasty. *Bone Joing J*. 2019; 101-B(1):7–14. https://doi.org/10.1302/0301-620X.101B1.BJJ-2018-0672.R1.

50. Zeppieri KE, Butera KA, Iams D, Parvataneni HK, George SZ. The role of social support and psychological distress in predicting discharge: a pilot study for hip and knee arthroplasty patients. *J Arthroplasty*. 2019;34(11): 2555–2560. https://doi.org/10.1016/j.arth.2019.06.033.

51. Halawi MJ, Chiu D, Gronbeck C, Savoy L, Williams VJ, Cote MP. Psychological distress independently predicts prolonged hospitalization after primary total hip and knee arthroplasty. *J Arthroplasty*. 2019;34(8):1598–1601. https://doi.org/10.1016/j.arth.2019.03.063.

52. Tang VL, Jing B, Boscardin J. Association of functional, cognitive, and psychological measures withing 1-year mortality in patients undergoing major surgery. *JAMA Surgery*. 2020;155(5):412–418. https://doi.org/10.1001/jamasurg.2020.0091.

53. Heger P, Probst P, Wiskemann J, Steindorf K, Diener MK, Mihaljevic AL. A systematic review and meta-analysis of physical exercise prehabilitation and major abdominal surgery (PROSPERO 2017 CRD42017080366). *J Gastrointest Surg*. 2020;24:1375–1385.

54. Zhong JX, Kang K, Shu XL. Effect of nutritional support on clinical outcomes in perioperative malnourished patients: a meta-analysis. *Asia Pac J Clin Nutr*. 2015;24:367–378.

55. Gillis C, Buhler K, Bresee L, et al. Effects of nutritional prehabilitation, with and without exercise, on outcomes of patients who undergo colorectal surgery: a systematic review and meta-analysis. *Gastroenterology*. 2018;155:391–410.

56. Hughes MJ, Hackney RJ, Lamb PJ, et al. Prehabilitation before major abdominal surgery: a systematic review and meta-analysis. *World J Surg*. 2019;43:1661–1668. https://doi.org/10.1007/s00268-019-04950-y.

57. Andersen BL, Lacchetti C, Ashing K, et al. Management of anxiety and depression in adjult survivors of cancer: ASCO guideline update. *J Clin Oncol*. 2023. https://doi.org/10.1200/JCO.23.00293.

58. Johnson J, Leventhal H, Dabbs J. Contributions of emotional and instrumental response processes in adaptation to surgery. *J Pers Soc Psychol*. 1971;20:55–64.

59. Johnston M, Vogele C. Benefits of psychological preparation for surgery: a meta-analysis. *Ann Behav Med*. 1993; 15(4):245–256. https://doi.org/10.1093/abm/15.4.245.

60. Powell R, Scott NW, Manyande A, et al. Psychological preparation and postoperative outcomes for adults undergoing

surgery under general anaesthesia. *Cochrane Database Syst Rev.* 2016;5. https://doi.org/10.1002/14651858.CD008646.pub2.

61. Freeman SC, Scott NW, Powell R, Johnston M, Sutton AJ, Cooper NJ. Component network meta-analysis identifies the most effective components of anesthesia. *J Clin Epidemiol.* 2018;98:105−116. https://doi.org/10.1016/j.jclinepi.2018.02.012.

62. Batchelor TJP, Rasburn NJ, Abdelnour-Berchtold E, et al. Guidelines for enhanced recovery after lung surgery: recommendations of the enhanced recovery after surgery (ERAS ®) society and the European society of thoracic Surgeons (ESTS). *Eur J Cardio Thorac Surg.* 2019;55(1):91−115. https://doi.org/10.1093/ejcts/ezy301.

63. McGinigle KL, Spangler EL, Ayyash K, et al. A framework for perioperative care for lower extremity vascular bypasses: a consensus statement by the Enhanced Recovery after Surgery (ERAS ®) Society and Society of Vascular Surgery. *J Vasc Surg.* 2023;77(5):1295−1315.

64. Nelson G, Bakkum-Gamez J, Kalogera E, et al. Guidelines for perioperative care in gynecologic/oncology: enhanced recovery after surgery (ERAS) Society recommendations—2019 update. *Int J Gynecol Cancer.* 2019;29(4).

65. Salzmann S, Salzmann-Djufri M, Wilhelm M, Euteneuer F. Psychological preparations for cardiac surgery. *Curr Cardiol Rep.* 2020;22(12):172. https://doi.org/10.1007/s11886-020-01424-9.

66. Andersen BL, Lacchetti C, Ashing K, et al. Management of anxiety and depression in adult survivors of cancer: ASCO Guideline update. *J Clin Oncol.* 2023. https://doi.org/10.1200/JCO.23.00293. Apr 19:JCO2300293.

CHAPTER 13

Framing Theoretically Informed Social Determinants of Health Research Questions

NAMRA QADEER SHAIKH, MBBS • ADIL H. HAIDER, MD, MPH, FACS

BACKGROUND

Advances in medicine have revolutionized patient care over the past decades, with improved patient outcomes and life expectancy. This is particularly true for surgery where the advent of minimally invasive and robotic techniques along with enhanced recovery pathways has led to significant reductions in surgery-related morbidity and mortality across the spectrum of surgical conditions.[1,2] The primary focus of these advancements has been on optimizing surgical care and management of diseases to improve patient outcomes. However, accumulating literature now demonstrates that medical care alone in itself cannot adequately improve overall health or limit healthcare disparities. Instead, health is more directly influenced by a complex interplay of social, psychological, and structural factors rooted in environments and systems that fundamentally shape downstream health indicators and determinants. It emphasizes the compelling role of certain social and dynamic factors (other than traditional "medical care") that directly influence patient outcomes and shape health across larger settings and populations. This is evidenced by widening mortality among social groups despite national health coverage programs permitting universal access to medical care suggesting prominent inequalities in health according to social class and economic status.[3] Moreover, literature suggests that only 10%–15% of preventable mortality can be accredited to the medical management of diseases. Instead, health outcomes and health-related behaviors are more significantly shaped by certain social, economic, and behavioral factors including income,

race, education, and occupational hierarchy.[4] Now widely recognized as social determinants of health (SDH), these dynamic characteristics have increasingly gained popularity as individual to systemic-level factors directly interacting with (and contributing to) adverse health outcomes and disparities in care.[5] These disparities have been shown to penetrate throughout the continuum of surgical care and range of health-related outcomes.[6-8]

With the increasing understanding of the overwhelming influence of SDH in shaping health outcomes, the medical community has called into question the appropriateness and importance of traditional health indicators. This has resulted in a growing emphasis on measuring impact of interventions to improve health through outcomes of populations at large. The importance of addressing SDH has been widely recognized in public health policy and practice in its crucial role in promoting health equity and reducing health disparities as a means to improving overall population health. In the context of surgery, a growing emphasis is being placed to understand the complex relation of these factors with healthcare, health seeking behavior, attitudes, and practices. Literature on SDH is replete with the impact of social, economic, and psychosocial factors on accessing surgical care, operative outcomes, and adherence to postoperative care.[9] It is now widely recognized that a considerable proportion of adverse surgical outcomes tends to cluster among individuals from underprivileged backgrounds, exhibiting interdependence between the two. Those who experience greater disadvantage from multiple SDH-related factors in multiple dimensions are more likely to experience poorer surgical outcomes including delayed access, low quality of care, more invasive operations, higher complications, and lower survival.[10] However, much of the research in this area has focused on describing the relationship between SDH and surgical outcomes, rather than developing cost-effective interventions aimed at mitigating them. To address the latter, targeted interventions to optimize their success requires a multidisciplinary approach and should be grounded in evidence-based research. These can then be leveraged to identify prevalence and distribution of health disparities, populations at the highest risk of these disparities, and shape evidence guided interventions to limit them. As such, ongoing research in this area is crucial to developing effective interventions aimed at improving outcomes. However, such efforts require an extensive understanding of the complex interplay of social determinants on daily life to ensure relevance and applicability of the findings and interventions developed in real-world settings. Therefore, in this chapter, we explore theoretical frameworks governing the relationship between social determinants and health outcomes with the aim to create a conceptual basis for identifying theoretically informed and relevant research questions.

THEORETICAL FRAMEWORKS

Theoretical frameworks have been widely used and implemented in public health research. Their primary purpose is to serve as a means to group interrelated concepts to understand the relationship between constructs and form hypotheses to understand behaviors and outcomes related to the theory or concept being studied.[11] Utility of such frameworks becomes imperative in exploratory work to understand abstract concepts, which are not very well understood. While conceptual models are more structured and explore a more specific topic, theoretical frameworks cast a wider net and explore broader ideas and theories. A significant advantage of theoretical over conceptual frameworks is their ability to allow public health experts to link related concepts to understand temporality and associations of a complex phenomenon. Since such phenomenon operate at various levels of systems and populations, these frameworks also allow the opportunity to understand associated factors at all levels, stages, and magnitudes of their effect.

Theoretical frameworks are not causal pathways. Instead, they serve as a conceptual lens through which the problem of interest can be viewed from multiple angles, each with the potential of forming a separate theory on its own. Each angle (theory) is then explored for its ability to explain a certain aspect of the complex, multifaceted problem, with each lens providing a different perspective. This allows all facets of the problem to be explored. Thereby, theories with a sound basis are then explored in the context of similar theories to understand their interaction with each other and combined association with outcomes. Theories found to be interrelated are then grouped into concepts, which are categorized based on their theme, structured and organized into models to understand temporal relations with the outcome. This results in the formation of theoretical frameworks, bringing together various abstract concepts related to an idea and organizing them into structured pathways, which can then be further explored to form hypothesis and propositions.

Theoretical frameworks also serve as guides for selection of appropriate research methodologies and techniques. Through laying a groundwork for selection of measures and outcome indicators most relevant to the theoretical constructs of interest, these frameworks ensure that the methods and data analysis techniques being used are consistent with the research questions being answered, facilitating real-world applicability of the research findings. Ultimately, theoretical frameworks serve as powerful tools that can aid in framing complex problems, understanding correlations, developing interventions, and guiding research to translate these hypotheses into evidence-based concepts.[12]

Role of Theoretical Frameworks in Understanding Social Determinants of Health in Surgery

Social determinants impact surgical outcomes through complex causal pathways mediated by a multitude of dynamic factors. Broad and multifaceted, these factors range from individual (genetics, lifestyle, health behaviors) to systemic levels (including infrastructure, hospital quality, and policies regulating access) and affect the entire continuum of surgical trajectory—from access to surgical care, intra- and postoperative outcomes to rehabilitation. In the context of surgery, theoretical frameworks accomplish two major purposes. Firstly, they serve as powerful tools providing a unique conceptual lens through which the complex interplay between (and influence of) nonmedical factors on surgical outcomes can be viewed from multiple levels (from individual to systemic). For example, racial and ethnic minorities are known to have lower access to surgical care and hence, postoperative outcomes and recovery. While the larger association has been established between race and surgical outcomes, there are a multitude of intermediary factors that mediate this effect. A large proportion of Black and Latino populations reside in economically disadvantaged neighborhoods with poor access to both healthcare and education.[13] Accumulating literature demonstrates that patients with low health literacy have difficulty understanding postoperative care instructions and poor follow-up retention, hence increasing their risk of complications and negative outcomes.[14] Additionally, neighborhoods with high crime and suicide rates also impact the residents' psychological well-being, with the resulting mental stress directly influencing their disease course and recovery. Through providing a structured and systematic model to conceptualize these various determinants, theoretical frameworks can help cluster related factors into meaningful categories, allowing the study of interaction between these determinants and their influence on surgical outcomes.

Secondly, the temporal relationships defined in these frameworks can help identify critical junctures in the causal pathways that are crucial to achieving the desired health outcomes. When leveraged appropriately, these standpoints can be targeted to optimize effectiveness of such interventions and shape policies governing the determinants of health. Examining the temporal relationship from a broader perspective also allows public health experts to identify critical gaps in current health policies and interventions, providing windows of opportunities to refine and/or renew policies to improve health equity and outcomes. Continuing the aforementioned example, incorporating the social and economic disadvantage of racial and ethnic minorities into urban housing, income, and employment policy development can target the root cause of poor surgical outcomes in these populations. Thus, identifying key standpoints in causal pathways can also help maximize the success of such interventions, while simultaneously boosting their cost-effectiveness. However, developing such interventions to mitigate surgical disparities first requires a thorough understanding of the mechanisms that cause them. Hence, understanding SDH through evidence-based research rooted in conceptual grounds is crucial to improving surgical outcomes and reducing health disparities on a systemic level.

RESEARCH ON SOCIAL DETERMINANTS OF HEALTH

Over the past three decades, there has been a growing realization that the dramatically rising health problems across the entire spectrum of healthcare conditions cannot be treated with medical care alone. Hence, awareness around social determinants and their overwhelming influence on surgical outcomes has led to various efforts grounded in evidence-based research to establish an understanding of their causal pathways,

mechanisms of action, and interplay with health. Since most of the research has been exploratory, various theoretical frameworks (including the ones discussed above) have been employed by public health experts to gain a comprehensive understanding of this broad and complex topic, with a focus on social justice and health equity. In the following, we discuss types of research surrounding SDH across the globe.

Types of Research
Epidemiological research
Epidemiological research is focused around understanding the prevalence and distribution of health disparities across populations. In doing so, it helps identify populations at the highest risk of worsened outcomes from systemic inequalities. This area of research explores the patterns of diseases and their outcomes in different populations. Epidemiological research has been gaining traction across the globe for identifying health disparities across socioeconomic, racial, and ethnic groups. Focusing efforts on vulnerable populations through population-level interventions can allow effective and equitable distribution of resources. Another area of focus in epidemiological research is to identify risk factors among these populations that make them vulnerable to adverse health outcomes. Thereby, health differences observed between populations and reasons accounting for these differences can be studied, allowing opportunities for improvement both within and between populations across the globe. Over the years, a robust body of evidence has accumulated aimed at understanding the impact of various social determinants on specific health outcomes such as cardiovascular health, diabetes, trauma, etc. among individuals, citizens, and nations. Table 13.1 illustrates examples of epidemiologic studies exploring SDH and their relation to patterns of diseases, differences in behaviors, and outcomes.

Sociological research
An important field in studying SDH, this discipline explores the interplay of social and economic factors in influencing health outcomes. Understanding social and economic inequalities allows health advocates and public health experts to identify mechanisms, leading to inequalities between individuals and across population to address and mitigate health disparities. Research in these areas targets individualistic factors (such as poverty, education, and social support) along with broader, systemic constructs including structural racism, discriminatory behaviors toward population subsets, and societal segregations. The compounding effect of racial/ethnic identity and socioeconomic status

TABLE 13.1			
Epidemiological Studies on SDH			
Name	**Study Details**	**Outcome Measures**	**Findings**
Shields et al.[15]	National study to assess sociodemographic and behavioral factors influencing health.	Predictors of life expectancy, disability-free life expectancy, and the presence of fair or poor health among residents.	Percentage of minority population, unemployment rate, older populations, average income, and education were stronger predictors of health compared with behavioral factors such as smoking, obesity, infrequent exercise, and heavy drinking.
Paro et al.[16]	National study of 853,449 medicare-insured patients on impact of social vulnerability on surgical outcomes.	Perioperative complications, 30-day readmission, mortality, and length of stay.	Despite insurance coverage, patients with higher social vulnerability had higher risk of complications, extended length of stay, readmission, and mortality rates from commonly performed surgeries.
Son et al.[17]	National study of 3142 US counties.	Trends and disparities in cardiovascular disease (CVD) mortality.	Rural counties with higher proportion of Black residents had higher CVD mortality accounted for by differences in income, food, and housing.
Haider et al.[18]	National study of 429,751 trauma patients on impact of race and insurance status.	Mortality from trauma.	African America, hispanic, and uninsured patients had the highest mortality from trauma.
Diaz et al.[19]	National study of 299,583 patients from high social vulnerability US counties.	Postoperative outcomes.	Black and minority patients residing in high socially vulnerable counties had up to 68% higher odds of serious complications from surgery.
Dhillon et al.[20]	Data analytical study to assess disparities and quantify disease burden in Southeast Asia Region (SEAR).	Trends of morbidity, mortality, risk factors, social determinants, research capacity, health education, workforce, and systems.	SEAR countries had the highest proportion of global mortality. Disparities within these countries and when compared globally were linked to inequalities in education, poverty, political conditions, and other social determinants.

has taken center stage in medicine over recent years, with wider and extensive implications across the spectrum of healthcare conditions. Literature is replete with evidence stressing on the inverse relation of both with health outcomes—where racial/ethnic minorities and individuals from underprivileged backgrounds face worsened health outcomes despite controlling for other important factors. Table 13.2 highlights a few

examples of sociological research exploring the effect of social and economic factors on health outcomes. By understanding and linking these structural factors and social mechanisms through which social determinants affect health outcomes, this crucial area of research enables experts to develop policies and interventions targeting the root causes of health disparities while promoting health equity.

TABLE 13.2 Sociological Studies on SDH			
Name	**Study Details**	**Outcome Measures**	**Findings**
Avendano et al.[21]	Longitudinal study on the effect of wealth, income, and education on stroke.	Incidence and mortality from stroke.	Low wealth and income were important risk factors for socioeconomic and social disparities in stroke identifying inequalities in access for economically disadvantaged groups.
Dedman et al.[22]	Cohort study of 1073 children on impact of childhood housing conditions on health outcomes.	Adult all-cause mortality.	Children with poorer household conditions reflecting low socioeconomic background had significantly increased risk of later adult mortality from common diseases.
Reyes et al.[23]	Cohort study of 80,312 patients on racial and ethnic differences in access to surgical care.	Delayed diagnosis of appendicitis.	Non-hispanic Black patients had higher rates of delayed appendicitis diagnosis.
Kim et al.[24]	National large database study on influence of socioeconomic factors on health outcomes.	Poor health and obesity.	Higher rates of poor health in low-income and education populations signifying a steep socioeconomic gradient.
de Jager et al.[25]	National large database study on impact of income on emergency General surgery outcomes.	Incidence of adverse events in rural and urban populations.	Patients from low-income quartiles in urban areas had higher adverse events from disparities in access to high-quality care.
Lamm et al.[26]	Cohort study of 96,990 patients on influence of socioeconomic status on gastric cancer outcomes.	Mortality and unplanned readmissions after gastric cancer surgery.	Patients with low income and low education had 57% and 48% higher mortality, respectively. Privately insured patients had lower mortality rates.

Health economics research

Disparities in healthcare result in higher costs of care and a preventable burden on already fragile healthcare structures. As interventions are being implemented and tested to reduce health disparities in the context of social determinants, there is a need to understand the cost-effectiveness of these interventions to estimate the social and economic benefits of reducing health disparities. Economic research explores the costs of health disparities and their effect of individuals, communities, populations, and healthcare systems. Another area of focus in economic research is to investigate the impact of healthcare interventions addressing social determinants such as healthcare programs for improving access, interventions to protect income, improving poverty, living conditions or educational interventions on improving individual to population health. However, the field is not solely limited to monetary benefits but also extends to the broader social and economic impact of such interventions. Examples include improved welfare, economic growth, and productivity. Another crucial arm of this disciple is policy implementation and assessing their success with the aim to inform strategies that are both effective and affordable. Such studies are crucial in shaping future policies and identifying priorities for further interventions to optimize their impact and utility. Table 13.3 describes some notable examples of economic research on SDH in surgery.

TABLE 13.3
Health-Economic Studies on SDH

Name	Study Details	Outcome Measures	Findings
Mohan et al.[27]	Systematic review on SDH guided interventions on breast, cervical, and colorectal cancer screening.	Intervention cost, incremental cost per additional person screened, and/or quality-adjusted life-year (QALY).	Interventions were found to be cost-effective, resulted in increased screening rates, and were associated with earlier diagnosis resulting in improved outcomes and significant gains in QALYs.
Zafari et al.[28]	Cost-effectiveness analysis of housing policy for low-income populations.	Long-term health and economic benefits.	Restricted housing vouchers resulted in lower overall cost, improved health, and increments on QALYs compared with traditional vouchers.
LaVeist et al.[29]	Cost–benefit analysis of eliminating health disparities for minority populations.	Direct medical costs, indirect costs (number of lost workdays due to an illness or disability), and cost of premature deaths.	Reducing health disparities for minority populations would save $230 billion from direct medical costs and $1 trillion from indirect loss, illness, and premature death.
Chaudhary et al.[30]	Data analytical study on incidence of racial disparities in universally insured patients.	Outcomes and healthcare utilization after trauma.	Universal insurance and equal access to care resulted in mitigation of disparities in outcomes of Black patients with overall lower odds of mortality and readmissions.
McGowan et al.[31]	Umbrella review on the effectiveness of place-based interventions in improving public health.	Health behaviors, personal and community well-being, living conditions, and access to resources.	Interventions aimed at improving physical environments had positive impact on health outcomes and were cost-effective. Patients living in proximity to the interventions had greater improvements than those living at a distance.
Brilliant et al.[32]	Field trial to assess the effectiveness of health education and economic incentive interventions on cataract surgery acceptance in rural India.	Awareness and acceptance of cataract surgery.	Interventions covering total cost of surgery and house to house visits had the highest acceptance rates.

Knowledge Gaps in Current Literature and Priorities for Further Research

Despite ongoing efforts to understand the wider implications, impact, and applicability of SDH in influencing health outcomes, several challenges and knowledge gaps continue to exist in the field. While causal pathways and upstream fundamental factors have been extensively identified along with potential interventions to address them, these concepts have yet to proportionally penetrate governmental policies and national surgical care planning. This can largely be attributed to the continuous individualistic approach of public health endeavors rather than shifting toward a structural approach to incorporate broader implications of such determinants on surgical outcomes. While health disparities research is now more widely recognized than ever in the surgical community, understanding of the source and perpetrators of these inequalities, along with factors enabling, sustaining, or removing them, remains limited. These issues can partly be traced back to the complex, dynamic, and interconnected nature of health determinants. Because these factors can take several decades or even generations to effect health and generate measurable outcomes, assessing their effects or designing interventions to address them necessitates longitudinal studies backed by vast financial and material resources, which are difficult to sustain. Additionally, these pathways pan out over long periods of time, and doing so becomes vulnerable to effect modification by various individualistic and environmental characteristics along causal pathways, adding to their complexity. This is further limited by lack of social, psychological, and other important nonmedical variables in large publicly available databases, making study of longitudinal relationships, patterns of disease, and outcomes difficult. Public health research is also often victim to political barriers in translating knowledge into outcomes, making implementation of designed interventions cumbersome. When compounded by the inverse graded relationship between socioeconomic status and health of both individuals and populations at large, implementing and assessing the effectiveness of such interventions in low resource setting becomes considerably difficult. Some aspects of these determinants also remain unexplored. As an example, while the effect of health determinants on illnesses and disease course has become apparent, their effect on recovery and rehabilitation remains limited.

A STEP-BY-STEP GUIDE ON FRAMING THEORETICALLY INFORMED RESEARCH QUESTIONS ON SDH

In light of the aforementioned, continuous research exploring the dynamic and continuously evolving pathways of social determinants; their outcomes on health at a microlevel (mechanism by which social structures influence individual health) and macrolevel (power dynamics and geopolitical influences that shape these social constructs); and testing multidimensional interventions to gather evidence on real-world applicability of interventions is needed to bridge these gaps and expand our understanding on the topic. It is imperative to ensure that this research is framed by theoretical and conceptual frameworks, allowing public health researchers to prioritize and explore the most relevant determinants to optimize the success and impact of

their work. Additionally, selecting frameworks relevant to the scientific area being explored also helps identify key gaps in current knowledge, highlight areas in need for further exploration, and guide the selection of the most appropriate methodological and analytical techniques. As a whole, frameworks in research offer a window through which planning and execution of health equity-related research can be structured and organized to maximize the impact and success of interventions.

However, it is also equally important to develop the right research questions. Research questions (the question developed to identify what information is being obtained by the study) are developed based on the problem at hand and area of interest being explored, and ultimately determine the relevance and effectiveness of the study. Since the topic of social determinants is extensive and encompasses several social, ecological, biological, and behavioral realms, a clear and well-formulated research question is crucial to help the researcher focus on the specific aspect of determinant at hand and prevent them from getting side-tracked by several other confounders and covariables that influence the pathways. In doing so, they enhance the chances of reaching meaningful conclusions and generating significant results, while ensuring the applicability of findings on wider public health and health policy development endeavors. With that understanding, we now explore how the aforementioned knowledge can be applied to frame theoretically informed research questions on SDH.

Identify the SDH Relevant to Your Research Idea/Question (Step 1)

Ever since the concept of SDH surfaced in the medical community, decades-long evidence has accumulated documenting various factors that have been identified. This has led to the understanding that an individuals' genetic and behavioral risks for diseases and their resulting effect on health outcomes operate under the influence of social, political, and environment factors. These factors (individually or in combination through layers and magnitudes of effect) govern access to fundamental resources including security, food, education, income, employment, housing, and finances. Together, they shape disease courses and health outcomes over an individual's lifetime and populations at large—hence termed the SDH. The first step in formulating a research question on SDH is to understand the various SDH reported in literature and identify the ones most relevant to the topic of interest. For ease of understanding, SDH can be broadly categorized as follows.

Individual-level determinants

- **Genetics**: Inherited and biological factors, along with familial traits observed through generations.
- **Health behaviors**: These include food, physical activity, lifestyle, smoking, and alcohol consumption.
- **Socioeconomic status**: These include income, occupation, education, and financial resources. Reverse causal relationships of these factors have also been identified where an individual's income and finances are affected by their health, e.g., financial loss or inability to work due to poor health.[33]

Community-level determinants

- **Neighborhood and physical environment**: These encompass sanitary food, living conditions, clean water and air, climate, safe housing, transportation, geography, and climate. While these factors have a direct influence on health, they also indirectly govern access to healthcare and other determinants such as health systems, communities, and social support.
- **Community and social context**: These include social integration, support systems, community engagement, and communal behaviors. These also include racism, discrimination, and stress. Literature suggests communities and neighborhoods with high anxiety, depression, suicide, and crime rates have a negative influence on individuals' health, while those that are collectively motivated to promote public health and well-being participate in health-promoting behaviors such as constructing parks and recreational activities.[34,35]

System-level determinants

- **Healthcare systems**: These include insurance coverage, provider availability, linguistic and cultural competency, availability of primary and preventative services, and overall quality of care.
- **Policy, welfare, and governance**: These include political stability, health policy advocacy, national policies, and state funds to support and promote health.

Review Relevant Theories and Identify the Right Theoretical Framework (Step 2)

Since social determinants affect all aspects of individuals and systems, research related to SDH is broad and encompasses multiple disciplines including epidemiology, sociology, psychology, and economics. Since the introduction of the concept, several attempts have been made to understand the complex, interconnected, and codependent relationship between these nonmedical factors and their correlation with health-related outcomes to understand and address health disparities. Subsequently, several models have been reported in literature that incorporate various theories to understand mechanisms by which SDH exert their effect. In the following, we describe a few commonly used theoretical frameworks in epidemiology, sociology, psychology, and economics to understand SDH and their implications on surgical outcomes.

Commonly used theoretical frameworks in SDH research

Social–ecological model. The social–ecological model emphasizes the interrelation between environmental conditions and human behavior and has two distinct dimensions. One aspect of the model grounds the health-promotive capacity of the environment in various physical, social, cultural, and biological factors with a direct influence on health outcomes. In doing so, the model takes away the individualistic effect of specific environmental factors such as air quality and suggests a cumulative effect of multiple factors, which may compound or negate each other. The other aspect of the model recognizes the influence of various individualistic attributes on human health. These include psychosocial behaviors, genetics, familial dispositions, and lifestyle patterns. By combining the two, this framework studies the complex and dynamic interplay between these various environmental and personal attributes to assess their compatibility and combined effect on health outcomes.[36] In doing so, the model describes the temporality of the effect. In the context of SDH, the model recognizes the complex interplay between various factors at multiple levels in shaping surgical outcomes. It also emphasizes the multifold and interactive impact of these factors including individual (personal lifestyle), interpersonal (social relationships), community (work and living environments), societal (cultural norms, polices, economics) and environmental (physical and ecological) factors. Hence, interventions designed based on this framework are multitiered and target several aspects simultaneously to mitigate disparities in surgery.

Life course perspective. This perspective is grounded in timing of exposures to explore their relationship with outcome occurrence, both within an individual's lifetime and to assess trends at a population level.[37] The model highlights the importance of timing, duration, and strength of exposure to SDH, and their significant impact on health outcome. It recognizes that such factors operate on all levels across an individuals' life course—from early development to old age—and can both have immediate health effects and form a foundation for disease occurrence later in life. However, it particularly stresses on the importance of early-life exposures and their role in shaping outcomes over an individuals' entire life course.

The temporal relationships described in these models can identify potential lag periods between exposures and outcomes where interventions can be targeted to limit disparities. In the context of surgery, this model can be used to understand the long-term impact of adverse childhood exposures (such as trauma, abuse, or neglect) on disease courses, recovery, and complications from surgery occurring later in life.[38,39] The model can also be extrapolated to study diseases across larger populations (to assess trends) and across generations (through biological transmission of risk factors) to contextualize exposures and outcomes on a broader level.

Health belief model. This model implies that an individuals' health-related behavior is influenced by their perception of the health problem. Described as a "value-expectancy" model, this ideology suggests that an individual's readiness to address their condition is shaped by their perception of (1) the gravity of the situation and the anticipated level of threat associated with the problem, (2) the benefit and feasibility of accessing the health-related behavior, (3) the barriers to taking action, and (4) internal and external cues promoting their behavior including personal perceptions of their health and influence of mass media. These cues can promote health-seeking behavior when accompanied by similar perceptions and beliefs. Ultimately, the theory suggests that an individuals' general concern about their health governs their health-seeking behavior and treatment uptake. Over the years, accumulating literature using HBM model and its effect on a broad range of health behaviors has validated its applicability and predictive power across various populations and demographic age groups to understand the interplay of SDH and health outcomes.[40] Hence, this can be used to understand the influence of patients' beliefs about their health and surgical procedure on adhering to postoperative protocols. Interventions designed through this model focus on promoting health through targeting individual perceptions and addressing barriers to enable health-seeking behavior.

Fundamental causes theory. This theory attributes the social inequalities in health to disparities in access to resources vital to maintaining health including finances, social hierarchal structures, and education. Referred to as "fundamental causes"—these factors form the root causes of health inequality by paving way to multiple causal pathways rooted in inequalities in basic necessities to result in differences in health outcomes across social and population groups.[41] The theory traces all these factors back to socioeconomic status (SES) as the main driver for disparities in health outcomes and mortality. This is supported by the idea that SES acts as the "upstream" variable and operates through several downstream effects that interact more directly with diseases and health in causal pathways. Higher social standing allows individuals access to critical resources including power, social connections, money, knowledge, and influence, which allows certain individuals to avoid risks and adopt protective strategies, while the opposite becomes true for individuals who lack access to these resources, thereby creating fundamental inequalities in access to care rooted in social constructs. With the global economic downturn, this gap in health outcomes is increasing widening with the systematically disadvantaged populations (social and ethnic minorities, individuals with lower education or SES) receiving the brunt of it. This model can be used to study the effect of low socioeconomic status, education, and racial/ethnic minority background on access to primary preventative, screening, preoperative testing, and postoperative care access. Exploring mechanisms behind discriminatory behaviors of healthcare systems can inform interventions aimed at addressing social determinants through targeting systemic factors such as education programs, financial coverage schemes, and screening clinics for underserved communities, instead of focusing on individual health behaviors.

Commission on social determinants of health framework. Developed by the World Health Organization, and perhaps the most widely recognized framework used in SDH related research, this framework theorizes the interplay of social, economic, and political factors in stratifying populations into social hierarchies, where an individuals' position determines their specific status of SDH.[42] Hence, an individuals' health status is reflective of their differential exposures, vulnerabilities to conditions negatively impacting health, and their placement within social hierarchies. A key feature of this model that sets it apart from the others is conceptualizing the healthcare system itself as a separate social determinant in the context of access across the social, economic, and political health gradient. The basis for this theory is formed by the ability of health systems to enable equitable access to care and improve health status of populations through policies and public health programs. Broadly, the model dichotomizes health determinants into structural and intermediary types. Structural determinants are ones commonly perceived as the classic SDH, while intermediary determinants are factors through which structural determinants operate to influence health outcomes.

Structural determinants are governed by (1) structural mechanisms, (2) context, and (3) socioeconomic positions. Structural mechanisms are factors that stratify populations into social classes that define their hierarchies of power and hence access to resources. These include race, ethnicity, gender, income, social class, education, and occupation. These structural factors are rooted in systems and behaviors largely regulated by (and work under the influence of) socioeconomic and political contexts that maintain these social hierarchies—referred to as "context." These include political governance and regulations, education systems, labor markets, and social and cultural norms, influencing movement of people between social strata. These amalgamate to define socioeconomic classes with structural hierarchies in populations that indirectly regulate individuals' health and result in disparities in access to healthcare.

Structural determinants have broader implications rooted in systems and behaviors. Their effect on population health is, however, indirect and mediated through a set of individual-level factors termed as intermediary determinants of health. While these stem from the underlying social stratification, these factors have a more downstream affect and influence biological and causal pathways, resulting in differences in exposures, vulnerability of diseases, and severity of outcomes related to health-compromising behaviors at an individual level. The model identifies three broad categories of intermediary determinants. Material circumstances are determinants related to physical environment including neighborhood, housing, living conditions, resource consumption (ability to buy food, clothing medicine), and work environments. Psychosocial circumstances are determinants related to mental health with a direct biological influence on health outcomes, including stressor, interpersonal relationships, coping mechanisms, and social support. Finally, behavioral, genetics, and biological factors form the most proximal points of the causal pathways, which directly affect health. These include lifestyle (eating habits, physical activity, alcohol, and tobacco consumption), genetical predispositions, and familiar behaviors passed down through generations. Additionally, as discussed earlier, this model also recognizes health systems itself as an intermediary determinant. The framework emphasizes the interconnectedness of social, economic, and political factors in the context of SDH and can be used to guide research, develop policies, and design interventions to target social and economic inequalities.

Overall, these various frameworks help to conceptualize and operationalize the health determinants to be able to use them in context of research. It is important to ensure that the theoretical framework chosen is relevant to the research idea and the problem being explored. Since these frameworks are not mutually exclusive, multiple frameworks are often employed by researchers at a time to obtain a holistic understanding of the topic.

Define the Research Problem (Step 3)

After understanding various SDHs and theoretical frameworks that govern their mechanisms, the next step is to review knowledge base in existing literature to identify knowledge gaps and formulate relevant question to addresses these gaps. While doing so, it is crucial to be cognizant and specific about the population, setting, and context of the research being conducted to ensure that the findings are relevant and applicable to the population it is targeting. Another important factor to consider while identifying the research question to understand the levels of influence the research is trying to achieve. These range from individual-level determinants such as health and lifestyle behaviors to system-level determinants such as racism, policies, and healthcare systems. Additionally, understanding the context in which the problem is being explored (filling a knowledge gap related to the problem vs. designing an intervention to address the problem itself) is important in selecting research methodology and analytical technique. Being clear about the research problem allows the researcher to specifically focus on the problem at hand in the relevant context and capacity, augmenting their chances of achieving significant and relevant findings.

Formulate the Research Question (Step 4)

Based on the specific social determinants relevant to the topic, their framework of action, and the problem (knowledge gap) in the relevant context, research questions can be developed to help guide the researchers in addressing the problem and formulating their study by narrowing down a broad topic to a specific area of study.

Types of research questions

There are several types of research questions, and their language is largely dependent on the type of research being conducted. Quantitative research questions are precise and specific and usually aim to answer the "what" questions. On the other hand, qualitative research questions are broad and nondirectional and usually aim to "explore" or "explain" the topic.[43] Research questions may be as follows:

- **Descriptive**: These questions seek to assess the response of the study population to a specific variable.
- **Comparative**: These questions compare the difference between two groups for a specific outcome variable.
- **Relationship**: These questions aim to assess associations and trends between two or more dependent and/or independent variables.
- **Causal**: These questions seek to establish cause and effect relationships between variables.
- **Exploratory**: These questions are employed when researching topics on which little is known. The aim of these questions is to gather a broad understanding on a lesser known topic/phenomenon, which can then be used to guide further research.
- **Evaluative**: These questions seek to assess the effectiveness of interventions or programs.

Components of a research questions

To ensure that the research questions address all important elements of the study, two popular frameworks have been developed and are commonly employed to construct research questions. These include the following:

- **PICOT framework**: Developed in 1995, this framework emphasizes that research questions should address the population being studied (P), the intervention or indicator (I), the comparison group (C), the outcome of interest (O), and time frame of the study (T).[44]
- **PEO framework**: More commonly employed in qualitative research, this framework includes the population being studied (P), the exposure to pre-existing conditions (E), and the outcome of interest (O).

Assessing the quality of research question

When designing studies, researchers might develop several research questions on their topic of interest. However, it is important to ensure that the final question that will shape the study going forward is realistic, measurable, and applicable. Hence, a set of guidelines termed as the FINER criteria were developed in 2007

and can be used to assess the "soundness" of a research question.[45] The criteria suggest that the research questions should be as follows:

- **F (Feasible)**: This seeks to answer if the research is doable while fully addressing the scope of the topic. Feasibility assessment includes ensuring availability of the data and resources required to do the study, along with realistically assessing if the intended scale of the study can be achieved.
- **I (Interesting)**: This element seeks to assess if the topic of the study would be of interest to the academic community at large. This ensures that findings from the study would have an impact on the larger community and can be used to guide further research on the topic.
- **N (Novel)**: This element ensures that the study is not solely a repetition of already understood topics but rather adds to the current pool of knowledge, fills a gap in literature, and brings new perspectives to the topic of interest.
- **E (Ethical)**: A crucial component of research, this element emphasizes on the ethical soundness of the study and topic of interest. All academic research conducted must be either approved or exempted from approval by the review board and other appropriate authorities to protect the rights and welfare of research participants.
- **R (Relevant)**: It is important to ensure that the research topic being explored is relevant to both the peers in the scientific community and the larger area of study.

Adhering to these guidelines can help researchers screen and optimize their research questions, thereby preventing them from wasting valuable time and resources exploring unrealistic or unattainable research questions. These also help ensure that all research conducted is grounded in strong ethical principles and poses no harm to the research participants.

Refine and Finalize

Once a research question has been drafted and screened using the criteria discussed earlier, it is crucial to have the questions reviewed by experts in the field along with colleagues and key stakeholders involved to ensure the feasibility, relevance, and soundness of the study. Based on their feedback and review of literature, research questions can then be refined further to ensure the highest quality of research and knowledge being generated. An outline of the step-by-step guide can be found in Fig. 13.1.

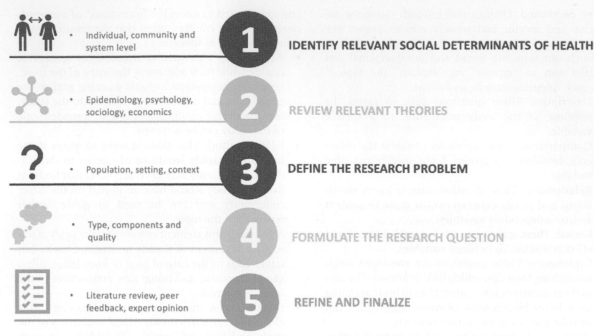

FIG. 13.1 Step-by-step guide to frame theoretically informed research questions on SDH.

CONCLUSION

SDH represent an important paradigm in healthcare research with dramatic implications for health of individuals and nations. As health systems navigate their way through numerous barriers, challenges, and loopholes toward equitable healthcare globally, substantial advancements have been made and continue to expand the scientific knowledge on the dynamic influence of these determinants on health outcomes. However, individual and systemic factors such as insurance, gender, racial and ethnic identity, neighborhood, and social hierarchal structures continue to drive surgical outcomes. While such challenges continue to rise, the compelling evidence supporting the existence and role of these factors in shaping surgical outcomes is no longer a point of contention. Instead, the question today is what are the most critical mechanisms by which these factors exert their effect and which mechanisms need to be targeted to mitigate their effect on health. With the passage of time, increasing awareness of new affect modifiers continues to add to the complexity of presently understood causal pathways by which these factors exert their effect on surgical trajectories of patients. As the evidence supporting the overwhelming influence of these factors has

become too compelling to ignore, the natural scientific progression is to now translate this knowledge into effective interventions and policies to limit their effect.

Continuing to explore these new frontiers in the field of surgical disparities while simultaneously addressing the emerging complexities of previously established concepts requires two things: (1) rigorous and ongoing scientific effort rooted in consistent and reproducible methodologies, allowing adaptability of methods and findings across various populations to obtain a nuanced understanding of these complex and multifaceted determinants; and (2) to develop translational strategies exploring new ventures of research to design and assess the effectiveness of multidimensional interventions to mitigate these inequalities. To address both, grounding innovative research strategies in theoretical frameworks is crucial to conducting rigorous and impactful research. While the process of designing theoretically informed research can be cumbersome, it is the necessary next step in creating successful SDH- based interventions aimed at modifying patient-specific risk to reduce inequalities in access to surgical care, paving way for equitable surgical systems that promote well-being of all individuals and nations.

Highlights

- Theoretical frameworks offer a conceptual lens through which the complex interplay between SDH and surgical outcomes can be viewed from multiple levels and can help identify critical junctures in the causal pathways that can be targeted to optimize effectiveness of interventions.
- Clear and well-formulated SDH research questions are crucial to reaching meaningful conclusions and generating significant results, while ensuring the applicability of findings on population health and policy development endeavors.
- To frame theoretically informed SDH research questions, first identify the SDH and theoretical frameworks most relevant to your research idea.
- Then review the knowledge base to identify specific gaps and priorities of your work. While identifying and defining the research problem, be specific about the populations, setting, and context of your study.
- Based on the aforementioned, develop your research questions. Clearly state the population, intervention, comparison group, outcome, and time frame of the study. Be cognizant of the language to ensure it reflects the type of research being conducted.
- Use the FINER criteria to optimize the feasibility, quality, ethical soundness of the study.
- Review, refine, and finalize the research question(s) based on expert opinion, peer review, and literature search.

REFERENCES

1. Ripollés-Melchor J, Ramírez-Rodríguez JM, Casans-Francés R, et al. Association between use of enhanced recovery after surgery protocol and postoperative complications in colorectal surgery: the postoperative outcomes within enhanced recovery after surgery protocol (POWER) study. *JAMA Surg.* 2019;154(8):725–736. https://doi.org/10.1001/JAMASURG.2019.0995.
2. Ripollés-Melchor J, Abad-Motos A, Díez-Remesal Y, et al. Association between use of enhanced recovery after surgery protocol and postoperative complications in total hip and knee arthroplasty in the postoperative outcomes within enhanced recovery after surgery protocol in elective total hip and knee arthroplasty study (POWER2). *JAMA Surg.* 2020;155(4):e196024. https://doi.org/10.1001/JAMASURG.2019.6024.
3. Mackenbach JP, Kunst AE, Cavelaars AEJM, Groenhof F, Geurts JJM. Socioeconomic inequalities in morbidity and mortality in Western Europe. *Lancet.* 1997;349(9066):1655–1659. https://doi.org/10.1016/S0140-6736(96)07226-1.
4. Stringhini S, Sabia S, Shipley M, et al. Association of socioeconomic position with health behaviors and mortality. *JAMA.* 2010;303(12):1159–1166. https://doi.org/10.1001/JAMA.2010.297.
5. Metzler M. Social determinants of health: what, how, why, and now. *Prev Chronic Dis.* 2007;4(4). /pmc/articles/PMC2099283/ . Accessed May 8, 2023.
6. Torain MJ, Maragh-Bass AC, Dankwa-Mullen I, et al. Surgical disparities: a comprehensive review and new conceptual framework. *J Am Coll Surg.* 2016;223(2):408–418. https://doi.org/10.1016/J.JAMCOLLSURG.2016.04.047.
7. Schoenfeld AJ, Sturgeon DJ, Dimick JB, et al. Disparities in rates of surgical intervention among racial and ethnic minorities in medicare accountable care organizations. *Ann Surg.* 2019;269(3):459–464. https://doi.org/10.1097/SLA.0000000000002695.
8. Haider AH, Scott VK, Rehman KA, et al. Racial disparities in surgical care and outcomes in the United States: a comprehensive review of patient, provider and systemic factors. *J Am Coll Surg.* 2013;216(3):482. https://doi.org/10.1016/J.JAMCOLLSURG.2012.11.014.
9. Braveman P, Egerter S, Williams DR. The social determinants of health: coming of age. *Annu Rev Public Health.* 2011;32:381–398. https://doi.org/10.1146/ANNUREV-PUBLHEALTH-031210-101218.
10. Ladin K, Rodrigue JR, Hanto DW. Framing disparities along the continuum of care from chronic kidney disease to transplantation: barriers and interventions. *Am J Transplant.* 2009;9(4):669–674. https://doi.org/10.1111/J.1600-6143.2009.02561.X.
11. Rocco ST, Plakhotnik SM. Literature reviews, conceptual frameworks, and theoretical frameworks: terms, functions, and distinctions. *Hum Resour Dev Rev.* 2009;8(1):120–130. https://doi.org/10.1177/1534484309332617.
12. Bergeron K, Abdi S, Decorby K, Mensah G, Rempel B, Manson H. Theories, models and frameworks used in capacity building interventions relevant to public health: a systematic review. *BMC Publ Health.* 2017;17(1):1–12. https://doi.org/10.1186/S12889-017-4919-Y/TABLES/1.
13. Rouse CE, Barrow LUS. Elementary and secondary schools: equalizing opportunity or replicating the status quo? *Future Child.* 2006;16(2):99–123. https://doi.org/10.1353/FOC.2006.0018.
14. Herrera-Escobar JP, Seshadri AJ, Rivero R, et al. Lower education and income predict worse long-term outcomes after injury. *J Trauma Acute Care Surg.* 2019;87(1):104–110. https://doi.org/10.1097/TA.0000000000002329.
15. (14) (PDF) The Health of Canada's Communities. Accessed May 8, 2023. https://www.researchgate.net/publication/261773754_The_health_of_Canada's_communities.
16. Paro A, Hyer JM, Diaz A, Tsilimigras DI, Pawlik TM. Profiles in social vulnerability: the association of social determinants of health with postoperative surgical outcomes. *Surgery.* 2021;170(6):1777–1784. https://doi.org/10.1016/J.SURG.2021.06.001.
17. Son H, Zhang D, Shen Y, et al. Social determinants of cardiovascular health: a longitudinal analysis of cardiovascular disease mortality in US counties from 2009 to 2018. *J Am Heart Assoc.* 2023;12(2):26940. https://doi.org/10.1161/JAHA.122.026940.

18. Haider AH, Chang DC, Efron DT, Haut ER, Crandall M, Cornwell EE. Race and insurance status as risk factors for trauma mortality. *Arch Surg.* 2008;143(10):945−949. https://doi.org/10.1001/ARCHSURG.143.10.945.

19. Diaz A, Hyer JM, Barmash E, Azap R, Paredes AZ, Pawlik TM. County-level social vulnerability is associated with worse surgical outcomes especially among minority patients. *Ann Surg.* 2021;274(6):881−891. https://doi.org/10.1097/SLA.0000000000004691.

20. Dhillon PK, Jeemon P, Arora N, et al. Status of epidemiology in the WHO South-East Asia region: burden of disease, determinants of health and epidemiological research, workforce and training capacity. *Int J Epidemiol.* 2012; 41(3):847−860. https://doi.org/10.1093/IJE/DYS046.

21. Avendano M, Glymour MM. Stroke disparities in older Americans: is wealth a more powerful indicator of risk than income and education? Stroke. *J Cerebr Circ.* 2008; 39(5):1533. https://doi.org/10.1161/STROKEAHA.107.490 383.

22. Dedman DJ, Gunnell D, Davey Smith G, Frankel S. Childhood housing conditions and later mortality in the Boyd Orr cohort. *J Epidemiol Community Health.* 2001;55(1): 10−15. https://doi.org/10.1136/JECH.55.1.10, 1978.

23. Reyes AM, Royan R, Feinglass J, Thomas AC, Stey AM. Patient and hospital characteristics associated with delayed diagnosis of appendicitis. *JAMA Surg.* 2023;158(3). https://doi.org/10.1001/JAMASURG.2022.7055. e227055-e227055.

24. Kim Y, Vazquez C, Cubbin C. Socioeconomic disparities in health outcomes in the United States in the late 2010s: results from four national population-based studies. *Arch Publ Health.* 2023;81(1):1−10. https://doi.org/10.1186/S13690-023-01026-1/FIGURES/2.

25. de Jager E, Chaudhary MA, Rahim F, et al. The impact of income on emergency general surgery outcomes in urban and rural areas. *J Surg Res.* 2020;245:629−635. https://doi.org/10.1016/J.JSS.2019.08.010.

26. Lamm R, Hewitt DB, Li M, Powell AC, Berger AC. Socioeconomic status and gastric cancer surgical outcomes: a national cancer database study. *J Surg Res.* 2022;275: 318−326. https://doi.org/10.1016/J.JSS.2022.02.004.

27. Mohan G, Chattopadhyay S. Cost-effectiveness of leveraging social determinants of health to improve breast, cervical, and colorectal cancer screening: a systematic review. *JAMA Oncol.* 2020;6(9):1434−1444. https://doi.org/10.1001/JAMAONCOL.2020.1460.

28. Zafari Z, Muennig P. The cost-effectiveness of limiting federal housing vouchers to use in low-poverty neighborhoods in the United States. *Publ Health.* 2020;178: 159−166. https://doi.org/10.1016/J.PUHE.2019.08.016.

29. Laveist T, Gaskin D, Richard P. Estimating the economic burden of racial health inequalities in the United States. *Int J Health Serv.* 2011;41(2):231−238. https://doi.org/10.2190/HS.41.2.C.

30. Chaudhary MA, Sharma M, Scully RE, et al. Universal insurance and an equal access healthcare system eliminate disparities for Black patients after traumatic injury. *Surgery.* 2018;163(4):651−656. https://doi.org/10.1016/J.SURG.2017.09.045.

31. McGowan VJ, Buckner S, Mead R, et al. Examining the effectiveness of place-based interventions to improve public health and reduce health inequalities: an umbrella review. *BMC Publ Health.* 2021;21(1):1−17. https://doi.org/10.1186/S12889-021-11852-Z/TABLES/4.

32. Brilliant GE, Lepkowski JM, Zurita B, Thulasiraj RD. Social determinants of cataract surgery utilization in South India. *Arch Ophthalmol.* 1991;109(4):584−589. https://doi.org/10.1001/ARCHOPHT.1991.01080040152048.

33. Muennig P. Health selection vs. Causation in the income gradient: what can we learn from graphical trends? *J Health Care Poor Underserved.* 2008;19(2):574−579. https://doi.org/10.1353/HPU.0.0018.

34. Morenoff JD, Sampson RJ, Raudenbush SW. Neighborhood inequality, collective efficacy, and the spatial dynamics of urban violence. *Criminology.* 2001;39(3): 517−558. https://doi.org/10.1111/J.1745-9125.2001.TB00932.X.

35. Ross CE. Neighborhood disadvantage and adult depression. *J Health Soc Behav.* 2000;41(2):177−187. https://doi.org/10.2307/2676304.

36. Stokols D. Translating social ecological theory into guidelines for community health promotion. *Am J Health Promot.* 1996;10(4):282−298. https://doi.org/10.4278/089 0-1171-10.4.282.

37. Ben-Shlomo Y, Kuh D. A life course approach to chronic disease epidemiology: conceptual models, empirical challenges and interdisciplinary perspectives. *Int J Epidemiol.* 2002;31(2):285−293. https://doi.org/10.1093/IJE/31.2.285.

38. Moeller TP, Bachmann GA, Moeller JR. The combined effects of physical, sexual, and emotional abuse during childhood: long-term health consequences for women. *Child Abuse Negl.* 1993;17(5):623−640. https://doi.org/10.1016/0145-2134(93)90084-I.

39. Mullen PE, Martin JL, Anderson JC, Romans SE, Herbison GP. The long-term impact of the physical, emotional, and sexual abuse of children: a community study. *Child Abuse Negl.* 1996;20(1):7−21. https://doi.org/10.1016/0145-2134(95)00112-3.

40. Harrison JA, Mullen PD, Green LW. A meta-analysis of studies of the Health Belief Model with adults. *Health Educ Res.* 1992;7(1):107−116. https://doi.org/10.1093/HER/7.1.107.

41. Link BG, Phelan JO. Social conditions as fundamental causes of disease.

42. Benach J, Friel S, Houweling T, et al. *A Conceptual Framework for Action on The Social Determinants of Health.* Geneva: World Health Organization; 2010. Published online.

43. Marshall C, Rossmann GB. *Articulating Value and Logic: Designing Qualitative Research*; 2010. Published online https://books.google.com/books/about/Designing_Qualitative_Research.html?id=qTByBgAAQBAJ. Accessed May 8, 2023.

44. Richardson WS, Wilson MC, Nishikawa J, Hayward RS. The well-built clinical question: a key to evidence-based decisions. *ACP J Club*. 1995;123(3). https://doi.org/10.7326/ACPJC-1995-123-3-A12.

45. Designing Clinical Research - Google Books. Accessed May 8, 2023. https://books.google.com.pk/books?hl=en&lr=&id=_7UWxJ5erSsC&oi=fnd&pg=PR13&dq=Hulley+SB,+Cummings+SR,+Browner+WS,+Grady+DG,+Newman+TB.+Designing+clinical+research.+3rd+ed.+Lippincott+Williams+and+Wilkins%3B+2007.&ots=YPVthRx5sI&sig=a0rjsEEjl0L0MJ_avVT3IArzqmA&redir_esc=y#v=onepage&q&f=false.

CHAPTER 14

Social Determinants of Health: Study Designs and Outcomes

BENJAMIN G. ALLAR, MD, MPH • HIBA DHANANI, MD, SCM • GEZZER ORTEGA, MD, MPH

INTRODUCTION

The social determinants of health (SDH) play a critical role in shaping how people access and interact with the healthcare system, subsequently impacting their health outcomes. A growing body of research demonstrates how SDH significantly shapes health outcomes and health disparities. This research is the result of thorough and thoughtful research designs and protocols, which aim to answer high-quality questions and whose results aim to improve health conditions on a population level. Studying the complex interplay between SDH and health is challenging due to its multifactorial nature and requires careful consideration of the chosen study design and outcomes.

When conducting research on addressing the SDH, it is essential to assess the *level* of the healthcare system at which the intervention or outcome will have an intended impact. At the systemic level, we investigate factors that influence policy and laws with widespread implications. Focusing on the hospital or community level, we are now focusing on social risk factors and, eventually, at the individual level, social needs.[1] A socioecological model is helpful to develop for your research problem to better comprehend all levels of influence for a desired outcome.

As we rethink how to conduct surgical disparities research to improve the science and promote health equity, this chapter will focus on the critical elements of study design and potential outcome metrics to evaluate in research. Of note, the language and terminology used in the health equity space continue to evolve. The authors intend to be as inclusive as possible and use terminology that is accepted practice and consistent with the views of those by which the terms may impact. SDH are inherently neutral—they are not dependent on a direction—but define an association between an exposure and outcome. Research often emphasizes how negative drivers of SDH are associated with worse disparities in outcomes. However, when a population's needs are adequately met, SDH surgical research can shift social and societal conditions in a positive direction to improve subsequent downstream health outcomes. The focus of this chapter is not to be exhaustive, as there are degree programs in Public Health as well as Epidemiology, but rather to highlight essential methods all researchers working to create positive drivers of SDH.[2]

IDENTIFYING THE RESEARCH QUESTION

The research question is so critical to study design, outcomes, and meaningful results that it should be briefly emphasized again. However, the previous chapter went into extensive detail on asking high-quality, impactful, theoretically informed SDH research questions. The research question is so foundational to the study design and designated outcomes that this chapter should always be read with others but only after researchers have read the previous chapter. SDH research questions are unique among surgical questions because they are framed within the context of community-level factors and public policy. Given this framing, the community of interest should be involved in asking surgical public health questions to involve all relevant stakeholders and ensure significance to the research population (see Community-Based Participatory Research section). This involvement can occur through a diverse research team, including diversity based on sociodemographic variables (race, ethnicity, gender, age, income, etc.) but also topic expertise. For example, a study on SDH and vascular surgery may include vascular surgeons. Still, researchers should also consider asking cardiologists, vascular medicine specialists, primary care physicians, nephrologists (if concerning vascular access for dialysis), and even vascular surgery patients. For example, a study developing a patient or surgeon survey should include psychometricians and pilot samples of patients/surgeons with subsequent interviews/focus groups. Like building a team for a survey, researchers should consider how they build their SDH research team. Including people with diverse perspectives can help develop specific and meaningful questions and solutions. Similarly, developing and supporting a diverse workforce is instrumental in promoting more equitable study design, as this workforce may have the lived experience to create meaningful questions.

The National Institute on Minority Health and Health Disparities (NIMHHD) Research Framework (Fig. 14.1) has an exemplar template for developing and expanding research questions focused on SDH.[3] This framework highlights five domains of disparities research: behavioral, sociocultural environment, healthcare system, physical/built environment, and biological. Each of these domains is then considered on multiple levels of influence: individual, interpersonal, community, and societal.[4] This resource can assist a researcher in evaluating potential levels and/or domains of influence when creating a research question,

selecting a study population, and utilizing subsequent confounders/exposures.

SELECT THE STUDY POPULATION

Defining the population is integral to the overall study because it informs the research's results, impact, and generalizability. The more purposefully diverse and inclusive research population will improve broad generalizability and impact. Admittedly, there are restraints in diverse inclusion due to research funding and the specific availability of special populations within the local communities, which can be discussed in a study's limitations. However, SDH research must reflect the community of interest with equity in mind. A thoughtful selection of study participants is necessary to ensure that diverse perspectives are included. However, care should be taken when studying vulnerable populations, including children, individuals with disabilities, and those who are incarcerated. Funders (National Institutes of Health, private foundations, societal groups, etc.) also require consideration be made for special populations with thorough explanations for their inclusion/exclusion.[5] Therefore, researchers should consider who

		Levels of Influence*			
		Individual	**Interpersonal**	**Community**	**Societal**
Domains of Influence (Over the Lifecourse)	**Biological**	Biological Vulnerability and Mechanisms	Caregiver–Child Interaction Family Microbiome	Community Illness Exposure Herd Immunity	Sanitation Immunization Pathogen Exposure
	Behavioral	Health Behaviors Coping Strategies	Family Functioning School/Work Functioning	Community Functioning	Policies and Laws
	Physical/Built Environment	Personal Environment	Household Environment School/Work Environment	Community Environment Community Resources	Societal Structure
	Sociocultural Environment	Sociodemographics Limited English Cultural Identity Response to Discrimination	Social Networks Family/Peer Norms Interpersonal Discrimination	Community Norms Local Structural Discrimination	Social Norms Societal Structural Discrimination
	Health Care System	Insurance Coverage Health Literacy Treatment Preferences	Patient–Clinician Relationship Medical Decision-Making	Availability of Services Safety Net Services	Quality of Care Health Care Policies
Health Outcomes		Individual Health	Family/ Organizational Health	Community Health	Population Health

National Institute on Minority Health and Health Disparities, 2018
*Health Disparity Populations: Race/Ethnicity, Low SES, Rural, Sexual and Gender Minority
Other Fundamental Characteristics: Sex and Gender, Disability, Geographic Region

FIG. 14.1 The National Institute on Minority Health and Health Disparities (NIMHHDs) research framework.

is included and who is also consciously or subconsciously excluded due to implicit or explicit biases.

Specific Populations

Diverse populations can help identify disparities and develop interventions toward health equity. There are common specific populations that need to be factored into study designs aimed at reducing health disparities due to SDH (Table 14.1). Caution should be taken when discussing such populations as identification with the below-mentioned groups does not convey homogeneous experiences or beliefs.[6,7] Furthermore, it is essential to recognize that within health-related research, race/ethnicity most likely serves as a proxy

for racism (internalized, interpersonal, institutional, structural) and discrimination.[8] Race is a crude proxy for the factors that mediate disparities in health outcomes.

Producing equitable research requires collecting data for these specific populations; you don't know what you don't measure. When using identity data, it should ideally be explicitly collected as self-identified. To implement health system change and enact new policies to promote equitable care, surgical researchers must recognize that this variable lacks construct validity and should seek to create targeted interventions that address true causes of disparities including, most notably, racism.

TABLE 14.1

Examples of Published Social Determinants of Health Research, Which Includes Specific Special Populations

RACIAL/ETHNIC	
Black/African American	Using the 2012–16 National Inpatient Sample, the authors found that compared with white women, black women who had mastectomy had longer length of stay, greater odds of complications, and were more likely to have autologous reconstruction.[9]
Hispanic/Latino/Latinx	Using HCUP State Inpatient Database in New Jersey, authors found that among 22,971 hispanic patients undergoing emergency general surgery operations, there were statistically significant differences in perioperative outcomes between hispanic subgroups (central/South American, Puerto Rican, Mexican, and Cuban).[7]
Asian	Using the 2004–18 surveillance, epidemiology, and End Results database, researchers found multiple significant sociodemographic and medical risk factors for increased specific mortality of prostate cancer among Asian American men.[10]
Indigenous	Given the low rates of cancer screening among American Indian men, these authors describe the Community-Based Participatory Research process and assessment of cancer screening while using text messaging among Hopi men. Researchers found that text messaging was more easily available than patient portals due to ease of access as well as decreased reliable internet.[11]
SEX AND GENDER	
LGBTQ+	Eleven patient-reported outcomes from the Patient-Reported Outcomes Measurement Information system (PROMIS) were administered to evaluate psychosocial outcomes after gender-affirming facial feminization surgery with reported improvement in anxiety, anger depression, and isolation.[12]
Women	Among 1.8 million patients in the Nationwide Inpatient Sample, researchers found a preference of endovascular over surgical revascularization among women, who were older and more likely to have critical limb ischemia versus intermittent claudication. They also found women are at increased risk of 30-day mortality and early complications.[13]
GEOGRAPHY	
Rural	This study demonstrated that rural geriatric surgical patients in New Hampshire are likely to receive care outside of their home county or be transferred, without differences in cost of care of unadjusted mortality. The researchers suggested further research into the specific reasons for transfers and which patients may benefit from remaining close to home.[14]

Continued

TABLE 14.1

Examples of Published Social Determinants of Health Research, Which Includes Specific Special Populations—cont'd

Immigrants, refugees, and asylees	This study interviewed 35 women who had immigrated from east Asia regarding perceptions of breast reconstruction. Themes included lack of information regarding reconstruction, desire to be cancer free and done with treatment, and perceptions of plastic surgery.[15]
Unhoused	Homeless patients living in Medicaid expansion states had lower rates of discharge against medical advice and decreased total index hospital charges after admissions for emergency general surgery.[16]
AGE	
Elderly	Mortality after major surgery was assessed among community-living older adults in the United States through the National Health and Aging Trends study data. Researchers found that 1-year morality rate was 12.4%, but three times higher for nonelective surgeries than elective surgeries, which can help guide patient discussions/expectations.[17]
Children	This study explored glycemic control in severely obese adolescents with type 2 diabetes who underwent medical therapy or surgical therapy, finding that compared with medical therapy, surgical treatment was associated with better glycemic control and reduced weight.[18]
OTHER	
Incarcerated or previously incarcerated	This article discusses the frequency of emergency general surgery or trauma visits within an incarcerated population across 12 centers. Patients were noted to have low follow-up after hospitalization, which was coupled with high rates of assault, mental health and substance use disorders, and self-harm.[19]
Adults with disabilities	This study compared rates of kidney transplant and its outcomes among adults with and without intellectual and developmental disabilities (IDDs). Adults with IDD were half as likely to be evaluated and more than half as likely to receive a kidney transplant despite similar outcomes.[20]
Veterans	Veterans who underwent total hip and knee arthroplasties at Veteran Affairs (VAs) health system had increased comorbidities overall compared with the general population (American college of Surgeons database matched), yet even after adjustment VA patients had increased postoperative complications, length of stay, and readmissions.[21]

Community-Based Participatory Research

Community-based participatory research (CBPR) is a research approach that relies on active community member participation in tandem with research teams throughout the entirety of the research process. CBPR enables community partners to provide insight into the unique landscape of local health systems and is intended to build equitable relationships with researchers. Moreover, CBPR ensures researchers are studying access and outcome measures important to the community and provides opportunities to analyze healthcare structures and processes, which in turn leads to the identification of patient-centered solutions. CBPR is not a singular method or research design but rather an approach that can be applied to multiple types of methods and research designs. Incorporating community members can take various forms, including community advisory boards (CABs), patient and family advocacy councils (PFACs), and partnerships with community organizations.

CBPR has been demonstrated to address healthcare disparities in decision-making and quality of care.[22,23] CBPR has recently been utilized to reduce socioeconomic status disparities in kidney transplantation access (RaDIANT protocol) and breast cancer decision-making (NCT03136367).[24,25] Researchers should consider adding community members to the authorship list and allow them to critically review/edit manuscripts/publications.

Recruiting Participants

To have a study population that will appropriately address the research needs at hand, participants must be recruited. There are a variety of mechanisms by which to recruit for study participation, including posters, video and radio advertisements, social media postings, mobile apps, handouts, emails, and brochures. Recruitment materials should be first and foremost approved by a local Institutional Review Board, but also culturally tailored with the help of community members (PFAC or CAB) to ensure that it effectively conveys the study's goal. Additionally, researchers should ensure that materials are translated appropriately or accessible for those with limited sensory capacity. Although over 8.7% of the US population has limited English proficiency (LEP), many research projects exclude patients with LEP due to systemic problems in communicating appropriately with patients with LEP.[26] These challenges, however, should never prevent researchers from attempting to recruit patients with LEP; if a researcher actively excludes 8.7% of the US population, this significantly limits the generalizability of public health studies. Beyond language considerations, specific plans regarding time away from work, transportation, childcare, caregiving, and translation needs should be made ahead of time to decrease the participant burden.

Unfortunately, within the United States and medicine overall, certain populations have been taken advantage of for research purposes. Infamous examples include the Tuskegee Syphilis Study, Henrietta Lacks' biologic content usage, and forced sterilization of Black women. Understandably, distrust in the medical system persists in part due to this legacy. More recently, there has been distrust related to the COVID-19 global pandemic that stems from rooted racism within healthcare.[27] To effectively recruit participants, the trustworthiness of the researchers and institution is paramount; PFACs and CABs may be particularly helpful surrounding systemic/institutional distrust.

Lived Conditions

The lived environment contextualizes the experiences of communities and patients and provides critical insight into health access and outcomes. The lived environment encompasses both human-made and natural environments where community members live that impact their health and well-being.[28] Environmental determinants of health can be divided into built (human-made environment such as walkability of a town, food deserts, green spaces, proximity to highways, proximity to hospitals, housing, transportation) and natural (not purposefully built by humans such as air quality, water quality, local pollutants, climate change, extreme weather). There are also distinct needs for urban and rural communities that should be defined and considered when developing a study.

Environmental conditions may be challenging to quantify, but different indices have tried to compile aspects of the neighborhood environment to provide context to healthcare outcomes. There are multiple publicly available sociodemographic indices available online (Table 14.2). One study from 2023 compared neighborhood deprivation index, social deprivation index (SDI), area deprivation index, and social vulnerability index on transplant populations, finding that "the choice of deprivation index affects the applicability of research findings across studies examining the relationship between social risk and clinical outcomes."[29]

STUDY DESIGN

If the research question is the foundation of any surgical SDH research project, the study design, covariate inclusion, and outcome measures form the structure on which the findings stand. SDH research within the field of surgery can focus on individual patient outcomes and their association with SDH variables. Still, the research can also be epidemiological in nature, capturing population data or outcomes to answer broader, population-based research questions. Public health problems that can be investigated using epidemiological research include environmental exposures, infectious diseases, natural disasters, etc. The exposure of interest within epidemiological studies will rely on the availability of the data and the level at which the data are collected (individual level vs. community level vs. state level). There are also multiple forms of bias and confounding that should be readjusted for or noted in the limitations of a research project. For example, a project may have confounding by personal preference, where even though neighborhood walkability may be associated with increased physical activity, people who live in those neighborhoods may also prefer walking/physical activity and therefore choose to live in those neighborhoods. In addition, there is the epidemiological challenge of compositional effects or ecological fallacy, where observations about a group are then transferred to individuals within that community. Just because soccer is the most popular sport in the world does not mean that John from Maine likes soccer (although he might!). The opposite of this is the aggregation fallacy, where relationships that exist at an individual level are assumed to hold at the group/community level.

TABLE 14.2
List of Publicly Available Sociodemographic Indices, Their Main Features, and Examples of Published Research

Index	Data source	Variables (Number)	Measurement Area	Example Surgical Study
Distressed Communities Index (DCI)	ACS 5-Y	7	ZIP	Researchers highlight how DCI improves American college of Surgeon's NSQIP risk-adjustment to predict perioperative outcomes and cost.[30]
Area Deprivation Index (ADI)	ACS 5-Y	17	Census block	Lower ADI was associated with improved outcomes across five major common surgeries. However, researchers found ADI disproportionately favored white patients.[31]
Social Vulnerability Index (SVI)	US Census Data	16	Census tract	Researchers found that increased SVI was associated with decreased "textbook" outcomes after hepatopancreatic surgery.[32]
Social Deprivation Index (SDI)	ACS 5-Y	7	County, census tract, ZCTA, and PCSA	Researchers adjusted for sociodemographic factors by using the SDI, finding black non-hispanic patients were more likely to undergo emergency surgery than white non-hispanic patients with colorectal cancer.[33]
Neighborhood Deprivation Index (NDI)[34]	UW School of Medicine and Public Health via ACS	13	9-digit ZIP	In a prospective longitudinal cohort study of bariatric surgery patients, researchers found that NDI level was not associated with differences in weight loss at 1 or 3 years.[35]

ACS, American Community Survey; *NSQIP*, National Surgical Quality Improvement Program; *UW*, University of Wisconsin; *ZCTAs*, ZIP Code Tabulation Areas; *PCSA*, primary census statistical area.

Data Collection

Data collection methods will depend on the study design and the research question. Data sources may include surveys, medical records, administrative data, and interviews. Researchers should ensure that the data collection methods are reliable and valid, and that they protect the privacy and confidentiality of study participants. Transparency in data utilization can also improve trust among research participants and the communities in which the research is being conducted. If institutional administrative data are collected, it should be confirmed also by looking at specific patient charts, if approved by the institution's IRB. If possible, data should be collected by multiple researchers, who can double-check each other's data collection to confirm accurate collection.

Quantitative Research

Observational and experimental epidemiological research studies should be selected based on the research question. Observational research is just that both exposure and outcomes are observed and then analyses are performed based on those observations. However, in experimental studies, the researchers influence the exposure before assessing the outcomes. Ultimately, the choice of study should be informed by the theoretical framework, research question, the availability of data, and the feasibility of conducting the study. Choosing the right study design, covariates, and outcome measures have implications for the study finding's generalizability and utility to improve the healthcare of the study population.

A cohort study splits the included subjects into control and exposure groups, and then the rate of the outcome is compared between the two groups, resulting in a relative risk (or risk ratio). Cohort studies can be prospective (following individuals forward in time, looking at incidence) or retrospective (looking back at historical data, looking at prevalence). For prospective studies, both groups start at a similar baseline, but then the control group is not exposed to the risk.

A case–control study involves comparing individuals with a particular health outcome (cases) to individuals without the health outcome (controls) to examine the relationship between SDH and the outcome. This study design is best for studying rarer diseases, as researchers do not need to wait for patients to acquire the disease as they would for prospective cohort studies. For case–control studies, researchers should then consider all potential factors (patient level, community level, etc.) and consider potential significant associations between risk factors and the outcome. The major difference between case–control studies and retrospective cohort studies is that cohort study groups are made based on exposures, while case–control study groups are based on outcomes. In addition, for case controls, if a whole subpopulation has a condition of interest, there may be an SDH driving this condition as well and should be factored into a causal analysis or adjusted for as a confounder.

A cross-sectional study involves the collection of data at a single point in time and is useful for examining the prevalence and distribution of SDH among a population. For these study types, exposures and outcomes are measured in one instance and there is no intervention. Although these can be easier to measure accurately and get a full dataset, cross-sectional study answers may often need follow-up studies or studies in different populations/cohorts to improve generalizability. The alternative to a cross-sectional study is a longitudinal study, which involves collecting data from the same group of individuals over an extended period and is useful for examining the long-term effects of SDH on health outcomes.

Although all the aforementioned studies can only focus on association, rather than causation, the strongest way for researchers to attempt to prove causation is through experimental studies, which includes randomized controlled trials (RCTs) and nonrandomized, field/community trials. RCTs place participants randomly into two groups, where one group receives an intervention and the other receives no intervention or standard of care. These are the most costly and complex research designs and are therefore completed less often. From an SDH perspective, they are relatively rare given that SDH can be challenging to "randomly" assign to one group or another and SDH cannot be blinded from a researcher or a participant, which is often a key step to RCTs to avoid placebo effect and researcher biases. It could be considered unethical to answer SDH research questions by randomizing into different groupings of SDH, such as randomly giving patients *worse* health insurance or randomizing interventions based on social identities. This makes performing RCTs on SDH work incredibly difficult. A method around the challenges with RCTs that is being more commonly used in surgery research is propensity matching. Propensity matching is where the two groups are attempted to be equalized in everything but the exposure through statistical maneuvers. There are other statistical methodologies used in surgery research as well, such as coarsened Exact Matching,[36] and researchers should consult with a biostatistician for further guidance to develop the most appropriate statistical model.

An ecological study involves examining the relationship between SDH and health outcomes at the population level, rather than the individual level. Ecological studies can be useful for identifying patterns and trends in health outcomes across different regions or populations. This may not be as applicable for surgical research, as surgery still happens on an individual person, and therefore, individual characteristics and variables should be included in the research, but it is critical to start thinking about how population-level SDH can impact individual presentations and outcomes for surgery, although researchers need to be cautious of ecological fallacy.

Qualitative and Mixed Methods Research

Quantitative studies provide valuable data and numbers behind SDH disparities within surgery, but it may not provide the depth of context necessary to design interventions that ultimately improve health equity. Qualitative research can also create new areas of research and develop new research questions that quantitative data cannot. Even more, as provider-focused outcomes after surgery continue to be maximized through effectiveness research, there is an increased emphasis on patient-focused outcomes—whether through patient-reported outcome measures (PROMs) or through qualitative research (semistructured interviews, focus groups, or ethnography). Mixed methods research is when qualitative and quantitative data are collected and analyzed within the same cohort/study. Mixed methods studies can give the most accurate overall picture of a problem and potential solutions within SDH research, as it combines quantitative data with other sources that are otherwise not traditionally gathered, strengthening the findings of the study.

Considering SDH Covariates

With the research design chosen based on the theoretical framework, research question, availability of data, and feasibility, researchers must also consider what additional variables need to be collected to describe the population and adjust for confounding.

For studies looking into SDH, multiple ecological levels should be adjusted for. For example, researchers should not just adjust for patient-level factors such as age, gender, race, ethnicity, or medical comorbidities, but also adjust for community-level factors (median household income, social vulnerability, proximity to food deserts, etc.) as well as hospital-level factors (bed size, academic-teaching status, joint commission certification, etc.). Hospital-level factors can be collected by researchers at those hospitals, or through administrative

databases such as the American Hospital Association database. If unavailable, researchers should still adjust for hospital level variation through mixed-effects modeling. Community-level factors are often best collected by the government and can be found on publicly available websites.

Prior chapters have already highlighted different measures of SDH, from finances and neighborhood to race and insurance status. However, the ability to use these measures depends on the research database you are using and its ability to connect to other databases. With a patient's ZIP code or FIPS code, researchers can connect to Centers of Disease Control and Prevention (CDC) level data and assign SDH measures to individual patients. However, this is still on a neighborhood level, as the CDC does not store data on individuals. In addition, it is critical to consider the implications of even using ZIP codes or FIP codes. ZIP codes can cross state lines and therefore may be less helpful when studying state-level policies. FIP codes, however, often cover a wider area because they cover a county, rather than ZIP codes, which are used for mail delivery routes that the USPS uses to organize/expedite mail delivery.

There are multiple variables to assess socioeconomic status, each with benefits and negatives. Income is a continuous variable that is comparable across time (adjusting for inflation). However, income can have a high reporting refusal rate, have a complex definition, unstable across years of health, and susceptible to reverse causation, and may have different implications based on household size. Education is less susceptible to reverse causation and is more routinely and accurately reported but has a more restricted range. In addition, education quality is variable and challenging to compare across different generations, where educational attainment is different. Occupation is another socioeconomic option, especially as it captures multiple dimensions of the SES experience (prestige, power, control) as well as physical and psychosocial aspects of work. Respondents are often honest about their responses, which makes bias less likely. Occupation, however, is susceptible to "Vice President" bias, where the title may not reflect actual occupation. In addition, occupation is susceptible to reverse causation, and it can be expensive/time-consuming to code. Finally, it does not capture students, retirees, and homemakers. The best marker may be personal wealth, as it captures intergenerational effects and people of all ages/careers as well as demonstrates debt (negative wealth). However, it is extremely difficult to measure and answer, especially in participant surveys/interviews. In addition, wealth is susceptible to reverse causation and confounding.

Data Sources

There are multiple potential data sources available to surgical researchers looking to investigate SDH. Administrative data are often a subset of demographic and clinical data and are frequently used to study healthcare outcomes and delivery. Within the United States, these data are often linked to national registries such as the oncologic Surveillance, Epidemiology and End Results (SEER) registry, National Cancer Database (NCDB), American College of Surgeons (ACS) National Surgical Quality Improvement Program (NSQIP), the National Trauma Data Bank (NTD), the Vascular Quality Initiative (VQI), and many others. Insurers such as Medicare and Medicaid also collect patient and hospital data through insurer claims and can include information such as procedures, diagnoses, and discharge information. Researchers should become familiar with potential and available (some cost money) databases before deciding which one to use, as each database has its known benefits and disadvantages.

Data Analysis

Data analysis should be guided by the research question and the theoretical framework. Statistical methods, such as regression analysis, can be used to examine the relationship between SDOH and health outcomes, while qualitative methods, such as content analysis, can be used to assess interviews and open-ended survey responses. Whatever the method is chosen, it is critical that the researchers describe their reasoning behind the method and be transparent about the data analysis methods to ensure validity, reliability, and reproducibility of the study findings. It is critical to bring early data findings to the team for informed discussion about ways to refine the protocol, develop sensitivity analyses, and discuss implications of the findings.

SELECT THE OUTCOMES

Clinical Outcome Measures

Clinical outcome measures in research are centered around clinical care and healthcare utilization. The AHRQ defines outcome measures as "[reflecting] the impact of the health care service or intervention on the health status of patients."[37] Some examples of this include survival and mortality after 30 or 365 days, inpatient mortality, length of stay, inpatient complications, and readmission. These clinical outcome measures may be easily comparable but may be limited to

the scope of healthcare systems. Furthermore, incentives to address such outcomes may be driven by cost and insurers. Clinical outcomes are the result of multiple factors that may be difficult to independently distinguish. Although "outcomes" may traditionally be seen as postoperative, surgical disparities research and SDH research also strongly emphasize access to high-quality care. The Metrics for Equitable Access and Care in SURgery (MEASUR)[38] categorizes access into four areas: Provider Access, Surgical Indication Detection, Progression to Surgery, and Receipt of Optimal Care. SDH can be mapped onto these categories in one of six "disparity domains," which include racial/ethnic, education, insurance, income, geography, and "other." Similarly, Loeher et al. (2018) asked how Medicaid expansion was associated with not just management of common surgical diseases ("receipt of optimal management") using hospital administrative data but also patient presentation (early uncomplicated disease vs. delayed/complicated disease).[39]

As population/public health research ultimately aims to improve local/state/federal policies, one method of assessing outcomes is through measuring outcomes before and after the implementation of a regulation/policy. This can be best performed with a difference-in-differences analysis, which can estimate the causal impact of a treatment or intervention on an outcome variable of interest. It can help researchers to isolate the causal effect of a treatment/intervention from other confounding factors that might also affect the outcome variable.

Evaluating heterogenous treatment effects (HTEs) of social policies is critical to determine how they affect health inequities. Knowing the HTE of specific policies enables researchers to determine how interventions affect different populations. For example, an intervention that disproportionately benefits individuals with worse health will reduce disparities, whereas an intervention that disproportionately benefits healthier communities will increase disparities. Unfortunately, methods for evaluating HTEs are varied with little consensus on which groups should be examined for HTE (geographic, education, age, gender, economic, race/ethnicity) and which studies should evaluate HTEs.[40]

Patient-Reported Outcome Measures

PROMs are patient centric and can better characterize experiences of patients with the healthcare system. In particular, they can elicit discrepancies between populations, particularly those who may face barriers to accessing high-quality care and optimal outcomes. These outcome measures enable researchers to investigate interpersonal racism and discrimination, which impact the patient experience and clinical outcomes. Quality of life is often an important component of PROMs. Qualitative methods can contextualize responses and also guide researchers in selecting outcomes. PROMs should be reportable in multiple languages and modalities to ensure that the population is appropriately reflected.[26] Several recording measures for PROMs exist across different clinical conditions (Table 14.3). PROMs may still be impacted by other factors including when they are administered postoperatively.[41] They also provide a method with which we can investigate how interpersonal racism and discrimination, which have been historically difficult to capture empirically, affect patient experiences and outcomes before, during, and after surgery. We have found that PROMs utilization can vary by patient language as well, which can lead to a noncomplete representative sample and reduce generalizability to all patients.[42] Researchers must also encourage the use of PROMs in multiple languages and modalities to ensure the measurements are reflective of the entire population. PROM implementation and research should include some minimum standard of collection.

Financial Outcomes and Cost-Effectiveness

As healthcare costs increase, there has been particular attention paid to outcomes regarding cost-effectiveness. Multiple components contribute to the cost of care including healthcare delivery via new technologies and high administrative costs. Value-based care has emerged to promote better clinical outcomes for patients in a cost-efficient manner. Ultimately, value-based healthcare may lead to lower patient expenditures particularly for those with chronic illness or recovering from surgeries.[43] Financial consequences for patients and caregivers can be devastating (also known as financial toxicity) so it is essential to ensure that efforts are made to reduce costs without compromising patient safety.

Implementation Science/Outcomes

Health services research has exposed disparities in access, cost, and outcomes. Yet, simply documenting disparities in these areas is not enough. It is crucial to turn these findings into implementation strategies that can improve outcomes. Surgical health services research needs to prioritize implementation science to move toward reducing disparities, rather than just elucidating and corroborating them. Implementation science research is unique and complementary to the predominantly observational nature of health services research. As SDH crosses multiple sectors, it will take multidisciplinary collaboration to create targeted interventions that address racism and its deleterious effects on outcomes for surgical patients.

TABLE 14.3
Type of Outcomes and Examples Within Social Determinants of Health Surgical Research

Type of "Outcome"	Example Outcomes
Clinical—Postoperative	Mortality, readmission rate, length of stay, complications
Clinical—Access	Emergency admission, rate of early uncomplicated disease
Patient-reported outcome measure (PROM)	Quality of life, functional status, symptoms (depression, pain), caregiving needs, trust in providers
Cost-effectiveness	Cost of stay, out-of-pocket cost, financial toxicity
Implementation	Acceptability, adoption, appropriateness, costs, feasibility, fidelity, penetration, sustainability

INTERPRETATION AND DISSEMINATION

In conducting surgical research that aims to address health equity, researchers must be mindful of the interpretation of their findings. As mentioned before, this discussion of interpreting the findings should be among a team of diverse researchers and include the populations that are impacted by the study. Considering how the outcomes will be interpreted by various stakeholders can provide context into how and where to share the findings of the study. Ultimately, the findings should answer the original research questions, and if a thoughtful theoretical framework was used, then it should make interpretation easier. The research team should consider the perspectives of the findings, for example, (1) What are the reference groups? (2) What are the comparisons that were made? (3) What are the potential headlines? (4) Could the findings cause potential harm to a group? Furthermore, what are the assumptions made during the research study? All projects have limitations, and variables such as race/ethnicity and median household income are social proxies that have discerning influences. Interpreting these proxies and addressing these questions *in advance* are vital to the narrative of the research study and the potential impact on mitigating the negative drivers of health outcomes.

Along with the interpretation of the findings, the dissemination of the research demands attention when working to improve health equity. A discussion on the dissemination plan should occur early on in the scope of a research project. Researchers may have a target journal for the research project, which is important for academic productivity, but they should also consider lay press and local newspapers or publications. One could consider printing their findings as an Op-Ed in a local newspaper. It could serve to support small media outlets with valuable content, strengthen and build trust with the local community, and share the findings with the populations who may be most impacted. Researchers may also consider community health fairs, radio advertisements, podcasts, websites, and other forms of media to share their findings. Building these relationships may also improve the capacity to recruit diverse individuals to research projects, which supports the imperative of equitable research endeavors. Additionally, identifying and investigating policies (beyond health, as we note, the SDH encompass many fields) can serve as a stimulant for areas of research investigations. This can lead to collaborating or partnering with local or national organizations and politicians who can assist in supporting findings that require policy reform. Lastly, researchers should consider a budget or plan for the continuity of their impactful findings. Upon completing a research project that has created a successful intervention for a population that can now receive more equitable healthcare or health outcomes, creating a succession plan to support this work beyond the budget timeline, through sponsorship of their local institution, philanthropy, government, or an organization that can take on the work to maintain the intervention. Nontraditional and multiple forms of dissemination can lead researchers to have the broadest impact possible, with the goal of reaching more people and thereby eventually influencing policies.

CONCLUSION

Studying the complex interplay between SDOH and health requires careful consideration of study design, which is developed based on a careful research question within the constraints of time, resources, and available databases. Researchers should identify a relevant and feasible research question, choose an appropriate study design (both in answering a question and in required resources), select a diverse and representative study population, choose outcome measures that are informed by a theoretical framework, collect reliable and valid data, analyze data using appropriate statistical and qualitative methods, and interpret results in the context of the limitations of the study design. Recruitment of participants should be thoughtful and may be more successful with community partnerships. Public health and population health research is unique compared with traditional comparative effectiveness research within surgery in that there are more factors than just individual patient characteristics—researchers must also consider the world/system that patients (and surgeons) live in. By following these key elements of study design, researchers can produce rigorous and meaningful research that equitably inform public health policy and practice.

Highlights

- SDH impact how people access and interact with the healthcare system.
- Factors have impact at different levels:
  - Systemic → policy and legal impact
  - Hospital or healthcare professional → social factors
  - Individual → social needs
- Five domains of disparities research:
  - Behavioral
  - Sociocultural environment
  - Healthcare system
  - Physical/built environment
  - Biological
- CBPR is a research method that emphasizes community participation throughout the research process (CAB, PFAC).
- CBPR can address healthcare disparities on multiple levels
- Many different populations exist within healthcare disparities research though care should be made to not treat groups as a monolith.
- Studies of the lived environment can provide insight into understanding contextual factors of healthcare, especially when adjusting for sociodemographic indices.
- Multiple research methods exist:
  - Quantitative
  - Qualitative
  - Mixed methods
- Covariates for SDH research should adjust for ecological levels.
- There are multiple types of outcome measures.
  - Clinical
  - Patient-reported (PROMs)
  - Cost-effectiveness
  - Implementation
- Thoughtful consideration of the interpretation and dissemination of the findings has the potential for broad impact of research.

REFERENCES

1. Zook KGM. *When Talking about Social Determinants, Precision Matters*. Health Affairs; 2019 (Health Affairs Forefront).
2. Staff N. *Social Drivers vs. Social Determinants: Using Clear Terms*; 2023. https://blog.nachc.org/social-drivers-vs-social-determinants-using-clear-terms/. Accessed April 5, 2023.
3. Disparities NIoMHaH. *NIMHD Research Framework*; 2017. https://www.nimhd.nih.gov/about/overview/research-framework.html. Accessed March 17, 2021.
4. Alvidrez J, Castille D, Laude-Sharp M, Rosario A, Tabor D. The national institute on minority health and health disparities research framework. *Am J Publ Health*. 2019; 109(S1):S16–s20.
5. Aging NIo. *Overview of the Office of Special Populations*; 2023. https://www.nia.nih.gov/research/osp/overview-office-special-populations. Accessed April 4, 2023.
6. Gore A, Truche P, Iskerskiy A, Ortega G, Peck G. Inaccurate ethnicity and race classification of hispanics following trauma admission. *J Surg Res*. 2021;268:687–695.
7. Maurer LR, Rahman S, Perez N, et al. Differences in outcomes after emergency general surgery between Hispanic subgroups in the New Jersey State Inpatient Database (2009-2014): the Hispanic population is not monolithic. *Am J Surg*. 2021;222(3):492–498.
8. Lett E, Asabor E, Beltrán S, Cannon AM, Arah OA. Conceptualizing, contextualizing, and operationalizing race in quantitative health sciences research. *Ann Fam Med*. 2022;20(2):157–163.
9. Sarver MM, Rames JD, Ren Y, et al. Racial and ethnic disparities in surgical outcomes after postmastectomy breast reconstruction. *J Am Coll Surg*. 2022;234(5):760–771.
10. Wu D, Yang Y, Jiang M, Yao R. Competing risk of the specific mortality among Asian-American patients with prostate cancer: a surveillance, epidemiology, and end results analysis. *BMC Urol*. 2022;22(1):42.
11. Batai K, Sanderson PR, Joshweseoma L, et al. Formative assessment to improve cancer screenings in American Indian men: native patient navigator and mHealth texting. *Int J Environ Res Publ Health*. 2022;19(11).
12. Caprini RM, Oberoi MK, Dejam D, et al. Effect of gender-affirming facial feminization surgery on psychosocial outcomes. *Ann Surg*. 2022. In press.
13. Lo RC, Bensley RP, Dahlberg SE, et al. Presentation, treatment, and outcome differences between men and women undergoing revascularization or amputation for lower extremity peripheral arterial disease. *J Vasc Surg*. 2014; 59(2):409–418.
14. Burney CP, Baumann L, Carlos HA, Briggs A. Impact of rurality on geriatric emergency general surgery patients in New Hampshire. *J Am Coll Surg*. 2022;236(6):1105–1109.
15. Fu R, Chang MM, Chen M, Rohde CH. A qualitative study of breast reconstruction decision-making among Asian immigrant women living in the United States. *Plast Reconstr Surg*. 2017;139(2):360e–368e.
16. Manzano-Nunez R, Zogg CK, Bhulani N, et al. Association of Medicaid expansion policy with outcomes in homeless patients requiring emergency general surgery. *World J Surg*. 2019;43(6):1483–1489.
17. Gill TM, Vander Wyk B, Leo-Summers L, Murphy TE, Becher RD. Population-based estimates of 1-year mortality after major surgery among community-living older US adults. *JAMA surgery*. 2022;157(12):e225155.
18. Inge TH, Laffel LM, Jenkins TM, et al. Comparison of surgical and medical therapy for type 2 diabetes in severely obese adolescents. *JAMA Pediatr*. 2018;172(5):452–460.
19. Bryant MK, Tatebe LC, Siva NR, et al. Outcomes after emergency general surgery and trauma care in incarcerated individuals: an EAST multicenter study. *J Trauma Acute Care Surg*. 2022;93(1):75–83.
20. Hand BN, Hyer JM, Schenk A, et al. Comparing kidney transplant rates and outcomes among adults with and without intellectual and developmental disabilities. *JAMA surgery*. 2023;158(4):386–392.
21. Frisch NB, Courtney PM, Darrith B, Copeland LA, Gerlinger TL. Veterans undergoing total hip and knee arthroplasty: 30-day outcomes as compared to the general population. *J Am Acad Orthop Surg*. 2020;28(22): 923–929.
22. Adler RR, Smith RN, Fowler KJ, et al. Community based participatory research (CBPR): an underutilized approach to address surgical disparities. *Ann Surg*. 2022;275(3): 496–499.
23. Moore Q, Tennant PS, Fortuna LR. Improving research quality to achieve mental health equity. *Psychiatr Clin*. 2020;43(3):569–582.
24. Durand MA, Yen RW, O'Malley AJ, et al. What matters most: randomized controlled trial of breast cancer surgery conversation aids across socioeconomic strata. *Cancer*. 2021;127(3):422–436.
25. Patzer RE, Gander J, Sauls L, et al. The RaDIANT community study protocol: community-based participatory research for reducing disparities in access to kidney transplantation. *BMC Nephrol*. 2014;15:171.
26. Allar BG, Eruchalu CN, Rahman S, et al. Lost in translation: a qualitative analysis of facilitators and barriers to collecting patient reported outcome measures for surgical patients with limited English proficiency. *Am J Surg*. 2022; 224(1 Pt B):514–521.
27. Best AL, Fletcher FE, Kadono M, Warren RC. Institutional distrust among African Americans and building trustworthiness in the COVID-19 response: implications for ethical public health practice. *J Health Care Poor Underserved*. 2021;32(1):90–98.
28. Davern M, Winterton R, Brasher K, Woolcock G. How can the lived environment support healthy ageing? A spatial indicators framework for the assessment of age-friendly communities. *Int J Environ Res Publ Health*. 2020;17(20).
29. Park C, Schappe T, Peskoe S, et al. A comparison of deprivation indices and application to transplant populations. *Am J Transplant: Off J Am Soc Transplant Am Soc Transplant Surgeon*. 2023;23(3):377–386.
30. Mehaffey JH, Hawkins RB, Charles EJ, et al. Socioeconomic "distressed communities index" improves surgical risk-adjustment. *Ann Surg*. 2020;271(3):470–474.
31. Diaz A, Valbuena VSM, Dimick JB, Ibrahim AM. Association of neighborhood deprivation, race, and postoperative outcomes: improvement in neighborhood deprivation is

associated with worsening surgical disparities. *Ann Surg.* 2022. In press.

32. Azap RA, Paredes AZ, Diaz A, Hyer JM, Pawlik TM. The association of neighborhood social vulnerability with surgical textbook outcomes among patients undergoing hepatopancreatic surgery. *Surgery.* 2020;168(5): 868−875.

33. Howard R, Hendren S, Patel M, et al. Racial and ethnic differences in elective vs. Emergency surgery for colorectal cancer. *Ann Surg.* 2023;278(1):e51−e57.

34. Kind AJH, Buckingham WR. Making neighborhood-disadvantage metrics accessible - the neighborhood atlas. *N Engl J Med.* 2018;378(26):2456−2458.

35. Drewnowski A, Hong BD, Shen E, et al. Neighborhood deprivation and residential property values do not affect weight loss at 1 or 3 years after bariatric surgery. *Obesity.* 2023;31(2):545−552.

36. Haider AH, David JS, Zafar SN, et al. Comparative effectiveness of inhospital trauma resuscitation at a French trauma center and matched patients treated in the United States. *Ann Surg.* 2013;258(1):178−183.

37. Agency for Healthcare Research and Quality R, MD. *Types of Health Care Quality Measures;* 2015. https://www.ahrq.gov/talkingquality/measures/types.html.

38. de Jager E, Levine AA, Udyavar NR, et al. Disparities in surgical access: a systematic literature review, conceptual model, and evidence map. *J Am Coll Surg.* 2019;228(3): 276−298.

39. Loehrer AP, Chang DC, Scott JW, et al. Association of the affordable care act Medicaid expansion with access to and quality of care for surgical conditions. *JAMA surgery.* 2018;153(3):e175568.

40. Cintron DW, Adler NE, Gottlieb LM, et al. Heterogeneous treatment effects in social policy studies: an assessment of contemporary articles in the health and social sciences. *Ann Epidemiol.* 2022;70:79−88.

41. Weick L, Brorson F, Jepsen C, Lidén M, Jensen EW, Hansson E. Giving meaning to patient reported outcomes in breast reconstruction after mastectomy - a systematic review of available scores and suggestions for further research. *Breast.* 2022;61:91−97.

42. Ortega G, Allar BG, Kaur MN, et al. Prioritizing health equity in patient-reported outcome measurement to improve surgical care. *Ann Surg.* 2022;275(3):488−491.

43. Barnett ML, Wilcock A, McWilliams JM, et al. Two-year evaluation of mandatory bundled payments for joint replacement. *N Engl J Med.* 2019;380(3):252−262.

CHAPTER 15

Interventions for Redressing Disparities Related to Social Determinants of Health in Surgery

YOSHIKO IWAI, MS • OLUWADAMILOLA M. FAYANJU, MD, MA, MPHS

BACKGROUND

The United States (US) Department of Health and Human Services defines social determinants of health (SDOH) as "the conditions in environments where people are born, live, learn, work, play, worship, and age that affect a wide range of health, functioning, and quality-of-life outcomes and risks."[1] SDOH include housing, transportation, education, literacy, employment, environment, discrimination, and violence domains within which individuals' demographic characteristics (e.g., race, country of origin) as well as provider-level and systemic biases contribute to differential access to resources and propagation of health disparities.

While SDOH have gained attention in research, quality improvement, and patient care in recent years, effectively identifying and intervening on barriers to equitable resource allocation and opportunity related to various SDOH remains challenging. In this chapter, we will discuss the current state of data collection on SDOH and address patient-, provider-, and system-level interventions reported in the literature with a focus on surgical care. We conclude the chapter with theoretical frameworks to guide development and implementation of equity-focused interventions.

DATA COLLECTION

To address health disparities in surgery and healthcare at large, we must first understand the state of social drivers, leading to downstream disparities in clinical outcomes and care quality. It is essential to maintain an up-to-date understanding of these drivers to develop meaningful research questions and subsequent interventions.

The "history and physical" is considered the backbone of a patient's medical record, the documentation that summarizes the clinical and social circumstances that led to an individual presenting for clinical care. However, there is significant provider variation with regard to the accuracy and completeness of clinical documentation.[2] For many providers, it is uncommon to complete a "social history" beyond tobacco, alcohol, or recreational drug use, and few ask about housing and food security or social isolation at clinic visits.[3,4] Even if electronic health record (EHR) systems have mechanisms for documenting health literacy, it is unclear how frequently this is recorded by clinicians or used to provide appropriately tailored documentation in after-visit summaries including perioperative instructions.[5] These type of data can theoretically be collected by outpatient primary care physicians, specialty care physicians, and clinic staff in the EHR or even by hand if time or resources are limited. However, temporal and financial pressures often prevent histories being taken that might reveal SDOH-related challenges and opportunity to address specific barriers to care.[6]

If SDOH-related data collection occurs at all, it is typically event-, procedure-, or screen-triggered and often without mechanisms for regular updating (e.g., smoking history often collected at initial establishment of care, but not at subsequent visits).[4] While some patients may choose to update these elements of their personal and social history using patient-facing EHR applications such as Epic's MyChart, many patients with limited technological access, bandwidth, or literacy may not. Furthermore, factors such as incarceration or residence in an assisted living facility may limit patient access to reporting mechanisms, and some SDOH such as environmental exposures may be unknown to patients themselves.

Several interventions can improve SDOH data collection processes. These include having standardized tools for SDOH data collection; dedicated, nonprovider individuals to collect SDOH-related data outside the clinical encounter; ensuring multiple modalities (e.g., patient portal, text message, paper and pencil) and opportunities (e.g., at home, in the clinic waiting room); and ensuring that both patients and providers feel the data are worth collecting by demonstrating real-time application and providing tangible assistance in response to patient-reported data.[7] In oncology, surgeons are often the first providers patients see after a new diagnosis of cancer, thus during or even prior to the initial surgical oncologic evaluation representing an important opportunity to capture and intervene upon these data.[8]

Finally, compliance with recommendations from government agencies and payers including the Centers from Medicare and Medicaid Services (CMS) may also encourage system-level commitment to standardizing SDOH data collection.[3,9] "Z codes" (i.e., Z55-Z65) are a set of International Classification of Diseases, Tenth Revision, Clinical Modification (ICD-10-CM) psychosocial risk and SDOH-related codes that can be used by providers including physicians and advanced practice providers as well as social workers to facilitate social history completion (Fig. 15.1A–B). Given increased promotion of Z code utilization by CMS and potential linkage of Z code usage to value-based payments, more widely adopted and consistent documentation of SDOH-related data may not only be desirable with regard to promoting health equity but also for the sake of these systems' own financial well-being.

PATIENT INTERVENTIONS

SDOH at the level of the patient are frequent targets of intervention and quality improvement. While there are many patient-level drivers of disparity, we have focused our discussion on interventions in the areas of technology, education, and health literacy.

With the surge in telemedicine usage necessitated by the COVID-19 pandemic, access to the Internet and smartphone devices has become a salient social determinant to consider. Smartphone ownership is associated with greater ability to obtain needed medical care and patient confidence in obtaining

medical information.[10,11] During the height of the COVID-19 pandemic, telemedicine usage and access are differed by patient demographics including age, race, and primary language, potentially widening health disparities.[12–14] Similar and sometimes starker differences were appreciated in telemedicine access among surgical patient populations.[15–18]

Several studies have reported on interventions to address these technology-based disparities in access to care. Most telehealth interventions have taken place in the context of primary care, such as diabetes management among racial/ethnic minorities or for the purpose of more generalized chronic disease prevention.[19,20] Telemedicine interventions to improve patient outcomes in surgery are underexplored, and the implications for addressing existing health disparities remain largely unknown. To date, evidence of telemedicine interventions that improve patient outcomes among all surgical patients are limited.[21,22] However, if implemented via an approach that prioritizes equitable access, telehealth still represents a promising option for mitigating transportation-related and geographic barriers to care, with effectiveness reported in fields requiring significant postoperative follow-up including plastic surgery, dermatology, burn management, and gender-affirming medical and surgical care.[23–27]

Patient education and literacy commonly overlap with technological access and hold abundant potential for research and intervention. Low health literacy is associated with poorer health outcomes and may partially explain some racial health disparities in the United States.[28] As with research in telehealth implementation, health literacy research has primarily focused on chronic medical conditions,[29] diabetes,[30] and cancer.[31] Health literacy research in surgical fields is relatively sparse. A 2020 systematic review by Chang et al. reported on a growing body of literature on health literacy in surgery where more than one-third of surgical patients were reported to have low health literacy.[32] Further, health literacy was lower among non-White and nonnative English-speaking patients and concentrated among patients with more comorbidities, lower education, and older age.[32]

As Chang et al. observed, interventions for addressing health literacy in surgical patients are emerging but remain small in number. A 2011 study implemented pictographs (i.e., simple line drawings) in discharge instructions for older patients undergoing hip replacement surgery and showed promising results with regard to elucidating aspects of the recovery period for patients with lower literacy.[33] Other studies have developed both tailored (e.g., for tubal ligation) and generalized surgical consent forms at grade-school

A

USING Z CODES:
The **Social Determinants of Health (SDOH)**
Data Journey to Better Outcomes

What are Z codes: SDOH-related Z codes ranging from Z55-Z65 are the ICD-10-CM encounter reason codes used to document SDOH data (e.g., housing, food insecurity, transportation, etc.).

SDOH are the conditions in the environments where people are born, live, learn, work, play, worship and age.

Step 1 Collect SDOH Data

Any member of a person's care team can collect SDOH data during any encounter.

- Includes providers, social workers, community health workers, case managers, patient navigators, and nurses.
- Can be collected at intake through health risk assessments, screening tools, person-provider interaction, and individual self-reporting.

Step 2 Document SDOH Data

Data are recorded in a person's paper or electronic health record (EHR).

- SDOH data may be documented in the problem or diagnosis list, patient or client history, or provider notes.
- Care teams may collect more detailed SDOH data than current Z codes allow. These data should be retained.
- Efforts are ongoing to close Z code gaps and standardize SDOH data.

Step 3 Map SDOH Data to Z Codes

Assistance is available from the ICD-10-CM Official Guidelines for Coding and Reporting.[1]

- Coding, billing, and EHR systems help coders assign standardized codes (e.g., Z codes).
- Coders can assign SDOH Z codes based on self-reported data and/or information documented by any member of the care team if their documentation is included in the official medical record.[2]

Step 4 Use SDOH Z Code Data

Data analysis can help improve quality, care coordination, and experience of care.

- Identify individuals' social risk factors and unmet needs.
- Inform health care and services, follow-up, and discharge planning.
- Trigger referrals to social services that meet individuals' needs.
- Track referrals between providers and social service organizations.

Step 5 Report SDOH Z Code Data Findings

SDOH data can be added to key **reports** for executive leadership and Boards of Directors to inform value-based care opportunities.

- Findings can be shared with social service organizations, providers, health plans, and consumer/patient advisory boards to identify unmet needs.
- A Disparities Impact Statement can be used to identify opportunities for advancing health equity.

CMS

For Questions: Contact the CMS Health Equity Technical Assistance Program

[1] https://www.cms.gov/medicare/icd-10/2022-icd-10-cm
[2] aha.org/system/files/2018-04/value-initiative-icd-10-code-social-determinants-of-health.pdf

B

Z code Categories

Z55 – Problems related to education and literacy
Z56 – Problems related to employment and unemployment
Z57 – Occupational exposure to risk factors
Z58 – Problems related to physical environment
Z59 – Problems related to housing and economic circumstances

Z60 – Problems related to social environment
Z62 – Problems related to upbringing
Z63 – Other problems related to primary support group, including family circumstances
Z64 – Problems related to certain psychosocial circumstances
Z65 – Problems related to other psychosocial circumstances

This list is subject to revisions and additions to improve alignment with SDOH data elements.

FIG. 15.1 ICD-10-CM "Z codes" for documenting social determinants of health data, Centers for Medicare and Medicaid services. **(A)** Using Z codes: The social determinants of health journey to better outcomes. **(B)** Z code categories. Centers for Medicare and Medicaid services. (Accessed at https://www.cms.gov/files/document/zcodes-infographic.pdf on March 30, 2023.)

reading levels to facilitate communication and found that patients with lower health literacy had a better understanding of the content with appropriately tailored paperwork (Fig. 15.2).[5,34] With the increasingly robust observational findings of the adverse effect that lower health literacy can have on equitable shared decision-making and patient–provider communication, future studies should consider developing evidence-based educational interventions for addressing disparate literacy among surgical patients.[35]

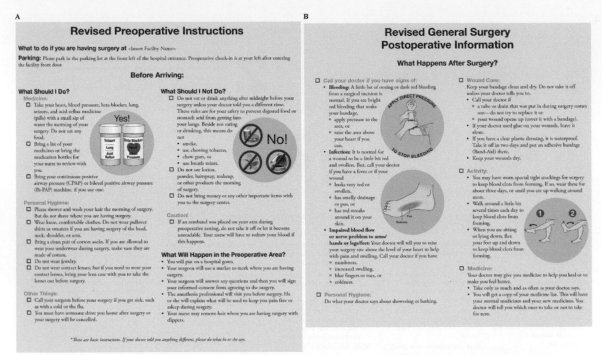

FIG. 15.2 Examples of pre- and postoperative instructions given to ambulatory surgical patients revised to optimize consumption by individuals with diverse health literacy levels. **(A)** Preoperative instructions—revised from twelfth- to fourth-grade level. **(B)** Postoperative instructions—revised from twelfth- to fifth-grade level. (Excerpted from Liebner, LT. "I can't read that! Improving perioperative literacy for ambulatory surgical patients." AORN J (Elsevier). 2015; 101(4):416–27. https://doi.org/10.1016/j.aorn.2015.01.016)

PROVIDER INTERVENTIONS

We often look to the patient for improving SDOH, but there is ample potential for intervention at the level of the physician and healthcare team. Most health disparities are multifactorial and often occur at the interstices of patient, provider, institutional, and societal factors that ultimately lead to poorer clinical outcomes. The goal of this section is to outline potential opportunities for physicians to make meaningful changes for their patients and their communities through direct patient care, professional development, and research.

For disease states where the role of screening is critical for early detection and improved outcomes, disparities in screening rates are often related to inequities in overlapping SDOH. In the case of mammography, Black women historically had lower frequency and quality screenings. Although screening rates have increased over recent years and are on par with those among white women, Black women are still more likely to be screened at nonaccredited or lower resourced facilities, leading to inferior image quality and potential delays in screening, diagnosis, and follow-up.[36] Timely and high-quality screening are critical for early detection of disease and mitigating disparities in cancer outcomes.[37,38] Barriers to mammography include fear of cost, mammogram-related pain, receiving bad news,[39] and cultural and immigration-related factors (e.g., community belief system or language barriers).[40] Interventions have focused on appropriately tailored patient education materials and community engagement, which reveals a potentially vital role that physicians can play in increasing screening rates and reducing patient-level psychosocial barriers.[41–43]

Community involvement is also essential in research. Community-based participatory research (CBPR) has gained prominence as a process for conducting ethical research to promote health equity, particularly in lower-income communities and communities of color, where trust for research and those who conduct research is often low.[44] A 2022 systematic review by McFarlane et al. reported that over 85% of CBPR studies appreciated statistically positive outcomes where CBPR was associated with increased community-partner participation across domains of data collection, study development, participant recruitment, and population-level outcomes (e.g., sustaining collaborative efforts).[45,46] Providers may not only increase direct patient care outcomes (e.g., screening practices) through community engagement but also incite further downstream change in SDOH by championing, participating in, and leading community-oriented research interventions.

Access to and participation in clinical trials represent additional areas for provider engagement. Clinical trials in the United States are rife with ethically fraught and racist history, from the development of the speculum on enslaved Black women by J. Marion Sims to the Tuskegee syphilis experiments.[47,48] Despite efforts to increase clinical trial participation among racialized minority groups starting with the 1993 National Institutes of Health Revitalization Act by US Congress,[49] participation among communities of color has remained low.[50] A 2022 study of US phase I therapeutic drug trials for metastatic cancer found that over the 18-year study period, disparities among racial/ethnic minority groups worsened, with overrepresentation of white participants and reductions in participation among people of color, particularly Black individuals.[51] The literature on disparities in participation among racial/ethnic minority groups in phase II and III trials is similar.[52−54]

Physicians do not offer clinical trials to patients equally for many reasons including perceived time constraints, administrative bandwidth, information gaps in eligibility criteria, and their own biases including perceived concerns about adherence by minoritized people.[55] Notably, studies have shown that disparities in clinical trial participation are reduced and sometimes eliminated when patients from minoritized backgrounds are given equal opportunities to enroll.[56−58] Interventions aimed at reducing disparities in clinical trial participation have found success in strategies that increase health professional engagement, formalizing processes for input

from racial/ethnic minority patients' and caregivers' on research studies, and increasing community stakeholder participation.[56,59] Differences in clinical trial accrual rates also depend on other, less quantifiable measures such as physician belief, attitude, and knowledge.[60] Programs that increase investigators' awareness and comfort in discussing clinical trials with all patients and standardizing trial recruitment and navigation processes can help improve equitable trial information access. An important example is Just Ask, a training program developed by Nadine Barrett, Ph.D., at Duke in 2017 that is now available as a joint offering of the American Society of Clinical Oncology (ASCO) and the Association of Community Cancer Centers (ACCC). The program uses interactive modules addressing diversity, equity, and health disparities and the role of implicit bias in clinical trial selection through vignettes with real-world examples. Notably, the program provides concrete strategies for mitigating disparities in recruitment in cancer research settings.[61,62]

SYSTEMIC INTERVENTIONS

We previously discussed the role providers can play in improving screening rates for breast cancer, but if a patient misses her appointment due to competing employment priorities, childcare needs, or other forms of financial instability, these issues cannot be solved by an individual physician. Systemic interventions for SDOH include local, state, and federal policies; incorporating sociocultural considerations into clinical practice; and institutional equity-centered reform. These interventions are often time- and resource-intensive, and it may be difficult to measure causal relationships due to their complex nature.

Federal policy interventions include the Affordable Care Act (ACA), which was passed in 2010 to expand health insurance coverage and access, thereby reducing various downstream health disparities across the United States. The ACA nearly halved the proportion of the US population without insurance coverage, particularly benefiting lower income, African American, and Hispanic communities.[63] However, despite the ACA, high cost-sharing (e.g., copays, deductibles, coinsurance) remains a source of financial distress for many. Further, several states that opted out of Medicaid expansion offered by the ACA have continued to relegate poorer communities to less accessible care.[63] Low-income individuals on Medicaid have reported difficulty accessing specialty care, though they have also reported better healthcare access and quality compared with individuals who were uninsured.[64]

Legislation at the level of the state is often contentious and has the potential to shape population health as evidenced by Medicaid expansion decisions.[65] Several key examples are worth noting in state policies that have far-reaching health consequences. In 2022, after the US Supreme Court overturned 50 years of protected reproductive rights under Roe, abortion laws were left to state decision-makers resulting in closure of abortion clinics and rapidly diminished access to reproductive healthcare for many women.[66,67] Firearm laws are well documented to be associated with fewer firearm-related deaths.[68-72] Notably, however, states with weaker firearm laws in neighboring states suffer from greater firearm deaths compared with states whose neighbors have similarly restrictive laws, suggesting the need for more geographically coordinated legislative action.[68,73] Similarly, oversight for medical aid-in-dying is legislated at the state level and has the potential to shape perspectives and processes of death and dying of local residents.[74,75]

More proximally, health professional societies have advocated for policy change through recommendations and guidelines for standards of care and future research directions. For example, ASCO published a policy statement itemizing strategies to reduce cancer disparities in the United States and prioritize improving equitable access to care, research, and information.[76] Other examples include revised perspectives on race-based medicine and development of evolving recommendations to change kidney function and transplant allocation guidelines.[77-79]

Institutional approaches to addressing SDOH can also encompass undergraduate medical education. To train a physician workforce that can recognize opportunities and promote efforts to address health disparities, medical education has prioritized training future physicians who are cognizant of the complexities of structural forces that disadvantage and prevent certain communities from accessing appropriate healthcare. Concomitantly, there is a growing body of literature on medical education curricula that equip future physicians with a foundation for addressing health equity. For example, the model of structural competence[80]—a pedagogical

approach built on five core competencies to ensure trainees can recognize socioeconomic forces of downstream health outcomes—has been instrumental in the development of curricula on interprofessionalism, antiracism, and empathy.[81-84] There is also rapidly expanding literature on education-based interventions to improve future physicians' commitment to health equity, using frameworks developed and led by students, trainees, and physicians across the country.[85-87]

FRAMEWORKS FOR IMPLEMENTATION OF EQUITY-FOCUSED INTERVENTIONS

Theoretical frameworks are increasingly recognized as providing an evidence-based structure for identifying, understanding, and intervening upon SDOH-related disparities. The Health Disparities Framework by Kilbourne and colleagues provides a research roadmap that can assist investigators engaged in this area of research.[88] They advocate for a multilevel—individual, provider, and organizational—approach that is attentive to selection bias in the populations studied and champions pragmatic study designs that are focused on inclusion of marginalized populations and are likely to yield generalizable, actionable data.

The tenets of implementation science are required to guide successful incorporation into practice interventions that ultimately reduce disparity and facilitate equity. Many of the commonly used implementation science frameworks (e.g., RE-AIM[89]) have been adapted for application in marginalized populations, while others have been developed de novo. The Health Equity Implementation Framework (HEIF[90]), for example, is a relatively new implementation framework that centers equity by incorporating the construct of power as a societal engine for disparity and also considering its impact on providers and patients within the clinical encounter (Fig. 15.3).[90] HEIF can be used to guide the design of survey materials and interpretation of results, tailor recruitment targets and methods, inform strategies for sampling groups historically underrepresented in research, and shape various other study design and data collection tools and types of analysis. Perhaps, most importantly, HEIF centers the potentially marginalized patient in the process of implementation to ensure that participant burden is minimized and equitable distribution of a given intervention is prioritized.

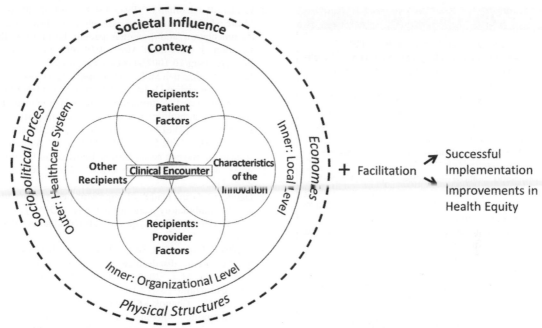

Fig. 1 The Health Equity Implementation Framework explains factors relevant to implementation and disparities in healthcare. In this framework, the innovation is delivered in the clinical encounter. We posit that the clinical encounter is an interaction between recipients (e.g., patient and provider) and the innovation itself (e.g., HIV prevention medication), although the interaction could occur in other settings (e.g., between patient and peer navigator). The Health Equity Implementation Framework identified healthcare system factors, broadly, which most closely aligned with the outer context in i-PARIHS. i-PARIHS specified two other levels within context: inner (local—clinic or unit or ward) and inner (organizational—hospital or network). In the Health Equity Implementation Framework, we highlight that societal influence is especially important to consider when assessing all other factors because of the impact society can have on healthcare disparities. Implementation facilitation, or facilitation, is an essential active process to ignite change to any of the elements or factors

FIG. 15.3 The health equity implementation framework. (Excerpted from Woodward, EN et al. The health equity implementation framework: proposal and preliminary study of hepatitis C virus treatment. Implement Sci. 2019; 14:26. https://doi.org/10.1186/s13012-019-0861-y. No changes were made to this figure, and its unrestricted use, distribution, and reproduction is permitted under the Creative Commons Attribution 4.0 International License: https://creativecommons.org/licenses/by/4.0/)

NEXT STEPS

Growing interest in and attention to SDOH, driven in large part by outsized disparities among racially minoritized groups during the COVID-19 pandemic, has prompted increased investigation on drivers of health inequity. This increasingly robust literature highlights the multifactorial nature of health disparities and their ubiquitous presence at all levels of healthcare, from patient to provider to systems. Yet, interventions that address these disparities remain sparse, particularly for surgical patients.

Future research must prioritize developing, implementing, and iteratively assessing interventions that aim to address identified disparities to make continued strides toward health equity and to institute durable, sustainable change. As highlighted in this chapter, these interventions must address the patient, provider, and structural forces that inform an individual's experience with the healthcare system and should be guided by equity-focused theoretical frameworks.

Highlights

- Increased interest in and attention to SDOH has prompted increased investigation on drivers of health inequity. Yet, interventions that address these disparities remain sparse.
- An important aspect of developing effective interventions to address SDOH-related disparities is optimizing data collection regarding unmet social need. Strategies to facilitate data collection include
  - having nonprovider individuals collect SDOH-related data outside the clinical encounter;
  - providing multiple modalities (e.g., patient portal, text message, paper and pencil) and opportunities (e.g., at home, in the clinic waiting room) for data to be collected; and
  - ensuring that both patients and providers feel the data are worth collecting by demonstrating real-time application and providing tangible assistance in response to patient-provided data.
- Patient-, provider-, and system-level interventions are required to effect meaningful improvement in SDOH-related health disparities.
  - At the patient level, equitable application of emerging health technology can bridge important gaps in care so long as care is made not to exacerbate extant disparities in technological access. Patient-facing communication tools and decision aids can also overcome challenges associated with differential health literacy.
  - At the provider level, training on recognizing and combatting bias as well as culturally adherent engagement with historically marginalized communities can help improve patient–provider communication and patients' trust in both healthcare and clinical research.
  - At the system level, coordinated state and federal legislation, equity-focused policies by healthcare systems and professional societies, and reconsideration of the role race should play in clinical care have the potential for significant reach as part of efforts to redress SDOH-disparities across multiple groups of patients and significant geographic distance.
- Equity-focused theoretical frameworks should guide both the development and implementation of interventions to redress SDOH-related disparities.

REFERENCES

1. U.S. Department of Health and Human Services, Office of Disease Prevention and Health Promotion. Social Determinants of Health. Healthy People 2030. Accessed March 23, 2023. https://health.gov/healthypeople/priority-areas/social-determinants-health.

2. Cohen GR, Friedman CP, Ryan AM, Richardson CR, Adler-Milstein J. Variation in physicians' electronic health record documentation and potential patient harm from that variation. *J Gen Intern Med.* 2019;34(11):2355–2367. https://doi.org/10.1007/s11606-019-05025-3.

3. Hatef E, Rouhizadeh M, Tia I, et al. Assessing the availability of data on social and behavioral determinants in structured and unstructured electronic health records: a retrospective analysis of a multilevel health care system. *JMIR Med Inform.* 2019;7(3):e13802. https://doi.org/10.2196/13802.

4. Chen ES, Manaktala S, Sarkar IN, Melton GB. A multi-site content analysis of social history information in clinical notes. *AMIA Annu Symp Proc AMIA Symp.* 2011;2011:227–236.

5. Liebner LT. I can't read that! Improving perioperative literacy for ambulatory surgical patients. *AORN J.* 2015;101(4):416–427. https://doi.org/10.1016/j.aorn.2015.01.016.

6. Fiscella K, Epstein RM. So much to do, so little time: care for the socially disadvantaged and the 15-minute visit. *Arch Intern Med.* 2008;168(17):1843. https://doi.org/10.1001/archinte.168.17.1843.

7. Lavallee DC, Chenok KE, Love RM, et al. Incorporating patient-reported outcomes into health care to engage patients and enhance care. *Health Aff.* 2016;35(4):575–582. https://doi.org/10.1377/hlthaff.2015.1362.

8. Fayanju OM, Ren Y, Stashko I, et al. Patient-reported causes of distress predict disparities in time to evaluation and time to treatment after breast cancer diagnosis. *Cancer.* 2021;127(5):757–768. https://doi.org/10.1002/cncr.33310.

9. Centers for Medicare and Medicaid Services. *Utilization of Z Codes for Social Determinants of Health Among Medicare Fee-For-Service Beneficiaries, 2019;* 2021. https://www.cms.gov/files/document/z-codes-data-highlight.pdf.

10. Oshima SM, Tait SD, Thomas SM, et al. Association of smartphone ownership and internet use with markers of health literacy and access: cross-sectional survey study of perspectives from project PLACE (population level approaches to cancer elimination). *J Med Internet Res.* 2021;23(6):e24947. https://doi.org/10.2196/24947.

11. Carroll JK, Moorhead A, Bond R, LeBlanc WG, Petrella RJ, Fiscella K. Who uses mobile phone health apps and does use matter? A secondary data analytics approach. *J Med Internet Res.* 2017;19(4):e125. https://doi.org/10.2196/jmir.5604.

12. Eberly LA, Kallan MJ, Julien HM, et al. Patient characteristics associated with telemedicine access for primary and specialty ambulatory care during the COVID-19 pandemic. *JAMA Netw Open.* 2020;3(12):e2031640. https://doi.org/10.1001/jamanetworkopen.2020.31640.

13. Hsiao V, Chandereng T, Lankton RL, et al. Disparities in telemedicine access: a cross-sectional study of a newly established infrastructure during the COVID-19 pandemic. *Appl Clin Inf.* 2021;12(03):445–458. https://doi.org/10.1055/s-0041-1730026.

14. Chunara R, Zhao Y, Chen J, et al. Telemedicine and healthcare disparities: a cohort study in a large healthcare system

in New York City during COVID-19. *J Am Med Inf Assoc.* 2021;28(1):33–41. https://doi.org/10.1093/jamia/ocaa217.

15. Eruchalu CN, Bergmark RW, Smink DS, et al. Demographic disparity in use of telemedicine for ambulatory general surgical consultation during the COVID-19 pandemic: analysis of the initial public health emergency and second phase periods. *J Am Coll Surg.* 2022;234(2):191–202. https://doi.org/10.1097/XCS.0000000000000030.

16. Darrat I, Tam S, Boulis M, Williams AM. Socioeconomic disparities in patient use of telehealth during the coronavirus disease 2019 surge. *JAMA Otolaryngol Neck Surg.* 2021; 147(3):287. https://doi.org/10.1001/jamaoto.2020.5161.

17. Chen EM, Andoh JE, Nwanyanwu K. Socioeconomic and demographic disparities in the use of telemedicine for ophthalmic care during the COVID-19 pandemic. *Ophthalmology.* 2022;129(1):15–25. https://doi.org/10.1016/j.ophtha.2021.07.003.

18. Xiong G, Greene NE, Lightsey HM, et al. Telemedicine use in orthopaedic surgery varies by race, ethnicity, primary language, and insurance status. *Clin Orthop.* 2021. https://doi.org/10.1097/CORR.0000000000001775. Publish Ahead of Print.

19. Anderson A, O'Connell SS, Thomas C, Chimmanamada R. Telehealth interventions to improve diabetes management among black and hispanic patients: a systematic review and meta-analysis. *J Racial Ethn Health Disparities.* 2022; 9(6):2375–2386. https://doi.org/10.1007/s40615-021-01174-6.

20. Pedamallu H, Ehrhardt MJ, Maki J, Carcone AI, Hudson MM, Waters EA. Technology-delivered adaptations of motivational interviewing for the prevention and management of chronic diseases: scoping review. *J Med Internet Res.* 2022;24(8):e35283. https://doi.org/10.2196/35283.

21. NIHR Global Health Research Unit on Global Surgery, GlobalSurg Collaborative. Use of telemedicine for postdischarge assessment of the surgical wound: international cohort study, and systematic review with meta-analysis. *Ann Surg.* 2022. https://doi.org/10.1097/SLA.0000000000005506. Publish Ahead of Print.

22. Fahey E, Elsheikh MFH, Davey MS, Rowan F, Cassidy JT, Cleary MS. Telemedicine in orthopedic surgery: a systematic review of current evidence. *Telemed E-Health.* 2022;28(5): 613–635. https://doi.org/10.1089/tmj.2021.0221.

23. Vyas KS, Hambrick HR, Shakir A, et al. A systematic review of the use of telemedicine in plastic and reconstructive surgery and dermatology. *Ann Plast Surg.* 2017;78(6): 736–768. https://doi.org/10.1097/SAP.0000000000001044.

24. Bashshur RL, Shannon GW, Tejasvi T, Kvedar JC, Gates M. The empirical foundations of teledermatology: a review of the research evidence. *Telemed E-Health.* 2015;21(12): 953–979. https://doi.org/10.1089/tmj.2015.0146.

25. Sohn GK, Wong DJ, Yu SS. A review of the use of telemedicine in dermatologic surgery. *Dermatol Surg.* 2020;46(4): 501–507. https://doi.org/10.1097/DSS.0000000000002230.

26. García-Díaz A, Vilardell-Roig L, Novillo-Ortiz D, Gacto-Sánchez P, Pereyra-Rodríguez JJ, Saigí-Rubió F. Utility of telehealth platforms applied to burns management: a systematic review. *Int J Environ Res Publ Health.* 2023;20(4): 3161. https://doi.org/10.3390/ijerph20043161.

27. Stoehr JR, Hamidian Jahromi A, Hunter EL, Schechter LS. Telemedicine for gender-affirming medical and surgical care: a systematic review and call-to-action. *Transgender Health.* 2022;7(2):117–126. https://doi.org/10.1089/trgh.2020.0136.

28. Berkman ND, Sheridan SL, Donahue KE, Halpern DJ, Crotty K. Low health literacy and health outcomes: an updated systematic review. *Ann Intern Med.* 2011;155(2): 97. https://doi.org/10.7326/0003-4819-155-2-201107190-00005.

29. de Melo Ghisi GL, da Silva Chaves GS, Britto RR, Oh P. Health literacy and coronary artery disease: a systematic review. *Patient Educ Counsel.* 2018;101(2):177–184. https://doi.org/10.1016/j.pec.2017.09.002.

30. Schillinger D. Association of health literacy with diabetes outcomes. *JAMA.* 2002;288(4):475. https://doi.org/10.1001/jama.288.4.475.

31. Oldach BR, Katz ML. Health literacy and cancer screening: a systematic review. *Patient Educ Counsel.* 2014;94(2): 149–157. https://doi.org/10.1016/j.pec.2013.10.001.

32. Chang ME, Baker SJ, Dos Santos Marques IC, et al. Health literacy in surgery. *HLRP Health Lit Res Pract.* 2020;4(1). https://doi.org/10.3928/24748307-20191121-01.

33. Choi J. Pictograph-based discharge instructions for low-literate older adults after hip replacement surgery: development and validation. *J Gerontol Nurs.* 2011;37(11): 47–56. https://doi.org/10.3928/00989134-20110706-03.

34. Zite NB, Wallace LS. Use of a low-literacy informed consent form to improve women's understanding of tubal sterilization: a randomized controlled trial. *Obstet Gynecol.* 2011;117(5):1160–1166. https://doi.org/10.1097/AOG.0b013e318213cbb1.

35. Walters R, Leslie SJ, Polson R, Cusack T, Gorely T. Establishing the efficacy of interventions to improve health literacy and health behaviours: a systematic review. *BMC Publ Health.* 2020;20(1):1040. https://doi.org/10.1186/s12889-020-08991-0.

36. Giaquinto AN, Sung H, Miller KD, et al. Breast cancer statistics, 2022. *CA Cancer J Clin.* 2022;72(6):524–541. https://doi.org/10.3322/caac.21754.

37. Bayard S, Fasano G, Chen Y, et al. Screening mammography mitigates breast cancer disparities through early detection of triple negative breast cancer. *Clin Imag.* 2021;80:430–437. https://doi.org/10.1016/j.clinimag.2021.08.013.

38. Chen Y, Susick L, Davis M, et al. Evaluation of triple-negative breast cancer early detection via mammography screening and outcomes in African American and white American patients. *JAMA Surg.* 2020;155(5):440. https://doi.org/10.1001/jamasurg.2019.6032.

39. Fayanju OM, Kraenzle S, Drake BF, Oka M, Goodman MS. Perceived barriers to mammography among underserved women in a breast health center outreach program. *Am J*

Surg. 2014;208(3):425–434. https://doi.org/10.1016/j.am jsurg.2014.03.005.

40. Miller BC, Bowers JM, Payne JB, Moyer A. Barriers to mammography screening among racial and ethnic minority women. *Soc Sci Med.* 2019;239:112494. https://doi.org/10.1016/j.socscimed.2019.112494.

41. Drake B, James A, Miller H, et al. Strategies to achieve breast health equity in the St. Louis region and beyond over 15+ years. *Cancers.* 2022;14(10):2550. https://doi.org/10.3390/cancers14102550.

42. Kamaraju S, DeNomie M, Visotcky A, et al. Increasing mammography uptake through academic-community partnerships targeting immigrant and refugee communities in Milwaukee. *WMJ Off Publ State Med Soc Wis.* 2018;117(2):55–61.

43. Gehlert S, Fayanju OM, Jackson S, et al. A method for achieving reciprocity of funding in community-based participatory research. *Prog Community Health Partnersh Res Educ Action.* 2014;8(4):561–570. https://doi.org/10.1353/cpr.2014.0054.

44. Ward M, Schulz AJ, Israel BA, Rice K, Martenies SE, Markarian E. A conceptual framework for evaluating health equity promotion within community-based participatory research partnerships. *Eval Progr Plann.* 2018;70:25–34. https://doi.org/10.1016/j.evalprogplan.2018.04.014.

45. Julian McFarlane S, Occa A, Peng W, Awonuga O, Morgan SE. Community-based participatory research (CBPR) to enhance participation of racial/ethnic minorities in clinical trials: a 10-year systematic review. *Health Commun.* 2022;37(9):1075–1092. https://doi.org/10.1080/10410236.2021.1943978.

46. Jagosh J, Bush PL, Salsberg J, et al. A realist evaluation of community-based participatory research: partnership synergy, trust building and related ripple effects. *BMC Publ Health.* 2015;15(1):725. https://doi.org/10.1186/s12889-015-1949-1.

47. Washington HA, ed. *Medical Apartheid: The Dark History of Medical Experimentation on Black Americans from Colonial Times to the Present.* 1st pbk. Harlem Moon; 2006.

48. Scharff DP, Mathews KJ, Jackson P, Hoffsuemmer J, Martin E, Edwards D. More than Tuskegee: understanding mistrust about research participation. *J Health Care Poor Underserved.* 2010;21(3):879–897. https://doi.org/10.1353/hpu.0.0323.

49. Freedman LS, Simon R, Foulkes MA, et al. Inclusion of women and minorities in clinical trials and the NIH Revitalization Act of 1993 — the perspective of NIH clinical trialists. *Contr Clin Trials.* 1995;16(5):277–285. https://doi.org/10.1016/0197-2456(95)00048-8.

50. Chen MS, Lara PN, Dang JHT, Paterniti DA, Kelly K. Twenty years post-NIH Revitalization Act: enhancing minority participation in clinical trials (EMPaCT): laying the groundwork for improving minority clinical trial accrual: renewing the case for enhancing minority

participation in cancer clinical trials. *Cancer.* 2014;120:1091–1096. https://doi.org/10.1002/cncr.28575.

51. Dunlop H, Fitzpatrick E, Kurti K, et al. Participation of patients from racial and ethnic minority groups in phase 1 early cancer drug development trials in the US, 2000-2018. *JAMA Netw Open.* 2022;5(11):e2239884. https://doi.org/10.1001/jamanetworkopen.2022.39884.

52. Grant SR, Lin TA, Miller AB, et al. Racial and ethnic disparities among participants in US-based phase 3 randomized cancer clinical trials. *JNCI Cancer Spectr.* 2020;4(5):pkaa060. https://doi.org/10.1093/jncics/pkaa060.

53. Owens-Walton J, Williams C, Rompré-Brodeur A, Pinto PA, Ball MW. Minority enrollment in phase II and III clinical trials in urologic oncology. *J Clin Oncol.* 2022;40(14):1583–1589. https://doi.org/10.1200/JCO.21.01885.

54. Loree JM, Anand S, Dasari A, et al. Disparity of race reporting and representation in clinical trials leading to cancer drug approvals from 2008 to 2018. *JAMA Oncol.* 2019;5(10):e191870. https://doi.org/10.1001/jamaoncol.2019.1870.

55. Hillyer GC, Beauchemin M, Hershman DL, et al. Discordant attitudes and beliefs about cancer clinical trial participation between physicians, research staff, and cancer patients. *Clin Trials.* 2020;17(2):184–194. https://doi.org/10.1177/1740774520901514.

56. Regnante JM, Richie NA, Fashoyin-Aje L, et al. US cancer centers of excellence strategies for increased inclusion of racial and ethnic minorities in clinical trials. *J Oncol Pract.* 2019;15(4):e289–e299. https://doi.org/10.1200/JOP.18.00638.

57. Simon MS, Du W, Flaherty L, et al. Factors associated with breast cancer clinical trials participation and enrollment at a large academic medical center. *J Clin Oncol.* 2004;22(11):2046–2052. https://doi.org/10.1200/JCO.2004.03.005.

58. Kemeny MM, Peterson BL, Kornblith AB, et al. Barriers to clinical trial participation by older women with breast cancer. *J Clin Oncol.* 2003;21(12):2268–2275. https://doi.org/10.1200/JCO.2003.09.124.

59. Mansfield LN, Nagy GA, Solorzano R, et al. Targeted strategies for recruitment and engagement of Latinx immigrants in longitudinal biobehavioral research. *Hisp Health Care Int.* 2022;3:154041532210836. https://doi.org/10.1177/15404153221083659. Published online March.

60. Somkin CP, Ackerson L, Husson G, et al. Effect of medical oncologists' attitudes on accrual to clinical trials in a community setting. *J Oncol Pract.* 2013;9(6):e275–e283. https://doi.org/10.1200/JOP.2013.001120.

61. Barrett NJ, Boehmer L, Schrag J, et al. An assessment of the feasibility and utility of an ACCC-ASCO implicit bias training program to enhance racial and ethnic diversity in cancer clinical trials. *JCO Oncol Pract.* 2023;19(4):e570–e580. https://doi.org/10.1200/OP.22.00378.

62. Association of Community Cancer Centers. *Just ASK^{TM} Increasing Diversity in Cancer Clinical Research.* An ACCC-

ASCO Training Program; 2019. https://courses.accc-cancer.org/products/just-ask-increasing-diversity-in-cancer-clinical-research#tab-product_tab_overview.

63. Gaffney A, McCormick D. The Affordable Care Act: implications for health-care equity. *Lancet.* 2017;389(10077):1442–1452. https://doi.org/10.1016/S0140-6736(17)30786-9.

64. Nguyen KH, Sommers BD. Access and quality of care by insurance type for low-income adults before the affordable care Act. *Am J Publ Health.* 2016;106(8):1409–1415. https://doi.org/10.2105/AJPH.2016.303156.

65. Status of State Medicaid Expansion Decisions: Interactive Map. Kaiser Family Foundation. https://www.kff.org/medicaid/issue-brief/status-of-state-medicaid-expansion-decisions-interactive-map/. Published February 16, 2023. Accessed March 25, 2023.

66. Lawmakers V. The scientific realities of human reproduction. *N Engl J Med.* 2022;387(4):367–368. https://doi.org/10.1056/NEJMe2208288.

67. Cohen IG, Murray M, Gostin LO. The end of *Roe v wade* and new legal frontiers on the constitutional right to abortion. *JAMA.* 2022;328(4):325. https://doi.org/10.1001/jama.2022.12397.

68. Liu Y, Siegel M, Sen B. Neighbors do matter: between-state firearm laws and state firearm-related deaths in the U.S., 2000–2017. *Am J Prev Med.* 2020;59(5):648–657. https://doi.org/10.1016/j.amepre.2020.06.022.

69. Lee LK, Fleegler EW, Farrell C, et al. Firearm laws and firearm homicides: a systematic review. *JAMA Intern Med.* 2017;177(1):106. https://doi.org/10.1001/jamainternmed.2016.7051.

70. Sabbath EL, Hawkins SS, Baum CF. State-level changes in firearm laws and workplace homicide rates: United States, 2011 to 2017. *Am J Publ Health.* 2020;110(2):230–236. https://doi.org/10.2105/AJPH.2019.305405.

71. Doucette ML, Crifasi CK, Frattaroli S. Right-to-Carry laws and firearm workplace homicides: a longitudinal analysis (1992–2017). *Am J Publ Health.* 2019;109(12):1747–1753. https://doi.org/10.2105/AJPH.2019.305307.

72. Díez C, Kurland RP, Rothman EF, et al. State intimate partner violence–related firearm laws and intimate partner homicide rates in the United States, 1991 to 2015. *Ann Intern Med.* 2017;167(8):536. https://doi.org/10.7326/M16-2849.

73. Liu Y, Siegel M, Sen B. Association of state-level firearm-related deaths with firearm laws in neighboring states. *JAMA Netw Open.* 2022;5(11):e2240750. https://doi.org/10.1001/jamanetworkopen.2022.40750.

74. Al Rabadi L, LeBlanc M, Bucy T, et al. Trends in medical aid in dying in Oregon and Washington. *JAMA Netw Open.* 2019;2(8):e198648. https://doi.org/10.1001/jamanetworkopen.2019.8648.

75. Emanuel EJ, Onwuteaka-Philipsen BD, Urwin JW, Cohen J. Attitudes and practices of euthanasia and physician-assisted suicide in the United States, Canada, and Europe. *JAMA.* 2016;316(1):79. https://doi.org/10.1001/jama.2016.8499.

76. Patel MI, Lopez AM, Blackstock W, et al. Cancer disparities and health equity: a policy statement from the American society of clinical oncology. *J Clin Oncol.* 2020;38(29):3439–3448. https://doi.org/10.1200/JCO.20.00642.

77. Gill JS, Kelly B, Tonelli M. Time to abolish metrics that sustain systemic racism in kidney allocation. *JAMA.* 2023;329(11):879. https://doi.org/10.1001/jama.2023.1076.

78. Levey AS, Titan SM, Powe NR, Coresh J, Inker LA. Kidney disease, race, and GFR estimation. *Clin J Am Soc Nephrol.* 2020;15(8):1203–1212. https://doi.org/10.2215/CJN.12791019.

79. Delgado C, Baweja M, Crews DC, et al. A unifying approach for GFR estimation: recommendations of the NKF-ASN task force on reassessing the inclusion of race in diagnosing kidney disease. *Am J Kidney Dis.* 2022;79(2):268–288. https://doi.org/10.1053/j.ajkd.2021.08.003.

80. Metzl JM, Hansen H. Structural competency: theorizing a new medical engagement with stigma and inequality. *Soc Sci Med.* 2014;103:126–133. https://doi.org/10.1016/j.socscimed.2013.06.032.

81. Caiola C, Nelson TB, Black KZ, et al. Structural competency in pre-health and health professional learning: a scoping review. *J Interprof Care.* 2022:1–10. https://doi.org/10.1080/13561820.2022.2124238. Published online October 20.

82. Godley BA, Dayal D, Manekin E, Estroff SE. Toward an anti-racist curriculum: incorporating art into medical education to improve empathy and structural competency. *J Med Educ Curric Dev.* 2020;7:238212052096524. https://doi.org/10.1177/2382120520965246.

83. Harvey M, Neff J, Knight KR, et al. Structural competency and global health education. *Global Publ Health.* 2022;17(3):341–362. https://doi.org/10.1080/17441692.2020.1864751.

84. Salhi BA, Zeidan A, Stehman CR, et al. Structural competency in emergency medical education: a scoping review and operational framework. *AEM Educ Train.* 2022;6(S1). https://doi.org/10.1002/aet2.10754.

85. Boatright D, London M, Soriano AJ, et al. Strategies and best practices to improve diversity, equity, and inclusion among US graduate medical education programs. *JAMA Netw Open.* 2023;6(2):e2255110. https://doi.org/10.1001/jamanetworkopen.2022.55110.

86. Afolabi T, Borowsky HM, Cordero DM, et al. Student-led efforts to advance anti-racist medical education. *Acad Med.* 2021;96(6):802–807. https://doi.org/10.1097/ACM.0000000000004043.

87. Keuroghlian AS, Charlton BM, Katz-Wise SL, et al. Harvard medical school's sexual and gender minority health equity initiative: curricular and climate innovations in undergraduate medical education. *Acad Med.* 2022;97(12):1786–1793. https://doi.org/10.1097/ACM.0000000000004867.

88. Kilbourne AM, Switzer G, Hyman K, Crowley-Matoka M, Fine MJ. Advancing health disparities research within the health care system: a conceptual framework. *Am J Publ Health.* 2006;96(12):2113–2121. https://doi.org/10.2105/AJPH.2005.077628.

89. Shelton RC, Chambers DA, Glasgow RE. An extension of RE-AIM to enhance sustainability: addressing dynamic context and promoting health equity over time. *Front Public Health.* 2020;8:134. https://doi.org/10.3389/fpubh.2020.00134.

90. Woodward EN, Matthieu MM, Uchendu US, Rogal S, Kirchner JE. The health equity implementation framework: proposal and preliminary study of hepatitis C virus treatment. *Implement Sci.* 2019;14(1):26. https://doi.org/10.1186/s13012-019-0861-y.

CHAPTER 16

Future Directions

SAMILIA OBENG-GYASI, MD, MPH • TIMOTHY PAWLIK, MD, PHD, MPH, MTS, MBA

Social determinants of health (SDH) have powerfully shaped disease incidence and mortality from antiquity until the present day. Consistently across time, studies have demonstrated that individuals facing social and economic marginalization continue to have poor health outcomes compared with individuals from socially and economically privileged groups.[1-4] For instance, racist and discriminatory governmental policies such as the Indian Appropriations Act of 1851 and Jim Crow laws have had adverse transgenerational effects on the health of American Indians and Black Americans, respectively.[5,6] Conversely, effective public health policies such as seatbelt laws, workplace smoking bans, and Medicaid expansion under the Patient Protection and Affordable Care Act have significantly improved health outcomes.[7-9] Nonetheless, despite significant gains in the diagnosis and management of disease, as well as increased awareness about the implications of SDH on health, there are continued disparities in health and clinical outcomes among minoritized and marginalized populations in the United States. Further, the politicization and polarization of conceptual and theoretical frameworks (i.e., critical race theory) that inform examinations of SDH complicate effective research efforts to describe, discuss, and resolve health and healthcare disparities rooted in SDH.

We hope this book has provided the reader with the necessary tools to move from first-generation health disparities research, which is mainly descriptive, toward fourth-generation health disparities research.[10] Specifically, research questions should be rooted in existing theory and conceptual frameworks (e.g., ecosocial theory), comprehensively evaluate multisystem (e.g., individual, institutional) SDH factors, and target interventions to address structural determinants of health inequities (e.g., racism) that are the major drivers of health inequality and health inequity.[10] Additionally, qualitative research frameworks such as intersectionality should be considered to understand comprehensively the intersection among social determinants of health, social identity, and health outcomes. Intersectionality examines the interplay between social categories (e.g., gender, race, class) and interactions with and access to power.[11] Furthermore, an intersectionality framework provides an avenue to synthesize and contextualize the impact of multiple SDH on the individual.

Chapters on the Conserved Transcriptional Response to Adversity (CTRA), allostatic load, and stress highlight the emerging literature on biological pathways from exposure to SDH to disease initiation, progression, and mortality. These concepts illustrate possible embodiment and weathering pathways by demonstrating the impact of SDH at the physiologic and molecular levels. Moreover, data noting that CTRA and AL can be mitigated with exercise and psychosocial support provide actionable targets for researchers to address the internalization of SDH.[12,13] As our understanding of the biological effects of SDH continues to evolve, additional work is needed to integrate these biological correlates into clinical practice.

The recent proliferation of health equity, health, and healthcare disparities literature has brought much-needed attention and funding to this area of research. In addition, there is a whole new era of seasoned and novice researchers who are thinking critically about SDH and its implications on health. The increased interest has led to concerns about "health equity tourism"—a practice defined by academic opportunism and self-interest with minimal regard for established research paradigms, scholarship, or the populations studied.[14] Consequently, we encourage researchers to include SDH within their research in ways that are not exploitative, but rather enrich and build on existing equity scholarship. Further, we recommend including health equity experts to ensure appropriate framing of research questions, as well as accurate interpretation of the data and results relative to SDH.

Social Determinants of Health in Surgery. https://doi.org/10.1016/B978-0-443-12366-5.00010-3

REFERENCES

1. Braveman PA, Cubbin C, Egerter S, Williams DR, Pamuk E. Socioeconomic disparities in health in the United States: what the patterns tell us. *Am J Publ Health*. April 1, 2010; 100(Suppl 1):S186–S196. https://doi.org/10.2105/ajph.2 009.166082.

2. Newman LA, Mason J, Cote D, et al. African-American ethnicity, socioeconomic status, and breast cancer survival: a meta-analysis of 14 studies involving over 10,000 African-American and 40,000 White American patients with carcinoma of the breast. *Cancer*. June 1, 2002; 94(11):2844–2854. https://doi.org/10.1002/cncr.10575.

3. Diaz A, Valbuena VSM, Dimick JB, Ibrahim AM. Association of neighborhood deprivation, race, and postoperative outcomes: improvement in neighborhood deprivation is associated with worsening surgical disparities. *Ann Surg*. July 7, 2022. https://doi.org/10.1097/sla.0000000000005475.

4. Azap RA, Paredes AZ, Diaz A, Hyer JM, Pawlik TM. The association of neighborhood social vulnerability with surgical textbook outcomes among patients undergoing hepato-pancreatic surgery. *Surgery*. November 2020;168(5): 868–875. https://doi.org/10.1016/j.surg.2020.06.032.

5. Krieger N, Jahn JL, Waterman PD. Jim Crow and estrogen-receptor-negative breast cancer: US-born black and white non-hispanic women, 1992-2012. *Cancer Causes Control*. January 2017;28(1):49–59. https://doi.org/10.1007/s105 52-016-0834-2.

6. Hutchinson RN, Shin S. Systematic review of health disparities for cardiovascular diseases and associated factors among American Indian and Alaska Native populations. *PLoS One*. 2014;9(1):e80973. https://doi.org/10.1371/jou rnal.pone.0080973.

7. Obeng-Gyasi S, Rose J, Dong W, Kim U, Koroukian S. Is Medicaid expansion narrowing gaps in surgical disparities for low-income breast cancer patients? *Ann Surg Oncol*. November 27, 2021. https://doi.org/10.1245/s10434-021 -11137-0.

8. *Policy Impact: Seat Belts*. Centers for Disease Control and Prevention; January 3, 2011. www.cdc.gov/transport ationsafety/seatbeltbrief/index.html.

9. *Smokefree Policies Reduce Secondhand Smoke Exposure*. Centers For Disease Control and Prevention; August 4, 2020. https://www.cdc.gov/tobacco/secondhand-smoke/protec-tion/shs-exposure.htm.

10. Thomas SB, Quinn SC, Butler J, Fryer CS, Garza MA. Toward a fourth generation of disparities research to achieve health equity. *Annu Rev Publ Health*. 2011;32:399–416. https:// doi.org/10.1146/annurev-publhealth-031210-101136.

11. Crenshaw K. Mapping the margins: intersectionality, identity politics, and violence against women of color. *Stanford Law Rev*. 1991;43(6):1241–1299. https://doi.org/10.2307 /1229039.

12. Ye ZJ, Qiu HZ, Liang MZ, et al. Effect of a mentor-based, supportive-expressive program, Be Resilient to Breast Cancer, on survival in metastatic breast cancer: a randomised, controlled intervention trial. *Br J Cancer*. November 7, 2017;117(10):1486–1494. https://doi.org/10.1038/bjc. 2017.325.

13. Bower JE, Crosswell AD, Stanton AL, et al. Mindfulness meditation for younger breast cancer survivors: a randomized controlled trial. *Cancer*. April 15, 2015;121(8): 1231–1240. https://doi.org/10.1002/cncr.29194.

14. Lett E, Adekunle D, McMurray P, et al. Health equity tourism: ravaging the justice landscape. *J Med Syst*. February 12, 2022;46(3):17. https://doi.org/10.1007/ s10916-022-01803-5.

Glossary of key terms

Ancestry

Genealogical ancestry: identifiable ancestors in one's pedigree or family tree.

Genetic ancestry: defines groups based on the proportion of an individual's genome inherited from the group of interest.

Genetic similarity: assigns group membership based on genetic similarity.[1]

Allostatic load

Allostatic load is an indicator of physiologic dysregulation in response to socioenvironmental stressors. High allostatic load indicates worsening physiologic dysregulation.[2,3]

Conserved transcriptional response to adversity

Conserved transcriptional response to adversity (CTRA) is defined by upregulated expression of genes involved in inflammation and downregulated expression of genes involved in type I interferon innate antiviral responses.[4,5]

Cultural humility

Described as the lifelong commitment to self-evaluation and critique of the patient–physician relationship. Further, this concept requires a commitment to remedy the power imbalances in the physician–patient relationship by fostering mutually beneficial and nonpaternalistic partnerships at the individual and community levels.[6]

Ecosocial theory

Ecosocial theory describes the internalization of social determinants of health. It comprises four key elements: embodiment, pathways of embodiment, the cumulative interplay of exposure, susceptibility, resistance, and agency and accountability.[7,8]

Ethnicity

A social construct based on shared "geography language, ancestry, or traditions."[9]

Financial toxicity

Describes the intersection of material resources, psychological worry, and patient coping behaviors secondary to the medical and nonmedical cost of treatment.[10]

Health disparity

The Centers for Disease Control describe health disparities as "preventable differences in the burden of disease, injury, violence, or opportunities to achieve optimal health that are experienced by socially disadvantaged groups."[11]

Health equity

According to the World Health Organization, health equity is "the absence of avoidable, unfair, or remediable differences among groups of people, whether those groups are defined socially, economically, demographically, or geographically or by other means of stratification. "Health equity" or "equity in health" implies that ideally, everyone should have a fair opportunity to attain their full health potential and that no one should be disadvantaged from achieving this potential.[13]

Health equity tourism

Lett et al. define health equity tourism as "The practice of investigators—without prior experience or commitment to health equity research—parachuting into the field in response to timely and often temporary increases in public interest and resources."[14]

Health literacy

The ability to "find, understand, and use information and services" for health decision-making.[15]

Healthcare disparity

Differences in healthcare access, health insurance coverage, affordability, utilization of healthcare, and quality of care between groups.[12]

Intersectionality

Describes the qualitative research framework that examines overlapping systems of oppression and discrimination individuals experience due to membership in groups based on social categories such as race, class, gender, etc.[16]

Race

A social construct where individuals are symbolically categorized "based on phenotype or ancestry and constructed to specific racial and historical contexts, that is misrecognized as a natural category." Racial categories are not rooted in genetic variation and are not biological classifications.[17-19]

Social determinants of health	The World Health Organization defines social determinants of health as "conditions in which people are born, grow, work, live, and age, and the wider set of forces and systems shaping the conditions of daily life. These forces and systems include economic policies and systems, development agendas, social norms, social policies, and political systems."[13]

REFERENCES

1. Mathieson I, Scally A. What is ancestry? *PLOS Genetics.* 2020;16(3):e1008624. https://doi.org/10.1371/journal.pgen.1008624.
2. McEwen BS, Wingfield JC. The concept of allostasis in biology and biomedicine. *Horm Behav.* 2003;43(1):2–15.
3. McEwen BS, Stellar E. Stress and the individual. Mechanisms leading to disease. *Arch Intern Med.* Sep 27 1993; 153(18):2093–2101.
4. Cole SW. Social regulation of human gene expression: mechanisms and implications for public health. *Am J Public Health.* Oct 2013;103(Suppl 1):S84–92. https://doi.org/10.2105/ajph.2012.301183.
5. Cole SW. Human social genomics. *PLoS Genet.* Aug 2014; 10(8):e1004601. https://doi.org/10.1371/journal.pgen.1004601.
6. Tervalon M, Murray-García J. Cultural humility versus cultural competence: a critical distinction in defining physician training outcomes in multicultural education. *J Health Care Poor Underserved.* May 1998;9(2):117–125. https://doi.org/10.1353/hpu.2010.0233.
7. Krieger N. Epidemiology and the web of causation: has anyone seen the spider? *Soc Sci Med.* 1994;39(7): 887–903. https://doi.org/10.1016/0277-9536(94)90 202-X.
8. Krieger N. Proximal, distal, and the politics of causation: what's level got to do with it? *Am J Public Health.* Feb 2008;98(2):221–230. https://doi.org/10.2105/AJPH.2007.111278.
9. Ford CL, Harawa NT. A new conceptualization of ethnicity for social epidemiologic and health equity research. *Soc Sci Med.* 2010;71(2):251–258. https://doi.org/10.1016/j.socscimed.2010.04.008.
10. Tucker-Seeley RD, Yabroff KR. Minimizing the "financial toxicity" associated with cancer care: advancing the research agenda. *J Natl Cancer Inst.* May 2016;108(5). https://doi.org/10.1093/jnci/djv410.
11. CDC. *Community Health and Program Services (CHAPS): Health Disparities Among Racial/Ethnic Populations.* Atlanta: U.S. Department of Health and Human Services; 2008.
12. *Disparities in health and health care: 5 key questions and answers, KFF;* 2023. https://www.kff.org/racial-equity-and-health-policy/issue-brief/disparities-in-health-and-health-care-5-key-question-and-answers/.
13. World Health Organization. Health equity. https://www.who.int/topics/health_equity/en/#:~:text=Equity%20is%20the%20absence%20of,by%20other%20means%20of%20stratification.
14. Lett E, Adekunle D, McMurray P, et al. Health equity tourism: ravaging the justice landscape. *J Med Syst.* 2022; 46(3):17. https://doi.org/10.1007/s10916-022-01803-5.
15. *Health literacy.* HRSA; 2022. https://www.hrsa.gov/about/organization/bureaus/ohe/health-literacy#:~:text=Personal%20health%20literacy%20is%20the,actions%20for%20themselves%20and%20others.
16. Crenshaw K. Mapping the margins: intersectionality, identity politics, and violence against women of color. *Stanf Law Rev.* 1991;43(6):1241–1299. https://doi.org/10.2307/1229039.
17. *Race Reporting Guide.* New York: Race Forward; 2015.
18. Desmond M, Emirbayer M. What is racial domination? *Du Bois Rev.* 2009;6(2):335–355.
19. Kittles RA, Weiss KM. Race, ancestry, and genes: implications for defining disease risk. *Annu Rev Genomics Hum Genet.* 2003;4:33–67. https://doi.org/10.1146/annurev.genom.4.070802.110356.

Index

'*Note:* Page numbers followed by "f" indicate figures, "t" indicate tables, and "b" indicate boxes.'